Sex-selective
Abortion
in India

For Prof. Wronba,

Hope we meet
again and talk
about each others' work
and explore further
in our studies.

Best wishes

Tulsi Patel
7/1/11

SEX-SELECTIVE ABORTION IN INDIA

Gender, Society and New Reproductive Technologies

Editor

TULSI PATEL

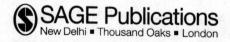

SAGE Publications
New Delhi ▪ Thousand Oaks ▪ London

First published in 2007 by

Sage Publications India Pvt Ltd
B-42, Panchsheel Enclave
New Delhi 110 017
www.indiasage.com

Sage Publications Inc
2455 Teller Road
Thousand Oaks, California 91320

Sage Publications Ltd
1 Oliver's Yard, 55 City Road
London EC1Y 1SP

Published by Tejeshwar Singh for Sage Publications India Pvt Ltd, typeset in 10/12 Calisto MT at InoSoft Systems, Noida, and printed at Chaman Enterprises, New Delhi.

Library of Congress Cataloging-in-Publication Data

Sex-selective abortion in India: gender, society and new reproductive technologies/Tulsi Patel, editor.

    p. cm.
  Includes bibliographical references and index.
    1. Abortion—India. 2. Sexism—India. 3. Sex distribution (Demography)—India. I. Patel, Tulsi.

HQ767.5.15S49   304.6'670954—dc22   2007   2006031234

ISBN: 10: 0-7619-3539-8 (PB)   81-7829-697-7 (India–PB)
        13: 978-0-7619-3539-1 (PB)   978-81-7829-697-5 (India–PB)

Sage Production Team: Manisha Jain, Swati Sahi, Sandeep Bankhwal and Santosh Rawat

For Kaki and Kakosa, my parents-in-law
(Smt. Jamuna and Shri Amrit Lal Patel)

CONTENTS

Part 3: Representation, Articulation and the State

LIST OF TABLES

LIST OF ILLUSTRATIONS

LIST OF ABBREVIATIONS

ANM	Auxiliary Nurse Midwife
ARI	Acute Respiratory Infections
BEE	Block Extension Educator
BIMARU	Demographically speaking, the sick states of Bihar, Madhya Pradesh, Rajasthan and Uttar Pradesh
CASSA	Campaign Against Sex-selective Abortion
CBR	Crude Birth Rate
CEDAW	Convention on the Elimination of All Forms of Discrimination Against Women
CEHAT	Centre for the Enquiry of Health and Allied Themes
CHC	Community Health Centers
CNAA	Community Need Assessment Approach
CPR	Couple Protection Rate, for contraception purposes
CSR	Child Sex Ratio
CSSM	Child Survival and Safe Motherhood Programme
CVARA	Coordinating Voluntary Adoption Resource Agency
CWDS	Centre for Women's Development Studies
DCCW	Delhi Council of Child Welfare
DEMARU	Daughter Eliminating Male Aspiring Rage for Ultrasound
DFPO	District Family Planning Officer
EPI	Expanded Program on Immunisation
FASDSP	Forum Against Sex Determination and Sex Pre-Selection
FGDs	Focus Group Discussions
FMR	Female Male Ratio
FPP	Family Planning Programme
FWP	Family Welfare Programme
GEI	Gender Equality Index
GWA	Guardians and Wards Act, 1890
HAMA	Hindu Adoptions and Maintenance Act, 1956
ICDS	Integrated Child Development Scheme
ICPD	International Conference on Population Development

IEC	Information, Education & Communication Activities
IMR	Infant Mortality Rate
IUD	Intra Uterine Device
JNU	Jawaharlal Nehru University
KAP	Knowledge, Attitude and Practice (surveys)
MASUM	Mahila Sarvangeen Utkarsh Mandal
MCH	Maternal & Child Health
MPW	Multipurpose Health Worker
MSS	Mahila Swasthya Sangh
MSS	Manuscript Sources
MTP	Medical Termination of Pregnancy
NFH	National Family Health Survey
NRI	Non-Resident Indian
NRT	New Reproductive Technologies
NSSO	National Sample Survey Organisation
ORT	Oral Rehydration Therapy
PBEF	Pre-Birth Elimination of Female
PHC	Primary Health Centre
PIL	Public Interest Litigation
PNDT	Pre-natal Diagnostic Techniques (Regulation and Prevention of Misuse, Act of 1994)
PP	Parliamentary Papers
RCH	Reproductive and Child Health Project
SC	Sub-centres
SCH	Subsidiary Health Centres
SDT	Sex determination test
SMP	Safe Motherhood Programme
SP	Sex Pre-selection
SRBG	Selections from Records of Bombay Government
SRG	Selections from Records of Government
TFA	Target Free Approach
TFR	Total Fertility Rate
UCI	Universal Child Immunisation
UIP	Universal Immunisation Programme
VCA	Voluntary Coordinating Agency
VHAI	Voluntary Health Association of India
VHW	Village Health Worker
VVIP	Very very important person

FOREWORD

No one can doubt the great importance of the subject that is addressed by this book—namely the decision by prospective parents to have a test conducted in order to determine the sex of a foetus, and the subsequent action to abort the foetus if the outcome points to the birth of a baby girl.

The results of the 2001 census of India have underscored just how big this problem has become in the country. The deficit of young girls—compared to young boys—is extremely pronounced in the states of Punjab, Haryana, and in western areas of Uttar Pradesh. However, it is severe as well in north-eastern Rajasthan, in western areas of Maharashtra, and throughout most of Gujarat. Census data for other parts of north India (for example, some districts in Bihar) also show incipient evidence of the practice of female specific abortion. And while in 2001 most districts in the country's south and east showed little sign of an abnormal deficit of young girls, this was not always the case. For example, data from the last four censuses reveal first for Salem district in Tamil Nadu, and later for adjacent districts, a disturbing trend towards an emerging deficit of young girls compared to young boys. The outward spread of the phenomenon from Salem resembles nothing less than the growth of a malignancy. It seems likely that this trend too partly reflects a rise in the practice of sex-selective abortion.

Of course, as many of the contributions to this volume attest, especially in areas of north India the modern practice of female specific abortion has been overlain on pre-existing discriminatory practices that have extremely deep historical roots. Thus in the 19th century and before, female infanticide was common in some sections of society, and as a result there were markedly fewer girls and women than would otherwise have been the case. While the overt practice of female infanticide diminished greatly during the 20th century, there remained very strong biases in patterns of childcare between the sexes. In particular, boys were *much* more likely to receive attention—medical and other—if they fell ill. Of course, such differences in childcare practices between boys and girls persist. And they mean that even today the death rates for young girls, especially in north India, are markedly higher than those for boys (a disparity that persists well into the reproductive years).

In sum, the fairly recent appearance of female specific abortion—reflecting the coming of new technologies—is occurring *on top of* deeply embedded practices that discriminate greatly against girls and women. Female infanticide, discrimination against girls, and sex-selective abortion—they all reflect the consequences of underlying social structures, especially in relation to fundamental concerns of marriage and inheritance.

The discriminatory practices against females—both before and after birth—that prevail in some parts of India are extreme by any standards. Yet it is important to remember that they do have echoes in other societies. For example, excess female child mortality was not unknown in parts of Europe in past times. And in Asia—especially East Asia—female infanticide and severely discriminatory treatment against girls and women were, and still are, very common. Of course, one upshot of this has been that the same new technologies that now make female specific abortion possible in India have also been taken up widely in countries like China and South Korea. It is worth remarking that—despite many other problems—a strong preference for boys over girls seems never to have characterized societies in sub-Saharan Africa. In part, this may ultimately have reflected greater land abundance in that region during previous millennia, compared to the constraints that were faced by the developing agricultural civilisations of Eurasia.

Returning to India, one wonders just where this invidious practice of female specific abortion is going. That is, what is likely to happen in the future? Clearly, for a country that is so vast and varied, there can be no simple answer to this question. However, in the end the matter will depend upon how people come to value the lives of girls and women relative to those of boys and men. And in this context there are both positive (i.e. encouraging) and negative (i.e. destructive) forces at work.

On the positive side, the fact of fertility decline raises the prospect that the lives of many Indian women will become increasingly freed from the concerns of the domestic domain, in particular childbearing and childcare. Largely as a consequence, the institution of marriage may itself come under increasing strain—something that would probably work to the benefit of women in the longer run. It is also possible that such beneficial developments could be strengthened by labour market changes that provide increasing opportunities for women compared to men (at least in some parts of society). And, of course, the state and sections of civil society will continue with efforts to improve the situation—although both the strength of such efforts and their impact are likely to be modest, at best. Perhaps a stronger positive force will come through the influence of the media on Indian society—reflecting the values and behaviour of the wider world which generally holds girls and women in appreciably higher regard. Also, one should not underestimate the potentially beneficial impact of visits to India by women of South Asian ancestry who have been brought up in the very different cultural milieu of North America, Europe and elsewhere.

Some commentators may doubt whether such positive forces will have much impact on the circumstances of Indian women—and therefore the extent to which practices like female specific abortion are resorted to. However, several of the developments noted above—perhaps especially the fact of low fertility, and the influence of new role-models for women's lives—could well have a transformative impact on the behaviour of urban middle class society over the next two or three decades. It should be recalled that social scientists have a rather indifferent record in foreseeing the speed at which such changes can occur. In this context it is noteworthy that the institution of marriage is being rapidly altered—nay, eroded—throughout much of Asia. Large parts of Indian society, especially the better off, will be no less influenced by these developments.

However, regarding the incidence of female specific abortion among the bulk of the country's population, the future looks rather dire. Particularly—but not only—operating through the marriage system, the pressures that work against the birth of a female appear to have the upper hand. Thus in common with many other societies, India is becoming more, not less, socio-economically differentiated as it develops economically. Therefore the pressures to marry off daughters and make a good match are increasing, not falling. In addition, as is noted by several of the contributors here, physical and economic access to the technology that makes sex-selective abortion possible will almost certainly rise in the coming years. When one looks at a map of district-level child sex ratios as revealed by the 2001 census, what strikes one are the huge areas of the country—especially in the south and east—where this invidious practice can yet spread, conditioned by essentially imported norms and patterns of behaviour. Alas, there is vast potential for these various negative processes to play out.

Of course, there are those who argue that the operation of the marriage market's 'hidden hand' will work to raise the value of the girl child in India in the long run, as shortages of potential brides emerge. There are several countries in Asia where shortages of women in the marriage market are being addressed partly through increased international migration. However migration of this sort certainly cannot have an appreciable influence on the dynamics of India's marriage market, and the same is likely to apply to internal migration. Those who have faith in the eventual operation of some beneficial 'hidden hand' neglect the distinct possibility that negative processes could become re-enforcing and self-sustaining in much of society. There are many examples in which the actions of individuals work against the collective interests of society as a whole. For example: who can doubt that India would be better in every way if men and women were held in equal regard? And in relation to the practice of female specific abortion, it is quite possible to envisage a future downward spiral in which this practice increases, making marriage more difficult, while at the same time marriage itself becomes an increasingly undervalued state.

Some thirty years ago, Ashok Mitra suggested that understanding the position of women in society was probably the single most important element in comprehending India's population. And despite all the changes that have occurred in the meantime, that observation surely retains its force.

So, to reiterate, this is a hugely important and challenging subject. The editor is to be commended greatly in making this volume possible, and the contributors are to be thanked for the insight that their writings contain. If there is any hope of influencing events so that the practice of female specific abortion disappears, then it must be based on increased understanding of the kind that is provided for us here.

TIM DYSON

PREFACE

My interest in the relationship between missing girls and female foeticide germinated on the margins of another study. This happened while I was doing a study for OXFAM, Lucknow, on domestic violence. The plan for the study took shape in 2002. The 2001 census of India, soon after the preliminary census results were out, had officially accepted the numerical female deficit in the child sex ratio figures as a serious cause for concern. It was in my meetings with NGO workers during the visits to Jhansi and other districts of Bundlekhand for the study that the processes operating toward the phenomenon of missing girls were gradually unravelled. By then the Pre-natal Diagnostic Techniques (Regulation and Prevention of Misuse) Act, 1994, commonly called (PNDT), initiated by women's groups and civil society organisations, had been a few years old and the service providers were all aware of the Act if not all the service seekers. Taking off from there, as I was persuaded by my personal interest, I explored more about the problem. And also reverted to a few stray cases I had fleetingly come across in towns in Rajasthan to gather more details. Subsequently, scholars and activists who had been working on this problem and fighting against its persistence participated in a workshop. The essays in this book are newer incarnations of those originally presented at the workshop I organised in the Department of Sociology, University of Delhi, at the end of October 2003. They mark out the various disciplinary orientations and vantage points from which the serious problem of missing girls in India is addressed. At that point, one was still hoping that the menace of sex-selective abortion, also called female foeticide, would subside and the tide would turn. I had not imagined that the problem will reach the steep level that it has today.

There was a great deal of social concern among social scientists and the media after the 2001 census reiterated its findings at various forums. In the public sphere, citizen's groups mobilisation had influenced the state apparatuses to revise the 1994 PNDT Act. It was an achievement that two amendments to the Act, those of 2002 and

2003 were passed. The theme of one of the three sections in this book, deals with the various layers and levels of interaction between the state and the society. It brings out the view that participation in, and defiance of different but intersecting systems of authority is, in itself a political phenomenon. Mobilisation of and by civil society groups in the public sphere regarding intimate, private and yet politically charged matters brings to light the conflict of ethics and interests. The life of the citizen as a person, revolves primarily around elements and mechanisms of the affective community. And the life of a person as a citizen is intertwined in multiple ways with the organs of the state at one level and those of the society and their representations at another.

The theme that sets out the book is the puzzle of positive indicators of development in modern India going gender-awry, especially as the society seems to turn against the female baby and foetus. Social inequities have been pegged on strata based on biological categories, such as age and sex in human society for long. But its traces persist in some societies, such as South and South-east Asia, while they are wiped out in others. This poses a serious challenge to social anthropology to study practices and processes that are not limited to small scale societies.

The political economy of emotions constitutes the theme running through most of the essays. It is on the micro-politics around socially shared consciousness regarding reproduction, progeny and parenting at several interrelated levels— the individual, the family and the society in everyday life. The meanings people assign to actions and consequences thereof are private and intimate political matters, but at the same time, they also are social and political matters for those very people. This reiterates the idea of personal as political. The subjectivity of people and the meanings they imbue to their and others' actions concretise politics at the private, individual as well as the social level, having micro- and macro level consequences. Politics as maternal agency, and passivity within and outside the family, is a complex play of individual and social groups' emotions and interests, of will and deed, and means and ends. The practice of sex-selective abortions is not uniform even within India. Certain high castes in India had had a tradition of female infanticide. Tradition in this book is not taken as a historical baggage or as a synonym for culture. It is a state of the mind, a state that provides meaning, embedded predispositions in thought and action to the present, in the light of mythology and a selective retrieval of the past in this specific context. The politics and economics of micro-power games are intertwined with the notions of prestige and esteem, which regularly nurse and draw upon the 'partially othering' ethos towards the daughter in North India. The daughter is for safekeeping in parental custody only for a time period; and this view is an important constituent for what it means to be a daughter's parents. Selective dislike for daughters, especially for the second and subsequent ones emerges in the essays, as they explore, the mindset along with other issues. They ask if an underlying layer of tradition is retrieved in a modern *avtaar* with its attendant structural considerations and meanings.

ACKNOWLEDGEMENTS

The book is an outcome of the efforts not only of the contributors and the editor. It also represents the contributions of the very many people who took part in the workshop of which this book is an incarnation, and who discussed the publication of this volume after the workshop. To the colleagues in the Department of Sociology whose questions I benefited from and to all those people therefore I would like to take this opportunity of expressing my thanks. Special mention may be made here for Janaki Abraham, Mahua Bandyopadhayay and Sudakshina Malik among others, who managed the organising of the workshop.

In preparing this volume, I have received much cordial support from colleagues in the Department of Anthropology, South Asia Institute, University of Heidelberg, Germany, where a great deal of editorial work for the volume was done. As Chair in India Studies for a semester, Professor William Sax willingly provided the requisite social and academic inputs. Dr Roland Hardenberg not only worked as a sounding board but also provided valuable inputs. Dr Gabriele Alex stood by her South Indian Vaghris who loved their daughters. Dr Elisabeth Shombucher-Kursterer and Professor Gita Dharampal-Fricke (Department of History) gave their critical inputs. Ferdinand Okwara's comments on one of my papers were helpful. Professor Ursula Sharma read two of my essays. I value her comments. Professor A.M. Shah's inputs have been of special importance at different junctures in the preparation of this volume. Dr Arima Mishra's comments on one of the essays were perceptive. I am grateful to all these people for cheerfully sharing what it takes to do such a task. For the forbearance they have shown at all times in the making of this volume, I take this opportunity to mention Radheshyam Patel, my husband who has been as usual the rock behind me, and Savita, my daughter whose inputs and experience have taught me many a lesson in the fruition of this volume's life.

All the contributors to this volume, unfortunately a couple of them could not find time to contribute their revised versions, I thank for their cheerful disposition, and for other support I needed from them, working across the continent. To Ms. Anamika Mukharji and Ms. Swati Sahi of Sage goes my admiration for prompt and careful handling of the publication. I am thankful to the anonymous reviewer for comments on the manuscript.

The production of this book has arisen out of the labour and interest of many researchers and concerned social scientists. The book has come at an enormous cost. It has seen the light of the day in the midst of a pathology. It has come at the cost of millions of girls who were not fortunate enough to be born. This need not be confused with taking a pro-life position. It is the selective genocide with which this effort engages. As I offer this volume to lost lives of those unborn girls, I share with the contributors of this volume the hope that the devaluation of the female sex is stalled.

Financial support through the University of Delhi was helpful in the participation of many scholars and students in the workshop in October, 2003. I am thankful to Delhi University for its support though it bears no responsibility for the views expressed here.

TULSI PATEL
30 April 2006

Introduction:
Gender Relations, NRTs and Female Foeticide in India

1

Tulsi Patel

> The real world consists not of numbers but shapes and sizes. It is topological rather than quantitative. Quantification for the most part is a prosthetic device of the human mind, though certainly a very useful one. Anyone who thinks that numbers constitute the real world, however, is under an illusion, and this is an illusion that is by no means uncommon. (Boulding 1980: 833).

This volume raises the emotive and touchy issue of millions of girls in India who fail to appear on the social scene, not figuratively, but in real demographic terms. The collection of essays on gender and new reproductive technologies, as they operate in India, is situated at the conjunction of several research issues. It locates the question of gender at a broader level, in the realm of western medical technological advancement as a harbinger of reproductive possibilities. On the one hand, it relates with the desirability of application of life-saving medical technologies on reproductive bodies. On the other, it sees that the hegemonic uniform rationality behind them translates differently at the local levels not only within the West but also within non-western societies. It is more than the relationship of application of benevolent neutral technology in the aid of biology. Social and cultural meanings of both technology and biology mediate in their interface. Human reproduction, like all other activities, is always imbued with cultural meanings. Gender is socially and culturally constructed and politico-economically situated. Caste, class, racial and religious categories are deployed in the construction of social and individual bodies. Thus specific subjective experiences, local responses, and human and societal costs of medical interventions into human reproduction are obtained.

Gender relations throw a spanner in the works. The parameter of gender complicates numerous explanations and analyses that may otherwise hold. What triggered the alarm bell was that despite the overall improvements in mortality situation, and a greater increase in life expectancy of women compared to that of men, the deficit of girls has increased over the past three decades. The conundrum here pertains to the statistic of sex ratio, with 35 million girls in India falling short of the expected number in the 2001 Census or 83 girls aged 0–6 years for every 1,000 boys of the corresponding age. It is ironical that in the last two decades the sex-ratio figures had to fall as low as they are now before arriving at a general agreement that sex-selective abortions are largely responsible for it.

It is widely agreed that sex ratio is a powerful indicator of the social health of any society. It conveys a great deal about the state of gender relations. Internationally speaking, socially as well as economically advanced societies have shown a sex ratio favourable to the female. But for many South and South-east Asian countries this relationship has not been so straightforward. Neither education nor affluence have brought about any significant change in attitudes towards women. The sex ratio figure, in 1921, of 972 women in India for every 1,000 men and its decline to 933 in the year 2001, questions the relationship between social development and sex ratio.

Since the early 1980s, India has witnessed a sharp decline in juvenile sex ratio, i.e. in the age group of 0–6 years, which became critical by serendipity. It was taken up for literacy analysis for, 2001 Census data in the first instance, when the decline in girl population appeared striking. Though not very satisfactory, the figure for 0–6 year population in India in 1961 was 976, which has sharply declined to 927 for every 1,000 boys in 2001. Since the early 1980s, the southern states of India that had relatively favourable sex ratio figures, have also been showing a decline in sex ratio. Do statistics convey what they project? Why and how has this trend of decline in the number of girl children occurred? Has the attitude towards the daughter altered? What is son preference and has it got heightened in the past couple of decades? Is the birth of a son the only way to increase parents', especially a mother's status in the household as well as in the society? How does one understand the political economy of emotions towards progeny and reproduction?

Is the sex ratio really an issue of numbers or is it reflective of the social behaviour towards the female? Sociological and hypothetical propositions need to be put forth in a comparative and historical perspective. The practice of legitimising pregnancy and birth within wedlock, and its inverse of abandoning babies born outside wedlock, existed alongside the institution of celibacy, which was as high as around 30 per cent in Ireland and between 19–30 per cent in colonial Malabar. A drastic reduction in fertility among the Japanese over the last 130 years as well as the strikingly high abortion rates in Eastern Europe, without any change in sex ratio at birth, pose the complexity of science–society relationship. Is the modern Indian culture and its corresponding mindset the culprit in leading to such abnormal sex ratios? Is culture the black box to which all explanations are attributable? Is it the active principle to whose tune people dance passively? Is culture a matter of analytical convenience, which is seen to make people desire a son to obtain a passport to heaven and make efforts to kill (sic) a female foetus, or be indifferent to such a practice? While acknowledging the empirical complexity of the matter, the essays here actually demonstrate a more widespread complexity of issues and dimensions with regard to many an unborn girl. These issues need theoretical interrogation and exploration. They need to be understood intertextually, across different fields and genres. In this volume, I have deliberately taken a range of different disciplinary genres to explore and demonstrate the usefulness of approaching the issue from different styles of analysis.

Demographic Behaviour and Gender Discrimination

Awareness of gender has become inescapable in recent years in studies of demographic processes, i.e. fertility, mortality and migration. As bearers of children, women have been the focus of attention both for demographers and policy makers. Gender formed an important category of interest in studies by Agnihotri (2000), Cassen (1978), Chen, Haq and D'souza (1981), Das Gupta and Bhat (1997),

Dyson and Moore (1983), Kishor (1993), Mason (1984), Mitra (1978), Mazumdar and Krishnaji (2001), Visaria (1971). Anthropologists interested in discriminatory behaviour and attitudes towards women and girls found gender as integral to their studies. Das Gupta (1987) and Miller (1981, 1984, 1991) had studied gender discrimination through sex differences in mortality and child survival, quite early. Besides Sen's (1990) famous 'missing women' phrase, economists had focused on gender discrimination, some of them being Agarwal (1988), Bardhan (1982), Cain (1984), Harriss (1989, 1999), V. Patel (1984), Sen (1984). Historians and other social scientists like Clark (1983, 1987, 1989, 1993), Greenough (1982), Pakrasi (1970), Pannikkar (1977), Vishwanath (2000), and the cultural anthropological work by Bhatnagar, Dube and Dube (2005) have provided archival, demographic, anthropological evidence and a cultural view of gender discrimination in India, especially of female infanticide. The historical practice highlighted during the colonial period in India, and presumed to have died out down time, resurfaced in pockets in India, not only before the new reproductive technologies (NRTs), particularly foetal-ultrasound came into the country, but even after their entry and popularity (Bumiller 1990). It would be worthwhile to trace the history of the practice and explore the institutional remnants, to connect the past with the present daughter discrimination, i.e. neglect and sex-selective abortion, and in some instances, even female infanticide practices in India. Historical evidence of a few caste groups and pockets in India practising female infanticide, raises the additional question of agency of these castes and communities in perpetuating the practice for politico-economic considerations as for the meanings they assigned to the category of the female, and to their births. Selective retrieval of mythology and history to suit the present is an Indian trait. And Nandy (1980) states that India is one society which refuses to dissociate history from myth.

Some demographers intend to emphasise the subordination of third world women and its profound ramifications on childbearing options. Women are portrayed as passive victims of patriarchal institutions where these women have little choice but to go for more children (Caldwell 1978, cited in Greenhalgh 1995). While there is a large element of truth in these portrayals, they paint too passive a picture of women in patriarchal societies. There are often instances where women are not just victims of oppressive systems but are also social actors who use the resources at their disposal to devise strategies that challenge and sometimes alter the systems. Gender is linked to agency and we shall take up the question of agency shortly.

Perspectives on Gender and Reproduction

Reproduction exists in closely intertwined social, material, political and cultural contexts. At the macro level, population has been seen as related with the politico-economic conditions. While the Marxian view is that population is dialectically related with mode of production, the Malthusian view sees it as an irresponsible and unrestrained indulgence on the part of the poor, leading to an impending doom. Poverty, inequality and population have been both internationally and nationally brought together for a long time (Patel and Purewal 2005) but the complexity of the issue remains as challenging. Marxist notions of household sustenance, social and biological reproduction of labour force and the related ideologies have been discussed by Eldohm, Harris and Young (1977), Mackintosh (1981), Morokvasic (1981). Looking at the micro level, anthropological and sociological studies have shown that gender relations are crucial in reproduction. Ginsburg and Rapp (1991) review the politics of reproduction in different parts of the world. In the Indian context, the question of gender politics in reproduction earlier, came through the demographic and policy formulation interest in fertility, population growth and non-acceptance of contraception, and subsequently on regional kinship and female autonomy differences between South and North India (Dyson and Moore 1983, Nag and Kak 1984, Mamdani 1972, Vlassoff 1979 and 1982, Vlassoff and Vlassoff 1980, Wyon and Gordon 1971).

Being associated largely with women, and seen as a women's issue, reproduction had not been central to anthropological research prior to the academic interest in gender issues, ensued by the second wave of feminist scholarship in the 1960s. Ethnographic interest in gender and reproduction in India emerged as parental status enhancement (Patel 1982), in the context of household political economy (Jeffery, Jeffery and Llyon 1989), fertility and status of women (Basu 1992), and the related domains of production and reproduction together with undervaluing of women's contribution in both of them (Sharma and Vanjani 1993), the processual view of fertility career over the women's life cycle in the socio-cultural, political and economic context (Patel 1994), female education and autonomy (Jeffery and Basu 1996) meaning and familial relations in the practice of reproduction (Saavala 2002). These ethnographic studies have located women at the centre of reproductive behaviour in situating them within households/families and communities. Though women are obliged to reproduce, they are not always passive reproducers of babies. Their agency and position in the household, family and community over their reproductive career, varies and so does their reproductive performance (Patel 2000). Supporting the practice approach to fertility, Greenhalgh (1995) stresses on the shift from societal norms to individual agency to seek the complex and mutually institutive relations between structure and agency.

Local and Global Forms of Power and Reproduction

Neo-Malthusian influence since the II WW has divided the world into two demographic blocks: those reproducing prolifically and those not reproducing enough. Anti-natalist and pro-natalist population policies respectively are applied to the two blocks (See Patel and Purewal 2005). Local and domestic reproductive relations are constituted by and resistant to national and global forms of power. Throughout history state power has directly or indirectly defined normative families and controlled populations (Donzelot 1979; Foucault 1977, 1978; O'Neil and Kaufert 1990. For a specifically gendered perspective, see Gandhi and Shah 1991 and several studies cited by them, and Jordanova 1980; for a gendered rendering of the racist pogroms of the National socialist regime of Hitler's Germany, Bock and Thane 1991, and for gender and international political economy, Rao 1998). The issue of the missing girls seen by an adverse sex ratio at the national and regional levels in India is an indicator of the politics of reproduction. It synthesises the two perspectives, the local and the global, as it links with the multiple and overlapping levels at which reproductive politics and practices take place. In this sense, it locates the problem of missing girls to sex-selective abortions as interconnected through various disciplinary perspectives whose application can throw light on the topic in a more comprehensive manner. In the field of technology, in particular, the local and global inter-relations are not at all difficult to observe in industrial production, consumption, services and communication, especially in the present day rapid globalisation process the world is experiencing. The use of new reproductive technologies (NRTs) is one of the illustrations of the experiences with globalisation.

Speaking in cultural terms, at the local level, gender and power differences have been reinforced through the binary opposition of purity and pollution. Female bodies have been shown in anthropological studies by Ardener (1975, 1992), Douglas (1960), McCormack and Strathern (1980), Reiter (1975), Rosaldo and Lamphere (1974), Yalman (1963) to have been assigned inferior values irrespective of their socio-economic contribution. Inability to have control on bodily functions, especially menstruation, has been structurally deployed to render women into the natural (biological and thereby inferior) vis-a-vis men into the cultural (superior) domain of life (Ortner 1974). In the Indian context in particular, Fruzzetti and Barnett (1976) and Fruzzetti and Ostor (1976) have paid attention to the representation of women's reproduction. Further, the commonly held view in India of the male and female reproductive substances in constituting human beings, is elaborated in the seed and earth (*beej-kshetra*) symbolism by Dube (1986, See Delaney 1991 for the monotheistic Islamic view of seed and soil symbolism in a Turkish village society). The seed-soil symbolism creates two highly unequal even if complementary possibilities of male and female contributions in biological conception and reproduction. The female (field) is inferior and more dispensable than the male (seed). It matters little if the field is provided by this or that woman; what is critical is the seed that determines social identity. The seed is the source of life, the field in turn merely nurtures that life. Semen is formed from blood, it is concentrated form of blood. Thus children carry father's blood and trace descent patrilineally, unlike in matrilineal societies studied by Nongbri (1988) and Weiner (1979). In the Indian context this symbolism is derived from the scriptural literature in the *vedas* as well medical texts, such as *Charak and Susrut samhitas* (See notes for more details in Dube 1986).

The deep rooted cultural understanding of unequal biological contribution of genders is linked to kinship, especially lineage, residence, right and control over children, and property, including questions of dowry (Agarwal 1994, Dube 1986 and 1997, 1984, Herschman 1981, Krygier 1982, Palriwala 1994, Patel 1994, Sharma 1981, 1984, Srinivas 1977, Vatuk 1975). Notwithstanding the variations between patrilineal and matrilineal kinship communities, male authority remained, be it in the critical importance of the father or the mother's brother (Dube 1973, Dumont 1961, 1964 and 1966, Goody and Tambiah 1973, Gough 1959, Schneider and Gough 1961, Inden and Nicholas 1977, Nongbri 1988). Avoidable dowry expenses as an argument justifying elimination of female foetuses, has gained common currency in both journalistic reporting and academic research. Among many middle and lower castes in India there has been a spur in adoption of the practice of dowry increasingly replacing that of bride price. This shift seems to have brought about the additional perception of the female as an economically expensive category overlapping with her more polluted though not inauspicious status as receiver and reproducer of the lineage seed. This area of research in Indian society is waiting to be studied. Kapadia (1995) mentions the unhappiness of lower caste parents of marriageable daughters in South India, owing to their inability to meet the increasing demand from prospective grooms, to 'put more gold' on brides. North India has, of course been infamous for dowry demands, the persistence lasting much after the wedding and even bride-burning for the purpose of dowry. The deep rooted consideration is, after all, the field is replaceable!

Anthropological studies on kinship, marriage, procreation and raising of children, found reproduction as socially and culturally organised, and sensitive to changes in domestic economies but at the same time involving power relations in society. Historically speaking, McLaren (1984 and 1990) has viewed the perception of fertility and contraception as political concerns. Taking a universal evolutionary frame of cultural materialism, Harris (1974) takes ecological adaptation rather than the functionalist position of a healthy organism as his model for institutional adaptation to the environment. He attributes primitive wars that place a premium on males who do most of the fighting, and female infanticide being a consequence of warfare, where females are killed overtly at birth or are allowed to die from neglect. MacLennan (1970/1865) refers to the practice of assigning higher value to the contribution of males compared to that of females, inter-tribal conflicts and tribal exogamy as reasons for female infanticide. Further, MacLennan refers to Macpherson (1852) who gives a religious explanation of female infanticide prevalent in areas of *boora*, a sect of the sun god in Orissa, alongside that of high marriage payments. The relationship between high marriage payments, tribal exogamy and female infanticide, however, needs a serious study. In their re-assessment of Engel's view on the historically determining role of relations of production and reproduction of immediate life and that of means of subsistence, anthropological studies, such as by Goody and Tambiah (1973), Goody (1976) and Yanagisako and Collier (1987) saw the mutual determination of the domestic and economic domains rather than a causal determination.

Closely related with the causal model, demographic studies on the value of children, the costs and benefits of children, were taken up by the human capital, micro-economic school (Becker 1981 and others) and by Fawcett (1972) and Arnold et al. (1975) for psychological values of children. Comparisons between fertility in societies at different stages of economic growth and between groups within societies in recent times have thrown up data that do not follow the predicted directions claimed by the theory of demographic transition. Fertility reductions were explained as a function of economic development, prosperity, education and reduced mortality through the demographic transition model. But this model is unable to explain recent fertility declines in developing countries (UNDP 2002). Women's status, autonomy and agency, emerged in this sequence, as research interests in order to grapple with the inability of the theory of demographic transition to explain many demographic changes in the world since the last quarter of the 20th century. There is evidence of women's negotiations with varying and contradictory forces within which their lives were embedded in the realm of their reproduction (for a review of this approach in demographic studies, especially in terms of questions and assumptions related with status and autonomy of women, see Madhok 2004 and Patel 2004). Unnithan-Kumar (2004) examines the intervention of state health policies with women's reproductive agency. In the context of female foeticide in India, the agency and passivity of women as reproducers remains an enigma as educated, gainfully-employed women prioritise their reproductive careers in unexpected ways. When it comes to the unrelenting desire to produce sons as against daughters, women's agency poses challenging questions. This feature of Indian society takes us beyond the issue of weaknesses of the theory of demographic transition as it baffles and contradicts the assumptions of status, position, autonomy and agency of women. Historically and culturally informed local ethnographies on this matter may be of much value.

Women's Movement and Reproductive Control

The common denominator for reproduction is that women bear babies. Yet, at once, the female reproducing body is assigned social meanings through race, class, ethnicity etc. While one race and class may be exhorted to reproduce more prolifically than it does, the other is discouraged to do so and even derided for it. Both the eugenic and the birth control movements have had some relationship in their understanding of and impact on the daily lives of women, either as active participants in the birth control or feminist movement or as groups subjected to population control-oriented contraception. Firestone (1971) cites Engels to examine the historic succession of events from which the antagonism between the sexes has sprung, in order to discover in the conditions thus created, the means of ending the conflict. The radical feminist view that biological reproduction is the primary enemy and source of women's oppression, found support in Sanger's birth control movement and the first feminist journal, *The Woman Rebel* in 1914. While the birth control movement stood for voluntary and common contraceptive provisions, the eugenics project remained dominant until it earned a bad name through the Nazi sterilisation drives in Hitler's Germany (Patel and Purewal 2005). Women in the US fought to get the ban on abortion removed in 1969 (See Ginsburg 1989, 1991 for the abortion struggle). This struggle stands in contrast with the legalisation of abortion in India in 1971, more as the state's measure for population control than for women's emancipation. The same applies to China and its single child policy of population control (Croll 1985). Struggles such as access to birth control, abortion, ending sterilisation abuse and rights of mothers are common, but they have not had uniform meanings and experiences across all societies. Women's struggles against invasive imposition of birth control by the anti-natalist policies of the state in India are discussed, among others, by Gandhi and Shah (1991). The location of women in states with different political, ideological, legal and religious leanings and in unequal economic conditions, impedes the same translations of rights, duties and experiences (Morgan 1989).

While white, middle-class women in the West gained through contraception and abortion rights, they soon realised that they had lost control over their bodies to the medical establishment as a marker of scientific practice and modernity (Foucault 1977). The woman's body was now not only dispensable as 'field', but was seen as deficient, requiring modern medicine's intervention (Martin 1987). These women soon realised that they were losing their recognition, even as reproducers, to obstetric domination in the medical system. Feminists objected to reducing birth to a mere mechanical, and physiological process of submitting the birthing body to modern medicine (Rich 1977, Oakley 1981, 1984). Reproduction was seen as an aspect of other contests for hegemonic control, such as the state eugenics policies. Globally, population policies had, as though in the spirit of the white man's burden, been linking women's status as child bearers with nationalist agendas. On the other hand, colonial policies imposed medicalisation of maternity in India (Ram 1998). The disregard of traditional birthing practices and practitioners continues as discussed in the pushing of training programmes of traditional birth attendants (Patel 2000), while many rural Indian women are themselves discontented with medicalisation and prefer home births (Patel 1998). Programmes of safe motherhood and maternal and child care, oriented towards modern medical birthing as the desirable practice, continue to be part of nationalist interest. There has been a cross national variation in medicalised births within western countries, especially striking variations with respect to anaesthesia during labour, birthing positions, postpartum and neo-natal care, etc. The explicitly cultural nature of western medicine, besides cultural variations between home and medicalised births is evident in the comparative birthing ethnographies (Jordan 1978, Laderman 1983, Shostak 1983, Patel 1994).

Between Priceless and Useless Babies

While multiple issues were raised regarding medicalisation of pregnancy and childbirth in different parts of the world, two further developments surfaced that had not been paid so much attention in earlier studies. While high fertility was focused, infertility was lost from the perception. Infertility is a curse and ruins many a woman's life in many parts of the world. Fertility and motherhood are critical for the identity and survival of a woman in Indian as in many other societies (Patel 1994, Inhorn 1995 and Inhorn and Balen 2002). It also provides the mother, especially that of a son, with the ability to negotiate from a position of stability in the family. Kinship structures are important in understanding inheritance, rights over children, authority and responsibility of members of the family or kin-group in India. The way the patriarchal family is structured is one of the major causes of inequality between men and women and of the understanding that motherhood is one of the major roles of a woman in society. Their need to have at least one son of their own encourages and/or forces many women to try new reproductive technologies that assist in producing a baby of their own. The second issue that surfaced in the mean time was not only that newer medical technology could assist infertile women, but new reproductive technologies (NRTs) could also identify 'welfare babies', i.e. those foetuses with chromosomal deformities in the West (Harpwood 1996). Rather than subjecting women to the medical profession, medical technology emerged as their saviour. Those women having babies in their mid-thirties or later could use amniocentesis and ultrasound tests to detect congenital deformities and were given the option to abort. On both counts, be it conceptive or for ante-natal care, the new medical technology, in principle, opened possibilities for women towards mothering their own normal babies (Stacey 1992).

Like means of contraception and abortion in the past, the NRTs were not uniform in their reception and effect. They translated themselves differently for women of different regions, classes and communities within and between countries (Ginsburg and Rapp 1995, Greil 1991, Gupta 2000, Widge 2001, 2002). For some, a child became priceless, while for others useless. The demand for technologically assisted conception and reproduction made the option of adoption more remote (Bharadwaj 2003). The possibility of 'one's own' biological offspring introduced new meanings and ready acceptance of the assisted reproductive technologies (ARTs). In India antenatal care technology of amniocentesis and, of late, ultrasound, has steered a revolution of sorts (Rao 2004). A hegemonic and unified rationality for pre-natal genetic testing is attributed to medical and

eugenic ideologies with unanticipated and even undesirable consequences (Rapp 1992). The experiences of women in India, though
not uniform, point to the consequences through the popularity of
sex-selective abortions. Infanticide has been studied as a continuum
in relationship with child survival as a postpartum form of reproductive control, child spacing, and determination of sex composition of
one's children as an investment strategy for privileging some offspring over others (See Scheper-Hughes 1987 for moving accounts in
Brazil). NRTs mediated the deeply interconnected processes of conception, pregnancy, birth, adoption and infanticide and foeticide
practices.

Public Sphere Discourses

In privileging of speech through the emergence of criticism in the
creation of public sphere in Europe, Habermas (1989) closely linked
the emergence of new social spaces in which rational individuals,
freed from political responsibility, could engage in the task of monitoring the exercise of power by the state. Civil society movements
through their organisations/groups, representations in mass media
and 'public interest litigation' have been publicly enunciating the
multiplex adversity in the wake of the India-specific use of NRTs
(i.e. amniocentesis and ultra-sonography). The local experiences and
ideologies are synthesised with the global/national ideologies in the
realm of reproduction. This is done especially through population
policies, practices, politics and western medical technology and its
alliance and/or resistance at the multilayered local level. The politics of gender and other hierarchies is essential in the understanding
of the complexity of reproductive experiences as they mediate through
ideologies and technologies spanning the global and the local. Some
of the issues are analysed in academic and activist circles and how
their influence has had an impact (See CEHAT 2003, Chhachi and
Sathyamala 1983, Mazumdar 1994, V. Patel 1984, and her essay in
this book).

This volume explores the questions and methods that have shaped
the experience and study of human reproduction with specific reference to the various notions, values and experiences related with
foetal sex determination technologies in India. Development,
globalisation and modernisation in India are not just contemporary

processes. Modernity incorporates several specific economic, political, social and cultural circumstances that inform and interact with family and gender relationships influencing and constituting reproductive practices. The discourses and representations around reproductive processes are rooted in local ways of relating with development, modernity and global technologies. The locally embedded modernity simultaneously generates discourses and practices viewed as common sensical in the realm of reproduction and gender relationships. The discourses around the issues have emerged from engagements of both feminist and social science scholars concerned with the demographic impact on Indian society in terms of devaluing of the female species as such. Second, and connected closely with the first concern, are the commercial and ethical dimensions through the profound and far-reaching impact made by the new medical technology from the west and its ready collaborators in local medical practice in India. As an effort to review and renew the scholarship on this multiplex topic, this volume has made a collaborative attempt with other related disciplines like social history, economics, demography, health sciences, and women' studies. It is hoped that such an integrative approach, drawn from different perspectives, will generate further questions about the gender principle and its reproductive dynamics across class, caste and other differences and move towards a critical policy evaluation in the experiences in varying local contexts that inform anthropological research.

Representation of Chapters in this Volume

The purpose of the volume has been to provide the reader with a multiplex approach to the issue of missing girls in India. It is characteristic of anthropology to tackle a given issue from various angles to get a holistic view. The authors in this volume, engaged in the study of gender and health related issues, contribute their understanding to the ongoing debates on the question of use/abuse of reproductive new medical technology in India. The essays analyse the specific empirical contexts studied by the authors or contexts in which they participated long enough and look afresh. The book shifts the controversial question of why millions of women do not survive in India to that of why millions of girls fail to take birth and are not wanted in India. The chapters are based on most authors' long-standing engagement with this and/or closely related research issues. The chapters are grouped into three topic areas which seem to emerge from the specific concerns they highlight and perspectives they represent. These are drawn from three dominant streams of scholarship that have been engaging with the issue of declining sex ratio in India in the last quarter of the century. Demographers, feminist scholars and health scientists (See Bose and Shiva 2003 for more studies) have focused their attention on the declining proportion of girls in the Indian population. This book attempts to sustain an inter-disciplinary focus with different perspectives informing one another on comparative realities and adds to others the social–anthropological perspective. As the problem at hand has an association with decline in fertility rate and family size engineered by the Indian state, it forms an important aspect of our focus.

In bringing together different disciplinary approaches to the rising deficit of girls in the population, this book takes an explicitly regional perspective in limiting itself to India. It is important to identify and contrast gender relations as they operate in India, which have assumed in the present day, a positive image of excellence in information technology skills the world over. In doing so, it locates gender across a whole spectrum of relations, from the most intimate and opaque, to those that are public and open. Between the most emotively intimate, sexual and reproductive domain to the public domain of the state, there operate a series of institutions, with specific meanings and a shared gendered consciousness about them. The chapters are based on fieldwork, survey data, archival records supported with fresh analysis of Census and NSS data.

The essays do not represent all the regions and communities of India. For instance, there is no essay on south Indian or north-east Indian data. Both the regions, south India more so, are gradually following the footsteps of north India in their child sex ratio figures. Also, pockets in south India are infamous for infanticide for a couple of decades now (Bumiller 1990). Relations of reproduction do not remain unchanged over time and region. Thus a comparative exploration of the northern region is made here. In this sense, the volume is not exhaustive enough for India as a whole. But hopefully this is the first effort and volumes on other regions might follow the theme, and inter-regional, comparative anthropological work might follow too. The essays in the volume are grouped under three broad but overlapping themes.

I. Depleting Child Sex Ratios: Ethical and Developmental Dilemmas

Numbers and inferences have an interdependence in science. Figures convey a great deal about their context, which comes from facts. From the declining child sex ratio (age 0–6) it is clear that girls are missing. How and why are they not there in the society? Is it that sex-selective abortion is responsible for the unfavourable female-male ratio asks Leela Visaria. Visaria eliminates under-enumeration, age misreporting, and sex-selective migration, but locates higher mortality of girls until recently (which more than offsets their natural immunity advantage over males) for the adverse sex ratio trends in India. For the past two decadal censuses (i.e. 1991 and 2001) the adverse sex ratio at birth signals the severity of this problem. What social factors are considered by a demographer to draw inferences, is seen in her discussion based on a large survey conducted in two districts, one each in the state of Haryana and Gujarat. The former had been showing declining sex ratios for two decades but the latter appeared on the blotted scene along with most other states in the Census decade between 1991–2001. Inter state and inter district comparisons, pointing to the increasingly unfavourable sex ratios in richer districts and more so in urban areas, pose serious questions to the trickle down and prosperity theses, notwithstanding differential calorie consumption, immunisation, health care, morbidity and mortality trends. Dagar's paper questions the development approach in this regard. The problem, argues Bose, based on his study in the three north Indian states of Punjab, Haryana and Himachal Pradesh, is not statistical alone but one of perceptions. The question worth raising here is what is son preference and how is it measured? Why are fewer daughters born to people as they get more prosperous and urban, making the prosperous, urban areas the epicentres of decline in female-male ratio? The clarity in the meaning of the usage of the terms 'son preference' and 'daughter dispreference', can render more fruitful, the use of demographic techniques of measurement. Bose likens the sex ratio decline to a civilisational collapse drawing from the survey conducted in three states. While Punjab and Haryana had registered an unfavourable sex ratio decades earlier, Himachal Pradesh like Gujarat, joined the downward spiral during 1991–2001.

The state-society inflection is discussed through the informal ties state officials have with medical establishments, obviating any booking of unlawful activity. Critiquing the perspective of development as a panacea for gender problems, Dagar argues that education, class and caste fail to support gender equity. Gendered notions of property and son as an essential offspring, prevail irrespective of developmental parameters. They transmigrate beyond national borders and persist among the Punjabi diaspora settled in the developed West. Dagar's paper is based on four large scale surveys conducted in rural and urban areas of the three cultural zones (Malwa, Majha, and Doaba) of Punjab. She includes data collected from interviews with non-resident Indians, including those of Indian origin (NRIs) from Punjab, who use sex-selective abortions and sex pre-selection technologies in Punjab. The data has also been collected from government health functionaries to critically examine the overall policy assumptions and norms held by the functionaries in their efforts to combat the depletion of female child population in the state. Critically relating the gender and developmental theoretical debates around technology and reproductive rights, Dagar provides some insightful policy suggestions.

II. Gender and Reproduction: Situating the Disappearance of Girls _____

In spite of the spread of schooling among girls in recent decades, the patriarchal social structure survives. Women derive value and status only as mothers of sons. Their happiness and social status in the conjugal homes is dependent on producing sons. Women have internalised these roles and values. Though they say that daughters take better care of parents or are more emotionally attached to the mothers, they desire to have more sons than daughters. In the pursuit of sons, they have become, with some pressure from the families, consumers of the new technology of ultrasound, which allows them to choose and bear sons. There is also an impression that husbands and their parents are pushing their wives and daughters-in-law to go for pre-birth sex determination tests and abortions. But everyone knows that many women themselves are interested in knowing the sex of the unborn child and they do not see any moral problem in undergoing these tests conducted by doctors. Most of the 11,000 volunteers for the AIIMS (All India Institute of Medical Sciences, New Delhi) experimental study of amniocentesis in 1974 carrying female foetuses had asked for abortion (Gandhi and Shah 1991).

The social context of the missing girl is seen in four essays in this part of the book. In the backdrop of a five year long study in a slum in Delhi, Sagar attempts unfolding the complexity of this issue. Female employment, poverty in the slum, and desperation to have a son, pose developmental dilemmas for Sagar both at personal and societal levels. These reveal the helplessness of those caught in this trap, as well as demonstrate the multiple levels at which this phenomenon operates. Through additional NSSO data, she demonstrates that while sex ratios are below unity in poor families, they are even lower in well-off families. She argues, while critically reflecting on the existing literature on women's development measures, for an ethical and gendered approach to development.

Bhatia's paper details the unity of meanings and thus the common purpose struck between the state health workers and the citizens around a Primary Health Centre in a district in Punjab that translates into a thriving business of sex determination tests and sex-selective abortions. Though some reservations were expressed on the contributory role of family planning programme measures in the use of sex determination tests and female foeticide, Bhatia's paper gives a rich ethnographic account of how the state health machinery, largely geared itself to meeting family planning targets, adapts itself to suit the requirements through sex determination tests and female foeticide in Punjab.

The experiential aspect of sex determination tests and resorting to female foeticide, shows how gender relations constitute the problem of sex ratio. The narrative of the every day and the ceremonial experiences in being a female and producing and raising one over her life cycle, provides meaning to numbers and to the adverse female-male sex ratio figures. Over the life cycle, the daughter syndrome is produced by a cluster of conditions and pre-existing networks. T. Patel's paper provides the narratives based on data from Rajasthan and Delhi on what it involves to raise and marry off a daughter. She further discusses the unfavourable view of daughters among the prospering middle and lower castes, who emulate the higher castes' customary (sanskritic) practices, which are clearly more adverse for women's status in and outside the household. The wife giver's honour syndrome implies a comparative low esteem, always being cautious, extra polite and holding their breath until the daughter produces a son in her conjugal family. The cluster of conditions such as these, connects with the sympathy a family receives upon the birth of a daughter. Those who suffer from it also support it in order to survive and prosper.

Among the middle and upwardly mobile lower castes too, more so in urban and metropolitan areas,[1] the insecurity and sexual violence on girls and women has been progressively rising. On the other hand, providing high professional education to daughters involves cost, which is clearly secondary (though not completely ignored) in the marriage market. When it comes to marriage, greater stress is laid on the institutions of family and marriage that mediate in constituting gender relations. This paper deals with how people come to see the daughter in a completely different manner compared with the son, and explores the working of the mindset that negotiates differently between the sexes of offspring. The seed earth symbolism and dowry burden are ethnographically unpacked in terms of their nitty-gritty in the everyday and the occasional in people's lives in the present times. While sex ratio is unfavourable for the girls in most parts of the country, Kapoor finds that there are far more girls than boys in an adoption home in Delhi which she has studied for nearly a decade. While women encounter enormous pressures on their fertility in the first instance, in contrast the pressure is on having a son, once fertility is proven through producing a baby. Even unwanted children face gender discrimination. More girls are disposed of and many land in adoption homes.

III. Representation, Articulation and the State

The goal of the state in reducing the family size to two children or even less per couple, is analysed through the duration of the family planning programme in India. The intervention of the state into society and its institutions and the response of the people mediated through institutional practices is discussed for the colonial period by Vishwananth and for the post colonial by T. Patel. In the former, it is the new land tenure system, while in the latter it is government of the family life through the state's policies and the norm of the small family. She analyses the state's success in providing contraception and abortion, and making these socially acceptable to a large majority of population in terms of various policies and interventions of the Indian family planning programme (FPP) for over half a century. The view of sex-selective abortion as horrifying, can have more than one interpretation, especially when seen in what light the medical termination of pregnancy (MTP Act, 1971) has been projected. MTP as a family planning and population control measure is projected by the state as a supportive and benign medical technological procedure, devoid of any emotional politics. In fact, the moral outrage against it was derided as backwardness. The conflicting views range from the religious right and pro-life on the one hand to the women's rights as human rights and the pro-choice liberal stand point on the other. Was MTP 1971 really introduced as a choice at a time when women in most of the advanced nations of the world had just about achieved the heavily conditional right to abort? Was it the highest expression of freedom of choice allowing control over one's body or was it a state-sponsored and state-organised eugenic strategy? It has the potential use against certain sections that are known for their disapproval of the state's small family norm, as is well known for the political emergency period in India (for ethnography of a resettlement colony in Delhi, See Tarlo 2000). T. Patel's journey through over half a century of state programmes to control population growth, shows how the thought style of people toward the family size norm has got modulated.

Vishwanath's very informed paper on female infanticide in colonial Gujarat and circumvention by higher castes of British policy interventions for perpetuating family honour and property, relates again with the state-society dynamics and constitution of instrumental rationality. The question whether modernisation is effective in improving women's condition remains to be explored. The high costs women have to pay for not conforming to society's expectations on the one hand, co-exist with the pressure on the authoritative male and the demand society makes on him to prove his masculinity on the other. The serious problem of the individual and society relationship needs addressing. What may be seemingly socially and reasonably advantageous to an individual may not be so for society. Does modern science offer choices or restrict choices for women and the family? The premonitions women's groups signalled in the 70s and 80s need not have been dismissed as wrong priorities or science fiction. Commercialisation of the medical profession as well as of human relations, propelled by large publicity in mass media, have spread their tentacles far and wide making desirable the use of sex determination tests and aborting the female foetus. It is all the more complicated when ultrasound as a technology cannot be banned and sex determination test too is not punishable unless it is done with the intent of aborting a female foetus, proving which is near impossible. The debate is hinged on a strong medical lobby and their claim that they are providing services highly in demand. Of course, the 1994 PNDT Act and its two amendments, one in 2002 and another in 2003, have muted the social service provision meaning given by medical professionals for a popular societal demand for sex determination tests and for lowering fertility growth. On the state-society inflection, V. Patel's account provides a picture of civil society's ongoing and long-drawn protest and use of democratic means to build pressure on the state to legislate and amend laws to curb what is seen as an unethical practice. The paper describes the zeal with which various organisations and groups have been protesting, impressing upon the state and seeking its intervention in this regard with the explicit purpose of preventing the commercially driven, unethical medical practices and the consequent depletion of the girl child population in India. She has been associated with the processes involved in getting the laws passed and amended since 1980s. Her paper speaks about the processes of obtaining state intervention as it also analyses the ethically questionable, strong, private profit motive of medical practitioners in this business. It is intriguing how abortion seeking was not brought into the public sphere as an ethical issue for a long time in India, unlike in the case of sex-selective abortions, which have occupied a great deal of public interest. A study of the discourse around the issue of abortion in the Indian context would certainly be of value, especially as there is little work available in this field, unlike a long drawn and continuing research on the abortion debate in the West.

Four appendices conclude this book. The first one, as mentioned earlier, is a case illustration of the experience between civil society and state interaction through a campaign in colleges in Delhi. The other three are full texts of the PNDT Act, 1994, its amendment in 2002 and the subsequent amendment of its rules in 2003.

Overview of some Common Issues

The papers, on the whole, attempt to provide an overview of the multiplex dimensions of the issue under consideration. Development, prosperity and urbanisation signalling unexpected gender responses, constitute a common link among most of the papers. The question of agency including women's agency, figured actively in several presentations, especially in Visaria (PNDT Act and choice), T. Patel (the differential care, caution and vigilance in raising daughters, and women eagerly accessing abortions among the upwardly mobile and urbanising groups, including OBCs emulating higher caste practices that go to convey what a mindset is, as an embodied concept, and how it gets strengthened), Sagar (women actively seeking doctor's help in achieving female foeticide), Vishwanath (archival records acknowledging the active role of communities in response to colonial land tenures), V. Patel (agency of feminists and their rather early warnings juxtaposed with the active participation of women in choosing to abort female foetuses in Maharashtra and elsewhere in India). Though not raised as an agency question, Kapoor's paper has at its back the agency of the mother who gives away/ abandons her undesirable babies, not unheard of in other parts of the world. Similarly, women in Bhatia's study exercise agency much against the state legislation. Bose's essay raises the issue of agency and passivity and this could be further investigated both analytically and empirically.

Why do women go for sex determination tests? Are they to blame for it? Women who have the choice, exercise it in favour of the son and against the daughter. How much choice do these women have? What forces work on them? Whether the pressure exerted on women to go for sex determination tests is to be construed as an exercise in choice, or is to be seen as their victimisation, would pose the problem in binary opposite categories, especially when the structural conditions are more grey than either black or white. Gaps in the law and its enforcement need addressing through campaign initiatives and commitment even while acknowledging the ongoing unresolved position on choice. Advocacy-induced legislation, such as the PNDT Act 1994, and two amendments of 2002 and 2003 were brought about to regulate and monitor the use of science and technology in this regard. The general syndrome to neglect the importance of law and treat it as a scapegoat, applies to sex determination tests and abortion of the female foetus. Redress as well as reversal in the impending chaos put a larger onus on advocacy (Nanda's report of a campaign in Delhi University in the appendix). Recently, there have been religious censures (by Sikh religious leaders). An inter-faith journey was also organised through the most affected north-western part of India in the first fortnight of November, 2005.

The strong medical lobby and their claim that they are providing services highly in demand which is instead claimed as an act of social work, comes in for strong criticism (V. Patel). Sagar posed the problem of irrational behaviour and the moral and ethical dilemma and the issue of internally unresolved and conflicting rights the medical professionals are confronted with. The ethically desirable medical regulation and reform have taken place only through external influence and it is not likely to change on its own through self-reflection. In the public health framework she suggests that structural conditions and policy interventions should create liveable and hopeful life. On the whole, the crucial question that needs to be raised here is the role and impact of privatisation and commercialisation of medical services in India, especially the spread of ultra-sonography and female foeticide in comparison with state/non-private medicine.

The above issues point to the role of the state and its relationship with society, with its citizens, be they parents—mothers and/or fathers, children—boys or girls, and other professionals as members of the society and the public sphere. State's policies, leadership, aims and objectives cherished and propagated by the leadership and influential officials percolate in a variety of ways anticipated and otherwise. Vishwanath's paper deals with the colonial state and people's experiences with it, regarding female infanticide. T. Patel traces the links between the population control and stabilisation goals in independent India and the thought styles it contributed in generating in the country through the family planning programme. V. Patel's paper brings to us the public sphere's role in relation with the state's role and responsibility in dealing with the complex, ethical and medical matters around reproductive technologies adopted in the country.

As stated above, clearly, south and north-east India need to be explored in their incipient stages, for this trend. Cultural and historical accounts of female infanticide in contemporary history and at present times, especially even after the popularity of NRTs is blurred from the view. It is only after the introduction of public debates on female foeticide, as discussed by V. Patel in her essay, that female infanticide has been reported in the mass media. Not much academic inquiry has gone into the prevalence of female infanticide. The question needs to be asked why does infanticide happen when foeticide is so prevalent? Though there is likely to be a denial on initial query on such a topic, there is a need to explore the institutional practice and practitioners in such a disappearance of the female child in India. The link between sonography and the technological deterministic perspective may be further probed in this regard. Regional sex ratio variations were found even in the 1872 Census of India. While Bengal, Madras, Mysore and Central Provinces had for every 100 males, females ranging from over 100 to 96.5, for Berar, Oude and Bombay from 93.5 to 91.5 and for NWP and Punjab 87.5 to 83.5.

It is widely acknowledged that female foeticide happens but little serious work is available on why do people resort to it. The volume tries to portray some threads of a larger tapestry. This tapestry needs to be on the wall. And hopefully its threads from other regional studies will perhaps join for the larger picture to emerge. Contemporary historical accounts and social–anthropological investigation need not be limited to regions other than North India, but also incorporate caste and communities historically not known for female infanticide. Surely, the female child population has not only depleted solely among those communities known for this practice in the past, but statistics of such a magnitude might convey the likelihood of a much wider spread of the practice among other caste groups and communities in India. Nevertheless, focus on caste groups and their sex ratios have a potential to inform a great deal about gender and caste relationship as it obtains at present in Indian society, as well as, among the Indian diaspora.

The spate of village studies of the 1950s and 60s threw up a great deal of data about rural life in India. There is a need for a revisit to see the rural world after half a century. Similarly, urban communities may be explored through intensive field studies which might be able to throw light on urban life in contemporary India. Such studies may retain the focus of how and what makes different caste groups and communities perceive and relate with NRTs, medical systems, legislation and the state in their everyday life. The peaks and troughs of sex ratio differences in communities obtained historically, may or may not continue to be similar. Studies such as the ones suggested above may show why and how the peaks and troughs are getting levelled or otherwise. The issue of women's, mother's and father's agency intertwined with the ongoing under-grounded practice of sex-selective abortions, calls for serious attention. With socio-economic development of the country, educational and employment indicators of the status of women improving, what is pulling women downward to the extent of female birth itself becoming an avoidable preference? Further, with globalisation and international opportunities increasing, especially for the middle and upper class urban Indians, why is this particular population showing greater dislike of female birth? Though surveys are important, they provide trends of the phenomenon and a picture of the larger canvas, micro-level ethnographic studies are needed for a closer view both for understanding the complexity of the issue and related questions of responsibility, reform and the state.

Practices existing at the margins of law may be taken up for investigation. The inflection of the state, through its policy measures and enforcement mechanisms are further linked with the medical system and the related legislation. An inquiry at the field level, into the social life of the community, may throw up newer dimensions of the inter-relationship between medical practice, its consumers and the state. Though the medical profession is rightly much maligned in this regard, except for the pure money-making logic that sustains the practice, which undoubtedly is a critical factor, social anthropological studies on the complex gamut of official and unofficial networks, how and why the practice continues to manage to thrive, are worth taking up. Issues of medical paternalism versus consumer autonomy and choice are among the most complex ones in this regard.

Note

1. Many girls in their early teens are being withdrawn from schools in Haryana as parents fear for their safety (reported by Saraswati Raju in response to my paper on Informal social networks and female foeticide presented at the Institute of Social Science in New Delhi September, 2003).

References

Agarwal, B. (ed.). 1988. *Structures of Patriarchy: State, Community and Household in Modernizing Asia*. New Delhi: Kali for Women.

―――. 1994. *A Field of One's Own: Gender and Land Rights in South Asia*. Cambridge: Cambridge University Press.

Agnihotri, S.B. 2000. *Sex Ratio Patterns in the Indian Population—A Fresh Exploration*. New Delhi: Sage.

Ardener, S. (ed.). 1975. *Perceiving Women*. London: John Wiley.

―――. (ed.). 1992. *Persons and Powers of Woman in Diverse Cultures: Essays in Commemoration of Audrey I. Richards, Phyllis Kaberry and Barbara E. Ward*. New York and Oxford: Berg Publishers.

Arnold, F., R.A. Bulatao, C. Buripakdi, B.J. Chung, J.T. Fawcett, T. Iritani, S.J. Lee and T. Wu (eds.). 1975. *The Value of Children: A Cross-National Study*. Vol. 1. Honolulu: East-West Population Institute.

Becker, G. 1981. *A Treatise on the Family*. Cambridge, MA: Belknap.

Bardhan, P.K. 1982. 'Little Girls and Death in India', *Economic and Political Weekly*, 17 (36): 1448–50.

Basu, A.M. 1992. *Culture, the Status of Woman, and Demographic Behaviour. Illustrated with The Case of India*. Oxford: Clarendon Press.

Bharadwaj, A. 2003. 'Why Adoption is Not an Option in India: the Visibility of Infertility, the Secrecy of Donor Insemination, and other Cultural Complexities', *Social Science and Medicine*, 56 (9): 1867–80.

Bhatnagar, R.D., R. Dube and R. Dube. 2005. *Female Infanticide in India: A Feminist Cultural History*. Albany: State University of New York.

Bock, G. 1991. 'Antinatalism, Maternity and Paternity in National Socialist Racism', in G. Bock and P. Thane (eds.), *Maternity and Gender Policies: Women and the Rise of European Welfare States*, pp. 233–55. London: Routledge.

Bose, A. and M. Shiva, 2003. *Darkness at Noon: Female Foeticide in India*. New Delhi: (VHAI.) Voluntary Health Association of India.

Boulding, K. 1980. 'Science: Our Common Heritage', *Science*, 207: 831–36.

Bumiller, E. 1990. *May You be the Mother of a Hundred Sons*. Fawcett Columbine: Ballantine Books.

Cain, M. 1984. *Women's Status and Fertility in Developing Countries: Son Preference and Economic Security*. World Bank Staff Working Paper Series No. 682, Washington D.C., World Bank.

Cassen, R.H. 1978. *India: Population, Economy, Society*. London: Macmillan.

CEHAT. 2003. *Sex Selection, Issues and Concern*. Mumbai: Centre for Inquiry into Health and Allied Themes.

Chen, L., E. Haq and S. D'Souza 1981. 'Sex-bias in the Family Allocation of Food and Health Care in Rural Bangladesh', *Population and Development Review*, 7 (1): 55–70.

Chhachhi, Amrita and C. Sathayamala 1983. 'Sex determination Tests: A Technology Which Will Eliminate Women', *Medico Friend Circle Bulletin*, 95: 3–5.

Clark, A. 1983. 'Limitations on Female Life Changes in Rural Central Gujarat', *The Indian Economic and Social History Review*, 20 (1): 1–25.

―――. 1987. 'Social Demography of Excess Female Mortality in India: New Directions', *Economic and Political Weekly*, 22 (17): WS12–WS21.

Clark, A. 1989. 'Mortality, Fertility and the Status of Women in India, 1881–1931', in T. Dyson (ed.), *India's Historical Demography: Studies in Famine, Disease and Society*, pp. 119–49. London: Curzon Press.

———. (ed.). 1993. *Gender and Political Economy: Explorations of South Asian Systems*. Delhi: Oxford University Press.

Croll, E. 1985. *China's One Child Policy*. London: Macmillan.

Das Gupta, M. 1987. 'Selective Discrimination Against Female Children in Rural Punjab, India', *Population and Development Review*, 13 (1): 77–100.

Das Gupta M. and P. N. Mari, Bhat. 1997. 'Fertility Decline and Increased Manifestation of Sex Bias in India', *Population Studies*, 51 (3): 307–15.

Delaney, C. 1991. *The Seed and the Soil: Gender and Cosmology in Turkish Village Society*. Berkeley: University of California Press.

Donzelot, J. 1979. *The Policing of Families*. NY: Pantheon.

Douglas, Mary. 1960. *Purity and Danger*. London: Routledge and Kegan Paul.

Dube, L. 1973. 'Caste Analogues among the Laccadives (Lakshdweep) Muslims', in I. Ahmad (ed.), *Caste and Social Stratification among Muslims in India*, pp. 195–231. Delhi: Manohar.

———. 1986. 'Seed and Earth: The Symbolism of Biological Reproduction and Sexual Relations of Production', in L. Dube, E. Leacock and S. Ardener (eds.), *Visibility and Power: Essays on Woman in Society and Development*, pp. 119–53. Delhi: Oxford University Press.

———. 1997. *Women and Kinship: Comparative Perspectives on Gender in South and South-East Asia*. Tokyo: United University Press; New Delhi: Vistaar.

Dumont, L. 1961. 'Marriage in India: The Present State of the Question: I', *Contributions to Indian Sociology*, 5 (October): 75–95.

———. 1964. 'Marriage in India: The Present State of the Question: II', *Contributions to Indian Sociology*, 7 (March): 77–98.

———. 1966. 'Marriage in India: The Present State of the Question: III', *Contributions to Indian Sociology*, 9 (December): 90–114.

Dyson, T. and M. Moore. 1983. 'On Kinship Structure, Female Autonomy and Demographic Behaviour in India', *Population and Development Review*, 9 (1): 35–60.

Eldohm, F., O. Harris and K. Young 1977. 'Conceptualising Women', *Critical Anthropology*, 9 (10): 101–30.

Fawcett, J. T. (ed.), 1972. *The Satisfactions and Costs of Children: Theories, Concepts and Methods*. Honolulu: East-West Population Institute.

Firestone, S. 1971. *The Dialectic of Sex: The Case for Feminist Revolution*. London: Cape.

Foucault, M. 1977. *Discipline and Punish: Birth of the Prison*, transl. A. Sheridan. NY: Pantheon.

———. 1978. *History of Sexuality*, Vol. 1, transl. R. Hurley. NY: Pantheon.

Fruzzetti, L. and S. Barnett. 1976. 'The Cultural Construction of the Person in Bengal and Tamil Nadu', *Contributions to Indian Sociology* (NS), 10 (1): 157–182.

Fruzzetti, L. and A. Ostor. 1976. 'Seed and Earth: A Cultural Analysis of Kinship in a Bengali Town', *Contributions to Indian Sociology* (NS), 10 (1): 96–131.

Gandhi, N. and N. Shah. 1991. *The Issues at Stake*. New Delhi: Kali for Women.

Ginsburg, F. 1989. *Contested Lives: The Abortion Debate in An American Community*. Berkley: University of California Press.

———. 1991. 'The "word-made" Flesh: The Disembodiment of Gender in the Abortion Debate', in F. Ginsburg and A. Tsing (eds.), *Uncertain Terms: Negotiating Gender in American Culture*, pp. 59–75. Boston: Beacon Press.

Ginsburg, F. and R. D. Rapp. 1991. 'The Politics of Reproduction', *Annual Review of Anthropology*, 20: 311–43.

———. and R. D. Rapp (eds.). 1995. *Conceiving the New World Order: The Global Politics of Reproduction*. Berkley: University of California Press.

Goody, J.R. 1976. *Production and Reproduction*. Cambridge: Cambridge University Press.

Goody, J. R. and S. J. Tambiah. 1973. *Bridewealth and Dowry*. Cambridge: Cambridge University Press.

Gough. K. 1959. 'The Nayars and the Definition of Marriage', *Journal of Royal Anthropological Institute*, 89 (1): 23–34.

Government of India. 2002. *Handbook on PNDT Act, 1994*. New Delhi: Department of Family Welfare, for use by Appropriate Authorities in States/ Union Territories.

Greenhalgh S. 1995. 'Introduction', in S. Greenhalgh (ed.), *Situating Fertility: Anthropology and Demographic Inquiry*, pp. 3–28. Cambridge: Cambridge University Press.

Greenough, P. R. 1982. *Prosperity and Misery in Modern Bengal*. New York: Oxford University Press.

Greil, A. L. 1991. *Not Yet Pregnant: Infertile Couples in Contemporary America*. New Brunswick: Rutgers University Press.

Gupta, J.A. 2000. *New Reproductive Technologies, Women's Health and Autonomy: Freedom or Dependency?* New Delhi: Sage Publications.

Habermas, J. 1989. *The Structural Transformation of the Public Sphere: An Inquiry into a Category of Bourgeois Society*. Cambridge: Polity Press.

Harpwood, Vivienne. 1996. *Legal Issues in Obstetrics*. Aldershot: Dartmouth.

Harriss, B. 1989. 'Differential Child Mortality and Health Care in South Asia', *Journal of Social Studies*, 44: 2–123.

Harriss-White, B. 1999. 'Gender Cleansing', in R. Sunder Rajan (ed.), *Gender Issues in Post Independent India*, pp. 124–153. New Delhi: Kali for Women.

Harris. M. 1974. *Cows, Pigs, Wars and Witches: The Riddles of Culture*. New York: Random House.

Hershman, P. 1981. *Punjabi Kinship and Marriage*. Delhi: Hindustan Publishing Corporation.

Hatti, N., T.V. Sekhar and M. Larsen. 2004. 'Lives at Risk: Declining Child Sex Ratios in India', Lund Papers in Economic History, No. 93. *Population Economics*. Department of Economic History, Lund University.

Inden, R. and R. Nicholas. 1977. *Kinship in Bengali Culture*. Chicago: University of Chicago Press.

Inhorn, M. C. 1995. *Infertility and Patriarchy: The Cultural Politics of Gender and Family Life in Egypt*. Philadelphia: University of Pennsylvania Press.

Inhorn, Marcia C. and Balen Frank van (eds.). 2002. *Infertility Around the Globe: New Thinking on Childlessness, Gender, and Reproductive Technologies*. London: University of California Press:

Jeffery P., R. Jeffery and A. Llyon. 1989. *Labour Pains, Labour Power: Woman and Childbearing in India*. London: Zed Books; New Delhi: Manohar.

Jeffery, R. and A.M. Basu (eds.), 1996. *Girls' Schooling, Women's Autonomy and Fertility Change in South Asia*. New Delhi: Sage Publications.

Jordon, B. 1978. *Birth in Four Cultures: A Cross-cultural Study of Childbirth in Yucutan, Holland, Sweden and the U.S.* Shelborne, VT: Eden Press.

Jordanova, L. J. 1980. 'Natural Facts: A Historical Perspective on Science and Sexuality', in C. MacCormack and M. Strathern (eds.), *Nature, Culture and Gender*, pp. 42–69. NY: Cambridge University Press.

Kapadia, K. 1995. *Siva and Her Sisters: Gender, Caste and Class in Rural South India*. Boulder: Westview Press.

Kishore, S. 1993. 'May God Give Sons to All: Gender and Child Mortality in India', *American Sociological Review*, 58: 246–65.

Krygier, J. 1982. 'Caste and Female Pollution', in M. Allen and S.N. Mukherjee (eds.), *Woman in India and Nepal*, pp. 75–104. Australian National University Monographs on South Asia, 8. Canberra: Australian National University Press.

Laderman, C. 1983. *Wives and Midwives: Childbirth in Rural Malaysia*. Berkeley: University of California Press.

Mackintosh, M. 1981. 'The Sexual Division of Labour and the Subordination of Women' in K. Young, C. Wallkowitz and K. McCullagh (eds.), *Of Marriage and the Market: Women's Subordination in International Perspective*, pp.1–15. London: CSE Books.

MacLennan, J. F. 1970 (1865). *Primitive Marriage: An Inquiry into the Origin of the Form of Capture in Marriage Ceremonies*. Chicago: University of Chicago Press.

McLaren, A. 1984. *Reproductive Rituals: the Perception of Fertility in England from the Sixteenth Century to the Nineteenth Century*. London, NY: Methuen.

McLaren, A. 1990. *A History of Contraception: From Antiquity to the Present Day*. London: Basil Blackwell.

Macpherson, 1852. 'An Account of the Religion of the Khonds in Orissa'. *Journal of the Royal Asiatic Society of Great Britain and Ireland*, 13: 216–74.

Madhok, S. 2004. 'Heteronomous Women: Hidden Assumptions in the Demography of Women', in Unnithan-Kumar, M. (ed.), 2004. *Reproductive Agency, Medicine and the State*, pp. 223–44. Oxford: Berghahn Books.

Mamdani, M. 1972. *The Myth of Population Control. Family, Caste and Class in an Indian Village*. New York: Monthly Review Press.

Martin, E. 1987. *The Woman in the Body*. Boston: Beacon.

Mason, K. O. 1984. *The Status of Women, Fertility and Mortality: A Review of Interrelationships*. New York: Rockefeller Foundation.

Mazumdar, V. 1994. '*Amniocentesis and Sex Selection*', Delhi: Centre for Women's Development Studies, Occassional Paper Series No. 21.

Mazumdar, V. and N. Krishnaji (eds.), 2001. *Enduring Conundrum: India's Sex Ratio*. Delhi: Rainbow Publishers.

McCormack, C. and M. Strathern (eds.), 1980. *Nature, Culture and Gender*. Cambridge: Cambridge University Press.

Miller, B. 1981[1991]. *The Endangered Sex. Neglect of Female Children in Rural North India*. Ithaca, NY: Cornell University Press.

Miller, B.D. 1984. 'Daughter Neglect, Women's Work and Marriage', *Medical Anthropology*, 8 (2): 109–25.

Mitra, A. 1978. *India's Population: Aspects of Quality and Control.* Vol. 1. New Delhi: Abhinav Publications.

Morgan, L. 1989. 'When Does Life Begin? A Cross-Cultural Perspective on the Personhood of Foetuses and Young Children', in E. Doerr and J. Prescott (eds.), *Abortion Rights and Fetal "Personhood"*, pp. 97–114. Long Beach, CA: Centerline.

Morokvasic, M. 1981. 'Sexuality and Control of Procreation', in K. Young, et al. (eds.), *Of Marriage and the Market: Women's Subordination in International Perspective*, pp. 127–43. London: CSE Books.

Nag, M. and N. Kak. 1984. 'Demographic Transition in a Punjab Village', *Population and Development Review*, 10 (4): 661–78.

Nandy, A. 1980. *At the Edge of Psychology.* Delhi: Oxford University Press.

Nongbri, T. 1988. 'Gender and the Khasi Family Structure: Some Implications of Meghalaya Succession to Self-Acquired Property Act, 1984', *Sociological Bulletin*, 37 (1 and 2): 71–82.

O'Neil, J. and P. Kaufert. 1990. 'Cooptation and Control: The Reconstruction of Innuit Birth', *Medical Anthropology Quarterly*, 4 (4): 427–42.

Oakley, A. 1981. *Woman Confined: Sociology of Childbirth.* New York: Schocken.

———. 1984. *The Captured Womb: A History of the Medical Care of Pregnant Women.* N.Y.: Basil Blackwell.

Ortner, S.B. 1974. 'Is Female to Male as Nature to Culture?', In M. Rosaldo and L. Lamphere (eds.), *Woman, Culture and Society*, pp. 67–88. Stanford: Stanford University Press.

Pakrasi, K. 1970. *Female Infanticide in India.* Calcutta: Editions Indian.

Palriwala, R. 1994. *Change and Continuity in Gender, Family and Kinship Relations.* Part I & II. Leiden: Women and Autonomy Center (VENA).

Panigrahi, L. 1972. *British Social Policy and Female Infanticide in India.* New Delhi: Munshiram Manoharlal.

Panikkar, K. N. 1977. 'Land Control, Ideology and Reform: A Study of the Changes in Family Organization and Marriage System in Kerala', *Indian Historical Review*, 4 (1): 30–46.

Patel, T. 1982. 'Domestic Group, Status of Woman and Fertility', *Social Action*, 32 (4): 363–79.

———. 1994. [2006]. *Fertility Behaviour: Population and Society in a Rajasthan Village.* Delhi: Oxford University Press.

———. 1998. 'Modern and Traditional Therapeutic Practices: The Case of Childbirth in Rural Rajasthan'. Paper presented at the Conference of Asia Pacific Social Science and Medicine Network, Yogyakarta, Indonesia, June 22–26.

———. 2000. 'Training of Traditional Birth Attendants in India: An Analysis.' Paper presented at the Conference of Asia Pacific Social Science and Medicine Network, Kandy, Sri Lanka, September 24–28.

———. 2004. 'Women in Fertility Studies and *In Situ*', in M. Unnithan-Kumar (ed.), *Reproductive Agency, Medicine and the State*, pp. 203–22. Oxford: Berghahn Books.

Patel T. and T. Purewal. 2005. 'Origins and Contours of the Population Debate: Inequality, Population Politics and the Population Debate', in M. Romero and E. Margolis (eds.), *The Blackwell Companion to Social Inequalities*, pp. 441–65. New York: Blackwell.

Patel, V. 1984. 'Amniocentesis—Misuse of Modern Technology', *Socialist Health Review*, 1(2): 69–71.

Ram, K. 1998. 'Maternity and the Story of Enlightenment in the Colonies: Tamil Coastal Women, South India,' In Ram, K. and M. Jolly (eds.), *Maternities and Modernities: Colonial and Postcolonial Experiences in India and the Pacific*, pp. 114–43. Cambridge: Cambridge University Press.

Rao, M. 1998. 'Quinacrine Sterilisation Trials: A Scientific Scandal', *Economic and Political Weekly*, 33 (13): 692–95.

———. (ed). 2004. *The Unheard Scream: Reproductive Health and Women's Lives in India*. New Delhi: Zubaan and Panos Institute.

Rao, V. 1993. 'The Rising Price of Husbands: A Hedonic Analysis of Dowry Increases in India', *Journal of Political Economy*, 101 (4): 666–77.

Rapp, Rayna. 1992.'Reproduction and Gender Hierarchy: Amniocentesis in Contemporary America', in B. D. Miller (ed.), *Gender Hierarchies: The Anthropological Approach*, pp. 108–26 Cambridge: Cambridge Press.

———. 1995. 'Accounting for Amniocentesis', in S. Lindenbaum and M. Lock (eds.), *Knowledge, Power and Practice: The Anthropology of Medicine in Everyday Life*, pp. 55–76. Berkeley: University of California Press.

Reiter, R.R. (ed.), 1975. *Towards an Anthropology of Woman*. New York. Monthly Review Press.

Rich, A. 1976. *Of Woman Born: Motherhood as Experience and Institution*. N.Y.: Norton.

Rosaldo, M. Z. and L. Lamphere (eds.). 1974. *Woman, Culture and Society.* Stanford: Stanford University Press.

Säävälä, M. 2002. *Fertility and Familial Power Relations: Procreation in South India*. Richmond. Curzon Press.

Scheper-Hughes. N. (ed.). 1987. *Child Survival: Anthropological Perspectives on the Treatment and Maltreatment of Children*. Dordrecht: Reidel.

Schneider, D.M. and K. Gough. (eds.). 1961. *Matrilineal Kinship*. Berkeley and Los Angeles: University of California Press.

Sen, A. 1984. *Resources, Values and Development*. Oxford: Basil Blackwell.

———. 1990. 'More than 100 Million Women are Missing', *New York Review of Books*, 20 December: 61–5.

———. 1991. 'Gender and Co-operative Conflicts', in I. Tinker (ed.), *Persistent Inequalities*, pp. 123–49. New Delhi: Oxford University Press.

Sharma, M. and U. Vanjani. 1993. 'Engendering Reproduction: The Political Economy of Reproductive Activities in a Rajasthan Village', in A W. Clark (ed.), *Gender and Political Economy: Explorations of South Asian Systems*, pp. 24–65. Delhi: Oxford University Press.

Sharma, U. 1980. *Woman, Work and Property in North-West India*. London and New York: Tavistock.

———. 1984. 'Dowry in North India: Its Consequences for Women', in R. Hirschon (ed.), *Women and Property, Women as Property*, pp. 62–74. Croomhelm: Beckanham.

58 | Tulsi Patel

Shostak, M. 1983. *Nisa: The Life and Words of a !Kung Woman*. New York: Vintage Books.

Srinivas, M. N. 1977. 'The Changing Position of Indian Woman'. *Man* (NS), 12 (2): 221–238.

———. 1984. *Some Reflections on Dowry*. Delhi: Oxford University Press.

Stacey M. (ed.) 1992. *Changing Human Reproduction: Social Science Perspectives*. London: Sage Publications.

Tarlo, E. 2000. 'Body and Space in a Time of Crisis: Sterilisation and Resettlement during the Emergency in Delhi', in V. Das, A. Kleinman, M. Ramphele and P. Reynolds (eds.), *Violence and Subjectivity*, pp. 242–70. Berkeley: University of California Press.

UNDP. 2002. *The Future of Intermediate Fertility Countries*. Expert Group Meeting on Completing the Fertility Transition. NY: UN Population Division Department of Economic and Social Affairs.

Unnithan-Kumar, M. (ed.), 2004. *Reproductive Agency, Medicine and the State*. Oxford: Berghahn Books.

Vatuk, S. 1972. *Kinship and Urbanization: White Collar Migrants in North India*. Berkley: University of California Press.

———. 1975. 'Gifts and Affines in North India', *Contributions to Indian Sociology* (NS), 9 (2): 155–96.

Visaria, P. 1971. *The Sex Ratio of the Population of India. Census of India 1961*. Monograph No. 10. New Delhi: Office of the Registrar General of India.

Vishwanath, L.S. 2000. *Social Structure and Female Infanticide in India*. Delhi: Hindustan.

Vlassoff, M. 1979. 'Labour Demand and Economic Utility of Children: A Case Study of Rural India', *Population Studies*, 33 (3): 415–28.

———. 1982. 'Economic Utility of Children and Fertility in Rural India', *Population Studies*, 36 (1): 45–59.

Vlassoff, M. and C. Vlassoff. 1980. 'Old Age Security and the Utility of Children in Rural India', *Population Studies*, 34 (3): 487–99.

Weber, M. 1949. *The Methodology of Social Science*. Glenco IL: The Free Press.

Weiner, A. B. 1979. 'Trobriand Kinship from Another View: The Reproductive Power of Women and Men', *Man*, 14 (2): 328–48.

Widge, A. 2001. *Beyond Natural Conception: A Sociological Investigation of Assisted Reproduction with Special Reference to India*, Unpublished Ph.D. thesis, Jawaharlal Nehru University, New Delhi.

Widge, A. 2002. 'Socio-cultural Attitudes towards Infertility and Assisted Reproduction in India', in E. Vayena, P. J. Rowe and P. D. Griffin (eds.), *Current Practices and Controversies in Assisted Reproduction*, pp. 60–74. Geneva, Switzerland: WHO Headquarters, http://www.who.int/reproductive-health/infertility/11. pdf

Wyon, J.B. and J.E. Gordon. 1971. *The Khanna Study*. Cambridge, Mass: Harvard University Press.

Yalman, N. 1963. 'On the Purity and Sexuality of Women in the Castes of Ceylon and Malabar', *Journal of the Royal Anthropological Institute*, 93 (1): 25–58.

Yanagisako, S.J. and J.F. Collier. 1987. 'Toward a Unified Analysis of Gender and Kinship', in J.F. Collier and S.J. Yanagisako (eds.), *Gender and Kinship*, pp. 14–50. Stanford: Stanford University Press.

PART **1**

*Missing Girls
and NRTs:
Ethical and
Developmental
Dilemmas*

Deficit of Girls in India: Can it be Attributed to Female Selective Abortion?

2

Leela Visaria

The deficit of women in India's population has been documented ever since the first decennial enumeration of people was conducted in the late 19th century. Over the span of more than 100 years, the deficit has progressively increased as evident from the sex ratio of the population; the number of women per 1,000 men steadily declined from 972 in 1901 to 933 in 2001.[1] India shares with China (and other South Asian countries with the exception of Sri Lanka) this phenomenon of deficit of women in the population. Both the large oriental societies of India and China are structurally patrilineal, exhibit strong son preference and here men enjoy higher status relative to women. Throughout the rest of the world, women outnumber men by 3 to 5 per cent. In India, according to the 2001 Census, there were 7 per cent more men than women.

The deficit of women in India and the possible factors responsible for it have aroused a lot of attention among demographers, social scientists and women activists who have tried to understand the phenomenon in terms of women being under-enumerated in the census counts, sex-selective migration, sex ratio at birth, as well as sex differentials in mortality. Historically, under-enumeration, especially of child brides in certain regions, where child marriages are customary, has found favour with many analysts of census data as one of the factors accounting for deficit of girls aged 10–14 years. On the other hand, there has been no evidence to support the likelihood of sex differentials in migration (implying greater out migration of women) or greater than the usual masculinity of sex ratio at birth.

What has been convincingly demonstrated is that the primary factor contributing to the deficit of women in India is the anomalous higher mortality among women compared to men (Visaria 1971). According to the data from the Sample Registration System of the past 30 years, Indian women have been experiencing higher mortality than men from the age of 12 months to almost up to the end of the reproductive period. Again, elsewhere in the world, women generally experience lower mortality than men at almost all ages such that the life expectancy at birth of women is greater by 5 to 8 years compared to that of men (Visaria 2002). In India, until 1980s, the life expectancy of women was lower by 2–3 years than that of men. It is only in the 1990s that the trend has begun to reverse.

The sex differential in mortality in India, resulting from the discriminatory treatment received by girls and women, more than offsets their natural or biological advantage over men. Within India, the social practices and cultural ethos that undervalue women are stronger in some regions than in others. In an almost contiguous belt extending from north-west of India to parts of Rajasthan, Gujarat and Maharashtra, the undervaluation of women is evident in the sex ratio of their population and in their juvenile sex ratio. In fact, an increase in the deficit of young girls noted in the three decennial Censuses of 1981, 1991 and 2001, is indicative of a strong possibility that the traditional methods of neglect of female children are increasingly being replaced by not allowing female children to be born.[2]

In this paper, I have attempted to estimate the magnitude of deficit of girls in India as a whole and in some of the female-disadvantaged states and have compared the situation in them with that in Kerala, which is considered a female-advantaged state. The Medical Termination of Pregnancy (MTP) Act and the Pre-Natal Diagnostic Technique prevention (PNDT) Act are discussed at some length because the recent manifestation of son preference and daughter non-preference needs to be understood in the context of these Acts. After briefly discussing some indirect evidence of female-selective abortion from primary data collected from one district each of Gujarat and Haryana, the voices of women are documented to understand what compels women or their families to abort female foetuses.

Magnitude of Deficit of Girls in Population

If all births in the country or a region were registered, one would be able to calculate the sex ratio at birth and surmise the extent to which female births are prevented from occurring, since sex ratio at birth is biologically determined and globally ranges between 102 and 107 male births to 100 female births. Unless there is a conscious effort at intervention by human beings, the sex ratio at birth is most unlikely to change even over a long time. However, in India except for states like Kerala, Tamil Nadu and Goa, where registration of births is nearly complete, elsewhere births are far from systematically or fully registered. A significant proportion of births occurring at home are missed from being registered.

In the absence of accurate information on vital events, we have to depend on other sources such as the decennial Censuses, which have provided in record short time after the conduction of each Census, data on number of children in the age group 0–6 by sex and region (up to district level) to estimate juvenile sex ratios. Other things being equal, the juvenile sex ratio also does not undergo significant changes over time.[3] In India, with a somewhat faster decline in female child mortality compared to male child mortality in the past 10–15 years, as evident from the Sample Registration System data, the juvenile sex ratio should have in recent years become more favourable to girls. However, contrary to this expectation, in the contiguous region from north to west of the country, the deficit of girls increased (and not decreased) between 1981 and 2001. This is also the region where historically the deficit of women in the total population is reported to be quite substantial. So the adverse juvenile sex ratio in itself was no surprise. What triggered the alarm bell was that in spite of the overall improvements in mortality situation, and a greater increase in life expectancy of women compared to that of men, indicating that the women have gained more than men from the improved health care, the deficit of girls increased. The states in question are: Himachal Pradesh, Haryana, Punjab, Rajasthan, Gujarat and Maharashtra. Delhi also very much falls in this league of states but it is not considered here because being a capital area, it experiences heavy in-migration that can vitiate our analysis to an unknown extent.

Table 2.1
Sex Ratio (FMR), All Ages and 0–6 Years for Select States, 1981–2001

State/Census year	All ages			Children 0–6 years of age		
	1981	1991	2001	1981	1991	2001
All India	935	927	933	971	945	927
Himachal Pradesh	973	976	970	971	951	897
Haryana	870	865	861	902	879	820
Punjab	879	882	874	908	875	793
Rajasthan	923	910	922	954	916	909
Gujarat	942	934	921	947	928	878
Maharashtra	937	934	922	956	945	917
Kerala	1038	1036	1058	970	958	963

Table 2.1 also gives figures of sex ratio of the population along with that of children 0–6 years of age. It is quite evident that between 1981 and 2001, the sex ratio of the total population at the all-India level as well as in the six states in the northern and western parts of the country, remained virtually the same with minor fluctuations. The exception was Gujarat where the deficit of women somewhat increased during this period. At the same time, the deficit of young girls, which was not at all evident in 1981 except in the traditionally and historically masculine states of Haryana and Punjab, became quite stark by 2001 in Himachal Pradesh, Gujarat, Rajasthan and also Maharashtra.[4] The sex ratio in Haryana and Punjab deteriorated even further.

In Table 2.2 estimates of the percentage of deficit of women in the total population and that of the girls in the 0–6 age group during 1981 to 2001 has been shown for the seven states including Kerala and for the country as a whole. The deficit is calculated in percentage terms of women or girls fewer in the total population in relation to the assumption that in the hypothetical situation the number of both sexes would be the same.

Two salient facts emerge from Table 2.2. One, among the selected states with the exception of Kerala where there were more women than men and therefore a deficit of men in the population, and in Himachal Pradesh where the percentage deficit of women in the total population was relatively small, a fairly high deficit of women was noted at the all India level and in the other selected states. The deficit of women ranged from 3 to more than 7 per cent in 2001. Two, in the 20-year period between 1981 and 1991, the percentage deficit of

Table 2.2
Per cent Deficit of Women and Girls (0–6 Years) by Select States, 1981–2001

State/Census year	Deficit of women in total population			Deficit of girls in 0–6 population		
	1981	1991	2001	1981	1991	2001
All India	3.4	3.8	3.5	1.9	2.8	3.8
Himachal Pradesh	1.4	1.2	1.5	1.5	2.5	5.5
Haryana	6.9	7.2	7.5	5.2	6.4	9.9
Punjab	6.5	6.3	6.7	4.8	6.7	11.6
Rajasthan	4.2	4.7	4.1	2.3	4.4	4.8
Gujarat	3.0	3.4	4.1	2.7	3.7	6.5
Maharashtra	3.3	3.4	4.0	2.2	2.8	4.3
Kerala	−1.6	−1.8	−2.8	1.5	2.1	1.9

women did not increase very much but the deficit of girls aged 0-6 years increased greatly in the country as a whole as well as in all the states for which data are shown in the Table, except for Kerala, the state to which the proportionate magnitude of deficit of women and girls is compared. In Haryana and Punjab there were 10 to 12 per cent fewer girls than boys.

In spite of the overall faster decline in mortality among women in India registered in the past two decades, the deficit of girls has progressively and dramatically increased in the last 20 years. Compared to 1981 when there were 1.9 per cent fewer girls than boys, the percentage doubled to 3.8 by 2001. The states of Haryana and Punjab enumerated 10 to 11.6 per cent less girls than boys in 2001, respectively, up from around 5 per cent in 1981. In three other states, the deficit of girls increased to close to or more than 5 per cent in 2001 from around 2 to 2.7 per cent in 1981. In absolute numbers, there were 23 million fewer women compared to men in 1981 but by 2001, the number increased to nearly 36 million. At the same time the absolute deficit of young girls increased by two and a half times; from 2.4 million in 1981 to 5.9 million in 2001.

In fact, according to the 2001 Census there were 49 districts in the country, where for every 1000 male children aged 0–6 years, there were less than 850 female children. Majority or 38 of these districts were located in just three northern and western states of Punjab, Haryana, and Gujarat (Census of India, 2001). The decline of 60 to 83 points in the juvenile sex ratio between 1991 and 2001 or in a span of just one decade observed in many of these districts cannot be explained solely by the discrimination against girls that has been practised in this region for several decades because at no other time in the history of census-taking of the region, has the sex ratio of children declined so drastically.

The distortion in the sex ratio was brought out starkly also by an analysis of the data from the second National Family Health survey (NFHS) conducted in 1998–99, undertaken by Arnold, Kishor and Roy (2002). They showed that at the all-India level, the male to female sex ratio of the last births was 1,434 (or 697 girls for every 1,000 boys), among currently married women who did not want any more children, which was much higher than the sex ratio of 1,069 (FMR of 935) for all the other births. However, there were significant inter-state variations and in the states of Haryana, Punjab and Gujarat. The strong son preference was manifested in the sex ratio of last births, which ranged between 1,752 and 2,173 implying that for every 1,000 girls who were last births, there were more than 1,750 boys who were last births, reflecting a strong effect of gender preference on the reproductive behaviour.

In a recently completed study in Mehsana district in Gujarat and Kurukshetra district in Haryana, undertaken with the support of Health Watch Trust, it was also observed that the last births had a stronger preponderance of boys than all other births.[5] Although more than twice as many boys as girls were reported among the last births by most groups of women, among those women who belonged to upper castes, whose families were landed, and who were literate, there were more than 240 males for every 100 girls in the last births (Visaria 2003). The overall assertion made by many that sex ratio is much more adverse to females among the better-off population groups in relation to others, does indeed hold true according to the study conducted in Gujarat and Haryana. This distortion is very likely due to the use of sex-selective abortions, which helps parents get rid of unwanted daughters before birth or due to avoiding having children once the minimum desired number of sons were born. In either case, the preference for sons was evident in the behaviour of the couples. The results for Gujarat are presented in Table 2.3 and for Haryana in Table 2.4.

As shown in Table 2.3, for Gujarat one of the noteworthy findings is that overall, the preponderance of male children increased as the birth order increased. Although the sex ratio of the first birth was greater than the normal acceptable range of 104–107 boys per 100 girls, by the time women have fourth or higher parity child, the

Table 2.3
Sex Ratio of Births and Birth Order by Women Surveyed in Gujarat Villages

Characteristics	Sex ratio of all live births	Sex ratio of first live birth	Sex ratio of second live birth	Sex ratio of third live birth	Sex ratio of fourth & higher order births	Sex ratio of the last birth
All	844	867	853	849	780	479
Age of women						
15–24	927	882	917	1098*	1072	732
25–34	860	983	841	722	824	460
35 +	799	716	839	974	730	353
Women's education						
Illiterate	900	892	993	947	783	557
Primary level	824	698	838	1143*	788	612
Upper primary level	767	887	707	562	944	366
Above upper primary level	742	893	659	618	286	360
Women's Activity						
Cultivator + animal husbandry	747	769	822	769	539	421
Agriculture/manual labour	931	891	926	949	972	598
Other misc. economic activity*	967	1053	1000	1100	714	360
Housework	820	928	787	772	667	431
Caste composition						
Upper caste	727	838	654	678	588	358
Other backward castes	886	883	952	935	773	565
SC + ST	971	889	1143	769	1138	524
Land ownership						
Yes	800	874	778	824	642	409
No	893	857	956	881	887	578

Notes: *The number of women with these characteristics was very few in the total universe and therefore the estimated sex ratios based on few cases are not likely to be stable and therefore cannot be considered as very dependable.

Table 2.4
Sex Ratio of Births and Birth Order by Women in Haryana Villages

Characteristics	Sex ratio of all live births	Sex ratio of first live birth	Sex ratio of second live birth	Sex ratio of third live birth	Sex ratio of fourth & higher order births	Sex ratio of the last birth
All	853	951	824	829	774	553
Age of women						
15–24	863	1020	742	560	800	755
25–34	836	962	833	716	716	434
35 +	866	935	848	859	824	385
Women's education						
Illiterate	870	903	883	906	782	483
Primary level#	852	–	–	–	–	500
Upper primary level	815	1168	649	482	947	404
Above upper primary level	854	887	934	583	–*	614
Women's Activity**						
Agriculture/manual labour	889	904	907	990	775	576
Housework	839	978	813	700	761	420
Caste composition						
Upper caste	801	973	792	571	686	414
Other backward castes	853	867	778	918	873	612
SC + ST	926	1067	935	903	789	443
Land ownership						
Yes	815	980	786	573	782	415
No	876	970	858	882	773	503

Notes: #In Haryana there were only a total of 50 births to 33 women whose level of education was up to primary level. Our data indicated (not shown here) that women in Haryana who enter the school system, continue to pursue education beyond primary level. As against only 3 per cent of all women having studied up to primary level, 53 per cent were reported to have studied beyond class IV. As a result, no stable estimates of sex ratio by birth order for women with primary level education are possible and are not estimated.

*There were no women in Haryana who were educated above upper primary level or class VIII who had given fourth or higher order birth.

**The number of women in the categories of cultivators-cum-animal husbandry and other miscellaneous activities was very small and hence the sex ratios of the children of these few women are not estimated.

chance of that birth being a male birth was greater by almost 30 per cent. The situation in Haryana is very similar to that observed in Gujarat. Sex-selective abortion during the first pregnancy was not practised, but by the time women had their second or third children, almost 50 per cent more boys were born compared to girls. This preponderance of males was observed more among those women who were better educated, who belonged to higher castes and whose families were landed. As in Gujarat, the Haryanvi women also belong to the dominant Chaudhury caste. Interestingly, the Chaudhury Patels of Mahesana district informed during the study that they migrated into this region from Haryana area some 200 years ago. They brought some of the social practices and customs, and till today have adhered to their caste-specific traditions. The similarity between the two groups as far as treatment of women is concerned is striking. The practice of female infanticide was known to exist in both the groups. With the advent of new technology, this inhuman practice has apparently been replaced by sex-selective abortion.

Sex-selective Abortion

The neglect of and discriminatory behaviour against girls leading to excess female mortality has been widely documented by several studies (Das Gupta 1987, Kishor 1995, Miller 1989, Visaria 1971). But the recent increase in the juvenile sex ratios discussed above has very likely resulted from the rapid spread of ultrasound and amniocentesis tests for sex determination in many parts of the country, followed by sex-selective abortions. Because of simplicity of the tests and their easy availability on the one hand and strong son preference on the other hand, female-specific abortions appear to have become popular and widely used.

It is important to understand the emergence of this phenomenon in a wider perspective. India pioneered in legalising induced abortion under the medical termination of pregnancy (MTP) Act, 1971 that specifies the reasons for which an abortion can legally be performed. The Act also clearly specifies who can legally perform the abortions and the kind of facilities in which they can be carried out. The stipulated conditions are such that abortions performed by trained doctors who are not registered in facilities not specifically approved for abortion services are termed illegal. According to

Chhabra and Nuna (1993), in India illegal abortions may be 8 to 11 times as high as legal abortions. While the intention is to provide women with safe, legal, timely abortion services, given the stringent nature of the Medical Termination of Pregnancy Act, many safe abortions may be classified as not legal. At the same time, the availability of and access to legal abortion services is so limited for a large proportion of women living in remote rural areas, that in the three decades since the passing of the Act, many abortions not only take place outside the ambit of the Act but are often performed in unsafe conditions leading to post-abortion complication and also to death.

Abortion can be legally availed if a pregnancy carries the risk of grave physical injury to a woman, or endangers her mental health or when pregnancy results from a contraceptive failure or from rape or is likely to result in the birth of a child with physical or mental abnormalities. Methods to detect deformities in the foetus such as amniocentesis and sonography that use ultrasound technology providing valuable and early information on a range of physical problems, have become available in the country, thanks largely private medical practitioners who are eager to use newer technologies for diagnosis. However, the technologies that help detect physical or mental abnormalities in the unborn child can also identify the sex of the foetus at no extra cost or effort.

There was increasing indirect evidence from some parts of India that termination of pregnancies was resorted not for the reasons stated under the MTP Act but because there is a strong son preference leading to female-selective abortions. The gender bias was flagrantly aided by a combination of medical technology that helped detect the sex of the foetus on the one hand and the liberal abortion law that helped couples to abort female foetus on the other. In view of this, the Indian government, responding to the petition made by non-governmental organisations and women's groups, passed an Act prohibiting the practice of pre-natal diagnosis of sex of the foetus (Pre-Natal Diagnostic Techniques [PNDT] Act of 1994). Under the Act, individual practitioners, clinics or centres cannot conduct tests to determine the sex of the foetus or inform the couples about it. However, in spite of putting monitoring systems in place, both at the state and the central levels, and with the Act in place for 6–8 years at the time of the 2001 Census, it is fairly evident that in many places the Act has been violated with impunity. Since the two activities of sex detection of the foetus and abortion need not be linked at the stage of using the services, it has become possible to evade the law in connivance with the clinics having ultrasound facilities and doing sonography.

Judging by the hoardings even in small towns and the regular advertisements in the local newspapers and magazines, before the passing of the PNDT Act in 1994, it was evident that clinics conducting sex determination tests had mushroomed in many towns in the states in the north-western belt. The open advertisements have now disappeared but the lucrative practice seems to flourish unabated by simply going underground as evident from the continued decline in the sex ratio of children 0–6 years of age. Anecdotal evidence suggests that a strong competition has reportedly led to a reduction in charges for availing these services, which has worked to the advantage of the potential clients. Easy access is, to a certain extent, a response to an increasing demand and female foeticide apparently has replaced the old tradition of culture of neglect of girl child, practice of infanticide among certain communities and sex differentials in the provision of medical care.

Although the release of the 2001 Census results has sparked serious concern about the widespread use of ultrasound and amniocentesis tests to detect the sex of the foetus, followed by sex-selective abortions, our understanding of many issues around this practice, at the level of the household or from the perspective of women who undergo such abortions, is extremely limited. It is also limited about what actually compels couples or their families to resort to such a practice, who the real decision makers in the family are, what impact does aborting female foetus have on the physical or mental health of the woman who typically undergoes abortion in the second trimester of her pregnancy. Our understanding of how the interlinkages of sex-selective abortion and decline in fertility or in the desired number of children are perceived and articulated is also very limited. The question often raised is: does the desire for fewer children compel parents to produce children of the sex that they want or that conform to the societal norms and regulate their fertility behaviour accordingly? The qualitative data collected by conducting 44 focus group discussions in which more than 400 women belonging to diverse socio-economic and educational groups in rural Gujarat and Haryana have provided insights on some of these issues.

Son Preference

During the discussions with women both in Gujarat and in Haryana, it was clearly indicated that majority of the women accepted the outcome of the first pregnancy—whether it was a boy or a girl. However, if the first-born child was a daughter, then the upper caste women were overtly or covertly pressurised to ensure that the second and or the third child was a boy and to take appropriate measures. Although the women from lower castes experienced this pressure from the family to a much lesser extent, many among them have started either emulating the women from the upper castes or have started thinking the same way.

Thus, the son preference was very evident among all social groups in both Gujarat and Haryana states even when the desired number of children had come down to two or three. No group of women indicated that they would want more than two or three children. They came up with fairly rational explanations about why many children are not desired in the present times and situation. However, in spite of wanting fewer children compared to their parents, women candidly admitted preference for male children. In order to minimise the influence of the other members of the family on the decision of women, women were asked to imagine a hypothetical situation of having all the freedom to choose the number and the sex composition of their children. Among those who indicated that they would like to have three children, the overwhelming response was for two sons and one daughter. However, some who indicated that they would like to have only two children preferred at least one of them to be a son. However, if the two children turned out to be girls then they would almost certainly opt for a third child with a hope that it would be a boy. Women did discuss the possibility that not all sons may support parents in their old age, and yet, the desire for a son was very strong among women of all social groups. As one backward community woman in Gujarat put it:

> Yes, we wait for the son. We must have a son, howsoever he may turn out to be. We would always hope for a son. After all, the daughter will go away after her marriage. The son will stay with us and take care of us.

Women from the upper castes that practise dowry (Chaudhary in Haryana and Chaudhary Patel in Gujarat) even voiced that if the first child born to them was a boy, then they would be satisfied with just one child. The menace not of the dowry system but of lifelong presents that have to be given to the girls from the day she marries to her death and also to her children, was a strong deterrent to having girls. Along with that a fear was articulated that the daughter might be sent back to the parental house if her in-laws were not satisfied with the presents that have been demanded or that she has been given on various occasions by her natal family or for any other reason.[6]

> There is trouble for daughters. They may find a good family or a bad family after their marriage. They [daughters] may come back home. If they have trouble with their in-laws, they may be sent back by their in-laws. In earlier times, the women used to do backbreaking labour, look after the cattle after their marriage. These days girls do not do that. If there is an economic problem, the in-laws will send the girl back to her parental home. So, a girl is always the reason for the tension of her parents. (Patel woman from Gujarat)

> A girl requires a dowry when she has to be married which is a cause for anxiety. Finding a suitable groom and hoping that she will settle down happily in her new home is always a source of worry for parents. (A woman from Haryana)

Sex Determination

This almost universal desire for more sons than daughters does get translated in actual behaviour as was evident from the sex ratio of live births that was discussed earlier. In the focus group discussions also, women from all communities categorically indicated that if the first-born child was a daughter, then the couples would want to and do find out the sex of the next child. Women knew where to go for sex determination tests, how much the tests cost, etc. They were aware that such tests were not done in public hospitals. One had to go to private facilities, majority of which according to them also provided abortion services. In fact, almost all women were able to describe the sex determination procedure quite accurately and in great detail.

Women also indicated that after the birth of a daughter, when they became pregnant again, there was some pressure from the elders in the family to ensure that the next child was a boy. Women themselves also wanted to produce a son. There is a deep internalisation of patriarchal values that are linked to their sense of security. The son preference was internalised to such an extent that women had no hesitation in saying that they would want the sex of the foetus to be known if they had already given birth to one daughter. Although almost all of them had to consult and get permission of their husbands (partly because the sex determination test involved a cost of few hundred rupees), they themselves saw nothing wrong in finding out the sex of the foetus. As articulated by a Kshatriya woman from Gujarat or a Chaudhary woman from Haryana:

> We have to go for the test if the first child is a girl. If we don't go for the test, we may end up giving birth to three or more daughters in the false hope of getting a son.

> Women definitely get the test done... if it is a girl they abort the foetus and if it is a boy, they keep the baby. Everybody knows about the test... the women themselves want to know whether they are carrying a male or a female child.

Although the parents or parents-in-law of the women very probably had given birth to several children, it appears that they do not wish their daughters-in-law to do so. As the women indicated, the facilities (for sex determination and abortion) did not exist in the earlier times and so the parents had no choice but to bear several children. But in present times, the mother-in-law herself often suggests that the daughter-in-law should get the sex determination test done, especially after producing one daughter. The parents of the woman, however, generally have no say in the matter, except for wishing that their daughters produce at least one son because their well-being and status in the families of the in-laws depends, to a great extent, on bearing sons.

> Mothers-in-law also have changed with the time. They are also aware of the price rise. They might have had raised their several children, but its difficult to raise more children today. (Backward caste woman from Haryana)

> If we already have one son and one daughter, the in-laws would ask us to go in for a test and if it were a daughter, they would even ask us to go in for abortion. (Chaudhary Patel woman from Gujarat)

Decision-making Process About Abortion

When women were asked about the decision-making process if the foetus was found to be that of a female child, the overwhelming response was that after one or two daughters, if the woman was found to be pregnant with another girl, the pressure on her to abort was enormous from her extended conjugal family. Women indicated that the decision to abort a female foetus was almost entirely that of their husbands and/or mothers-in-law. By themselves, women could not take the decision to go in for abortion. Women who had virtually no decision-making power, apparently accepted whatever was desired by her conjugal family, including husbands. They simply accepted and went along with the decision made for them by others. However, we observed some differences between women belonging to higher social groups and those who belonged to scheduled caste and other backward communities with regard to the influence of the in-laws in these matters. High caste women had to inform and consult their in-laws but low caste women had to obtain the consent of only their husbands for abortion. The influence of the extended joint family was not so strong on the decision of the women from lower caste groups.

> A woman cannot take a decision on abortion on her own. If the husband does not want a daughter then he would ask us to go in for abortion. And if he wants a daughter, then we keep the daughter. If the husband is ready to support us and stand by us, we can be firm and go for abortion or not for abortion. In any case we need to consult our husbands. (Backward caste woman from Gujarat)

> If the first two children are girls and the third one too is a girl then we need to take the permission of the elders to go in for abortion. We have to follow the advice of the elders. (Patel woman from Gujarat)

Women also reported that sometimes they themselves desire to abort a female foetus because they already have had one or two daughters. This feeling was stronger among women belonging to social groups such as Patel and Kshatriya, who valued sons much more than daughters. Although they themselves, without much hesitation, would opt for abortion, they still would have to get the permission of the elders of the family to exercise their wish.

Conclusion

The analysis clearly points to a collusion of culture or social norms and technology that is all pervasive. On the one hand the son preference is so strongly entrenched in Indian society especially in the north-western region and on the other hand the well-being and status of girls is so precarious once they are married, that couples avoid having girls at all costs. Facilities conducting sex detection tests with ultrasound machines have proliferated and are found even in some of the relatively large villages.

Despite the spread of schooling among girls in recent decades, the patriarchal social structure survives. Women derive value and status only as mothers of sons. Their happiness and social status in the conjugal homes is dependent on producing sons. Women have internalised these roles and values to such an extent that even when they say that daughters take better care of parents or are more emotionally attached to the mothers, these statements have a ring of hollowness because in spite of such feelings, more sons than daughters are desired. In the pursuit of sons, they have become, with some pressure from the families, consumers of the new technology of ultrasound, which allows them to choose and bear sons. The possibility of delinking availing legal abortion services from finding and revealing the sex of the foetus provides an opportunity to abort the child of an unwanted sex.

The shift to small family size, evident in India more recently, has not, however, been accompanied by a shift at the same time in the economic and social pressures to have sons and avoid daughters. As was stated by women in both Gujarat and Haryana, they desire and want few children while ensuring that at least one if not two of those children are sons. This has also led to increased acceptance and use of sex selection tests to achieve parental preferences to have sons while not exceeding the desired number of children.

At the same time, the awareness about a ban on sex determination tests is fairly widespread among women in our study area. Many women also felt that the ban should be removed and couples should have the choice to decide the sex composition of their children. Women were very well aware that the services are easily available from private providers and are within easy access. Government legislation against the use of ultrasound technology for sex detection has only driven it underground and raised the cost but it is extensively available and used for sex detection. The cost is still affordable and in any case, as many respondents indicated, the cost of the test and related abortion is much lower than the cost of providing dowry and other life-long presentations to a daughter after marriage. As one of our researchers pointed out: 'The alarm bells ringing in the corridors of power about the missing girls do not find an echo in the dusty by-lanes of the villages of these districts' (Chaudhury, 2003).

The patriarchal structure and values are ingrained for centuries and the practice of getting rid of daughters is known to exist in these regions such that certain social groups in both Gujarat and Haryana have started feeling the deficit of brides for their sons. According to some women, a few men are forced to remain bachelors and for some, brides are being brought or bought by paying bride price from scheduled tribes and other groups from far away places including other states. We have no hard evidence on the extent of this practice but it may become a lesson in social integration. However, in spite of the deficit of women, whose impact is being felt in procuring brides, the social norms do not yet seem to be responding.

As is evident, legislation banning the use of sex determination tests has thus far not succeeded in deterring couples from seeking these tests or preventing the medical practitioners from performing them. The prevalent social norms and practices do raise a number of questions. Is passing of a national legislation to regulate pre-natal diagnostic technologies and their misuse an answer? Thus far, the law has been largely ineffective but will regulatory mechanisms clamped at all levels or better implementation prevent its misuse? Will impounding ultrasound machines in unregistered clinics and to maintain detailed registers about their use in registered clinics help in reducing their use for sex detection of foetus? We believe, what is needed is a concerted effort to address the bias against girls at the source and changing the underlying conditions that promote sex-selective abortions. However, it is an uphill task and every action and every group that can address this would contribute to improving the status of women in our society.

Notes

1. The one exception in 1981, which recorded some improvement in the sex ratio in favour of women, was viewed as a beginning of a reversal of a trend. However, the 1991 Census belied the hope that the situation of women had begun to improve.

2. However, there is little evidence that the care and treatment meted out to those girls who are born or allowed to be born, has improved. Violence against women is reported in studies from many parts of the country. Dowry deaths continue unabated. We have little empirical evidence on the trends in violence and the recorded dowry deaths suffer from many limitations, to gauge whether there is decline in the incidence of such atrocities against women.

3. Sex differentials in misreporting of ages, can affect the estimated sex ratios; however, it is assumed that over the 20–30 year period, there are unlikely to be any significant changes in the age reporting of boys and girls.

4. Given the fact that at birth in every 1,000 live births, boys outnumber girls by about 50 births, and assuming that there are no significant sex differentials in mortality among children up to 6 years of age, the sex ratio of children aged 0–6 years would fall in the range of 935 and 960. Sex ratio above this would signify either female-selective misreporting of ages and/or significantly higher mortality among boys relative to girls. Sex ratio below this would signify the opposite of these phenomena.

5. In both Mehsana and Kurukshetra districts, listing of all the houses in three villages each was undertaken and lifetime pregnancy histories of all married women in the reproductive ages were recorded. These data form the basis of the estimates of sex ratios by birth order and of the last birth. The number of women interviewed was 2,500 from 12 villages.

6. The proverbial exchange marriage practised by the Patel community of North Gujarat known as *ata-sata*, has reportedly declined over the years. The educated youngsters do not always approve it and fathers of sons try and arrange marriages without receiving a daughter of another family in exchange. Substantial dowry and expensive marriages are believed to be the motivating factors. There is a move by some leaders of the community to encourage the exchange marriage once again that is believed to address the twin issues of eliminating dowry and reversing the deficit of girls. But the situation is very fluid and the reforms discussed to address them are still tentative among the Patels of Mehsana.

References

Arnold, F. S. Kishor and T.K. Roy. 2002. 'Sex-selective Abortions in India', *Population and Development Review*, 28 (4): 759–85.

Chaudhury, Manisha. 2003. 'Sex-selective abortion in Haryana', New Delhi: HealthWatch Trust, typescript.

Chhabra, R. and S.C. Nuna. 1993. *Abortion in India: An Overview*. New Delhi: Veerendra Printers.

Census of India. 2001. *Series-1, India, Provisional Population Totals, Paper 1 of 2001, Supplement, District Totals*. New Delhi: Office of the Registrar General of India.

Das Gupta, M. 1987. 'Selective Discrimination Against Female Children in Rural Punjab, India', *Population and Development Review*, 13 (1): 77–100.

Kishor, Sunita. 1995. 'Gender Differentials in Child Mortality: A Review of Evidence', in Monica Das Gupta, Lincoln C. Chen, and T. N. Krishnan (eds.), *Women's Health in India: Risk and Vulnerability*, pp. 19–54. Bombay: Oxford University Press.

Miller, B.D. 1989. 'Changing Patterns of Juvenile Sex Ratios in Rural India, 1961–1971', *Economic and Political Weekly*, 20 (2) June 2: 1229–36.

Visaria, L. 2002. 'Deficit of Women in India: Magnitude, Trends, Regional Variations and Determinants', *The National Medical Journal of India*, 15 (Supplement 1): 19–25.

———. 2003. 'Sex Selective Abortion in the States of Gujarat and Haryana: Some Empirical Evidence', New Delhi, HealthWatch Trust, typescript.

Visaria, P. 1971. *The Sex Ratio of the Population of India*. Census of India 1961. Monograph No. 10, New Delhi: Office of the Registrar General, India.

Female Foeticide:
A Civilisational Collapse

3

Ashish Bose

The most dismal data revealed by the results of the 2001 Census of India relate to the low child sex ratio (girls per 1,000 boys in the age group 0–6 years) in almost all the states of India. This could not have happened without the widespread use of pre-birth sex determination tests, followed by sex-selective abortion in case of female foetuses. This to our mind is a symptom of civilisational collapse.

We undertook a study of this tragic phenomenon at two levels: (i) through a detailed district-wise analysis of the 2001 Census data and (ii) through intensive fieldwork in the worst states of India, namely, Punjab, Haryana and Himachal Pradesh. For operational reasons, we left out Gujarat which should have been bracketed with the three north-western states. We present our findings in brief.

The districts with the lowest child ratios may be classified into three categories as follows:

D1: child sex ratio 850–900
D2: child sex ratio 800–850
D3: child sex ratio 750–800

Obviously the worst category is D3. All the states and districts in India can be classified according to the level of child sex ratio. D stands for our acronym—DEMARU—to indicate daughter eliminating male aspiring rage for ultrasound. The summary picture in the districts of three of the four worst states are as follows:

Demographic black holes: DEMARU States and districts (The child sex ratio in 2001 is given in brackets)

1. PUNJAB: Overall rating–D3 (793)
   Districts:

D1: nil

D2: Faridkot (805), Muktsar (807), Nawanshahr (810), Hoshiarpur (810), Ludhiana (814), Ferozepur (819), Moga (819)

D3: Fatehgarh Sahib (754), Patiala (770), Gurdaspur (775), Kapurthala (775), Mansa (779), Bhatinda (779), Amritsar (783), Sangrur (784), Roopnagar (719), Jalandhar (797). Note: All 17 districts are in the D Category, see Map 3.1 Sex Ratio in Punjab, 2001.

2. HARYANA: Overall rating–D2 (820)

Districts:

D1: Faridabad (856), Gurgaon (863)

D2: Jhajjar (805), Panipat (807), Karnal (808), Yamuna Nagar (807), Rewari (814), Mahendragarh (814), Jind (818), Sirsa (818), Hissar (830), Fatehbad (830), Panchkula (837), Bhiwani (838)

D3: Kurukshetra (770), Sonepat (783), Rohtak (796), Ambala (784), Kaithan (789). Note: All 19 districts are in the D category, see Map 3.2 Sex Ratio in Haryana, 2001.

3. HIMACHAL: Overall rating–D1 (897)

Districts:

D1: Hamirpur (864), Bilaspur (884), Solan (900)

D2: Kangra (836), Una (839)

Note: 5 of the 12 districts belong to the D category, see Map 3.3 Sex Ratio in Himachal Pradesh, 2001.

It will be seen that Fatehgarh Sahib in Punjab, Kurukshetra in Haryana and Kangra in Himachal Pradesh are the worst districts. Thanks to the Voluntary Health Association of India (VHAI), I could do a spell of fieldwork, along with Dr. Mira Shiva, a noted health activist (for details see, Bose and Shiva 2003). VHAI decided to take up intensive fieldwork in these districts to find out what was happening at the grass-root level. Our hypothesis was that if we could tackle the worst districts we could certainly improve things in other districts with suitable intervention strategies. VHA Punjab and VHA Himachal Pradesh joined us in undertaking our difficult fieldwork, which by virtue of the secrecy and sensitivity of the issues under consideration, called for tremendous tact and skills in survey methodology and data collection. Apart from our perception surveys of doctors and Panchayat members and interviews of married women, we had the benefit of a series of focus groups discussions and inter-action with village people, which gave us valuable insights.

Complexity of Re-constructing Attitudes and Bringing about Behavioural Change

One gets an impression from seminars and conferences on gender issues that husbands and their parents are pushing their wives and daughters-in-law to go for pre-birth sex determination tests and abor-tions. Our field surveys, focus group discussions and our own im-pressions do not lend support to this proposition. We find that many women *themselves* are interested in knowing the sex of the unborn child and they do not see any moral problem in undergoing these tests conducted by doctors: it is like getting blood tests for malarial parasites. And second, most women have an inherent son complex. They know for certain that their status—in the eyes of their family, extended family, community and the village as a whole—will go up with the arrival of a son. Gifts will flow in, there will be celebrations and relatives from far and near will call on them. On the other hand, if they give birth to a daughter, there is general gloom, no celebra-tions, no gifts and the image of the woman suffers badly. As one of our senior health activists in Punjab, Manmohan Sharma pointed out: 'women are conditioned by social norms and they do not have independent views, they tend to ditto what the husbands say or think and this is considered as proper behaviour for ideal wives'. In such a situation, enforcement of the PNDT Act becomes very difficult. We came across cases of collusion between doctors and clients. The modus operandi is as follows: A doctor from a city or even a small town goes to villages with his mobile ultrasound machine and in case the sex determination test shows a female foetus, gives the client an address in the nearest city where abortions are conducted in secrecy. There were cases in Punjab when the police arrested some women for undergoing sex determination tests while the doctors went scot-free. This led to an agitation by several health activists and ultimately the women were set free. In the villages we surveyed, there was a lot of apprehension about our study. Even though we conducted our survey with great tact, it was clear to us that women respondents were not telling the truth when they said that they were not aware of female foeticide. At a well-attended meeting for a focus group discussion in a village in Punjab, the district-level authorities pleaded helplessness with regard to enforcement of the PNDT Act. It was argued that doctors do not have any idea about the legal provisions of the Act and the Judicial Officer of the district, who has to interpret and implement the Act, is frequently transferred. Thus there is no continuity in following up cases and, as a result, nothing gets done.

Networking of Government Doctors, Private Doctors, ANMs and Dais

During our fieldwork we could sense a silent conspiracy between the government doctors, medical and paramedical staff and private doctors with regard to the illegal practice of sex determination tests leading to female foeticide. The dais and ANMs often act as go-betweens and collect their honorarium (roughly Rs 200 per case). We also suspect that medical representatives are a party to the game of making quick money. One does not have to go to big cities such as Chandigarh, Ludhiana or Shimla to undergo these tests and abortions. Within an ambit of 20–30 km one comes across clinics that undertake such work and have mushroomed under various cover names. The fact that an ultrasound machine is registered as required by law, does not guarantee that it is not misused. A tragic aspect of this is that very often doctors show utter disregard for medical ethics. They know very well that through ultrasonography it is not possible to determine the sex of a foetus within 12 weeks of conception and yet they conduct these tests and indicate the results (invariably 'it is a girl'). The doctors know that it is just speculation and not scientific observation. In fact, we have come across reports of cases when after abortion it was found that the foetus was male, much to the agony of the parents. One could draw a distinction between a woman agreeing on the suggestion of her husband or in-laws to undergo a test and a woman who, having undergone the test and finding that it was a female foetus, agrees to go in for abortion. Generally, this test is conducted only during the second and subsequent conceptions. But in Punjab, we were told about the recent tendency to go in for these tests *even for the first conception*. There were also cases of murder within the family when the young daughter-in-law refused to go for abortion after the very first conception. According to Dr Betty Cowen, who spent many years at the Christian Medical College (CMC), Ludhiana, 'there was a time in Punjab when the first daughter was welcome, the second was tolerated and the third was eliminated' (personal communication). We are now facing the tragic prospect of the first daughter being eliminated, what to say of the second and third. Demographers have worked out the sex ratio by order of birth and it is observed that the higher the order of birth, the lower is the sex ratio. Our field data also confirm this. There is no doubt that if this trend persists for another two decades, states such as Punjab and Haryana will face disastrous social consequences.

Mixing up Family Planning with Female Foeticide

As a result of 50 years of propaganda on the merits of a small family norm, there is today general awareness of family planning and the need for adopting a small family norm. Our fieldwork reveals that men and women in Punjab, Haryana and Himachal Pradesh do accept the idea of a two-child family and they are also aware of the technology of pre-birth sex determination tests. As in most parts of India, two sons constitute the cut-off point for accepting sterilisation (Patel 1994 reports the same trend for rural Rajasthan). The people seem to be quite puzzled that the government wants a small family norm to be practised yet opposes the conduct of these tests and subsequent abortions. They argue that since every family wants at least one son, if not two, the best way to ensure a small family, is to go for the test and act according to the results. A well-meaning and prominent doctor, having a flourishing private practice in Himachal Pradesh, told us that government hospitals should allow pre-birth determination tests only in cases where the first child is a daughter. His argument was that in case the second child is a son, the family will be satisfied and will opt for sterilisation. This will help in stabilising the population. The doctor argued that the merit of this formula was that it would reduce quackery and maternal mortality, and would also achieve the national goal of population stabilisation. This doctor had a large private practice and was not at all keen to take abortion cases, let alone conduct sex determination tests. In fact, he narrated how he was pressurised to conduct this test and abortions by several

VVIPs, whose names he could not divulge. In the eyes of the people, there is a dichotomy between the government's sustained advocacy of family planning and small family norm, with legislation prohibiting the conduct of sex determination tests and sex-selective abortions. This mix-up is the creation of circumstances and neither the government nor the people can be blamed. If an enlightened doctor, who commands great respect and is not a greedy person, genuinely believes that the government should allow such cases and abortions to be conducted on demographic grounds, his views deserve serious consideration. One must pause and think how best to counter such an argument. Under the PNDT Act, very often the appropriate authority is the Chief Medical Officer and it is very unlikely that a doctor will prosecute a fellow doctor. One must note the solidarity of doctors in remote areas where social life is confined to playing cards and/or drinking. Besides, it is often pointed out that since a person has to spend so much money in private medical institutions to get trained as a doctor, he is unlikely to forego efforts to make quick money; sex determination tests and abortions provide perhaps the best opportunity to make such money. According to rough estimates of people who are knowledgeable, in many places 90 per cent of the income of several doctors (mostly those in small towns) comes from these tests and abortions. It was clear to us that the legal machinery in the districts was not equal to the task of effectively implementing the PNDT Act, where higher-level officials are busy with pressing administrative problems.

Economic Prosperity and Social Backwardness

In states like Punjab, Haryana and Himachal Pradesh, which are economically prosperous, the attitude towards the girl child is alarmingly unprogressive. Our fieldwork leads to the conclusion that there are at least three pre-conditions for the spread of female foeticide: (i) easy access to medical facilities, in particular, ultrasound and abortion facilities; (ii) ability to pay the doctor and abortionist for the test and abortion; and (iii) a good network of roads to cut down the cost of travel and the time taken to travel. These conditions are fulfilled in our study areas, for example, in the Fatehgarh Sahib district of Punjab, which has the lowest child sex ratio in India (754): the villages are prosperous, the transportation network is very good and there is easy access to medical facilities, particularly in Ludhiana (Fatehgarh Sahib was once a part of Ludhiana district). Above all, the dominant Jat community is historically known for its son complex. On the other hand, in Kerala, even if these three conditions are fulfilled, it may not trigger off a spate of female foeticides because of the absence of the son complex, though of late, it has been observed that if a couple opts for one child they would rather have a son than a daughter. In the southern states, there is growing evidence that people would be content with one son and one daughter and would not go on with repeated pregnancies with the hope of getting sons as in the north. While doing this fieldwork we did come across tragic cases of numerous abortions among women desperately looking for a son, even after giving birth to five or six daughters. The adverse impact on the physical and mental health of mothers can be imagined. The 2001 Census data also reveal that in tribal-dominated districts, the son complex does not dominate the social ethos, and girls are valued. In the north-east India too, the son complex is less prevalent. One distressing question that arises in this regard is: with higher levels of economic growth, better income levels and better transportation networks, will all states in India follow the footsteps of the states like Punjab and Haryana.

Causes of Female Foeticide

We also tried to ascertain the causes of female foeticide through our surveys. The general perception is that the cost of marriage and dowry has gone up and so daughters have become greater financial liabilities. The dowry system is invariably blamed. We are not convinced that dowry alone is the main cause of female foeticide. Families that are well-off and do not have to depend on dowry to augment their income are also opting for female foeticide. The real reason seems to be the high status of families with several sons and the low status of families with no sons. Another interesting factor for the preference for sons is that the prospect of migration of sons to, say the Gulf or western countries, is much higher for men than for women (except in special cases such as Kerala from where nurses go all over the world). In the eyes of the local community, a family with children abroad has a higher status and certainly a higher income level than non-migrant families. Globalisation is thus adding to the miseries of the girl child.

In short, there are numerous causes for the spread of female foeticide and it will be unscientific to believe that dowry alone is the cause, as is the general perception. Nevertheless, our perception during the fieldwork did reveal that people are aware of the upward swing in dowry demand and the rising cost of marriage. Greed has increased in our society and numerous TV channels and endless advertisements increase this greed further.

Female foeticide is a symptom of increasing crime against women. It would be manifestly wrong if we conclude that female foeticide is a matter of medical technology alone. There is no doubt that easy access to ultrasonography has been largely responsible for the spread of female foeticide throughout the country. As Mira Shiva (2002) maintains, many women opted for female foeticide not because they were heartless but because they were genuinely concerned about the fate of girls who are being increasingly subjected to eve-teasing, molestation and sexual harassment and, after marriage, exposed to the risk of bride burning and dowry death, in the unending demand for dowry from our emerging consumerist society. This calls for a good look at gender issues in all their ramifications in our increasingly dysfunctional society.

References

Bose, Ashish and Mira Shiva. 2003. *Darkness at Noon—Female Foeticide in India.* VHAI: New Delhi: VHAI (Voluntary Health Association of India).

Census of India. 2001. *Provisional Population Totals, Series 1, Paper 1 of 2001.* New Delhi: Registrar General of India.

Patel, T. 1994. *Fertility Behaviour: Population and Society in a Rajasthan Village.* New Delhi: Oxford University Press.

Shiva, Mira. 2002. *Skirting the Issue: The Girl Child Seen but not Heard.* New Delhi: VHAI.

Map 3.1
Sex Ratio in Punjab, 2001

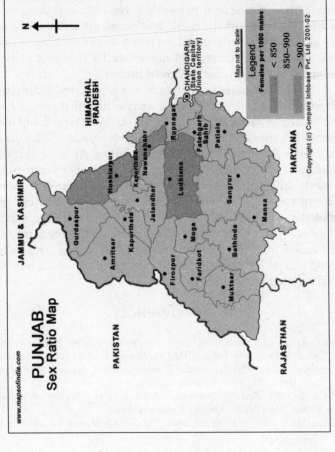

www.mapsofindia.com

PUNJAB
Sex Ratio Map

N

PAKISTAN

JAMMU & KASHMIR

Gurdaspur

Amritsar

Kapurthala

Hoshiarpur

Kapurthala

Jalandhar

Nawanshahr

Firozpur

Faridkot

Moga

Muktsar

Bathinda

Ludhiana

Mansa

Sangrur

Rupnagar

Fatehgarh
Sahib

Patiala

CHANDIGARH
(State Capital/
Union territory)

HIMACHAL
PRADESH

HARYANA

RAJASTHAN

Map not to Scale

Legend
Females per 1000 males

< 850

850–900

> 900

Copyright (c) Compare Infobase Pvt. Ltd. 2001-02

Map 3.2
Sex Ratio in Haryana, 2001

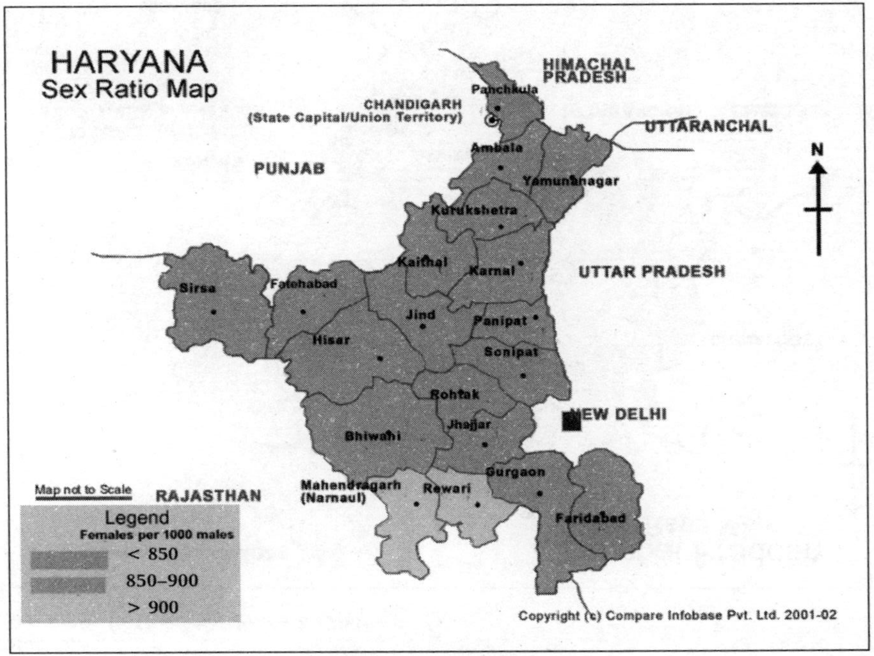

HARYANA
Sex Ratio Map

Map 3.3
Sex Ratio in Himachal Pradesh, 2001

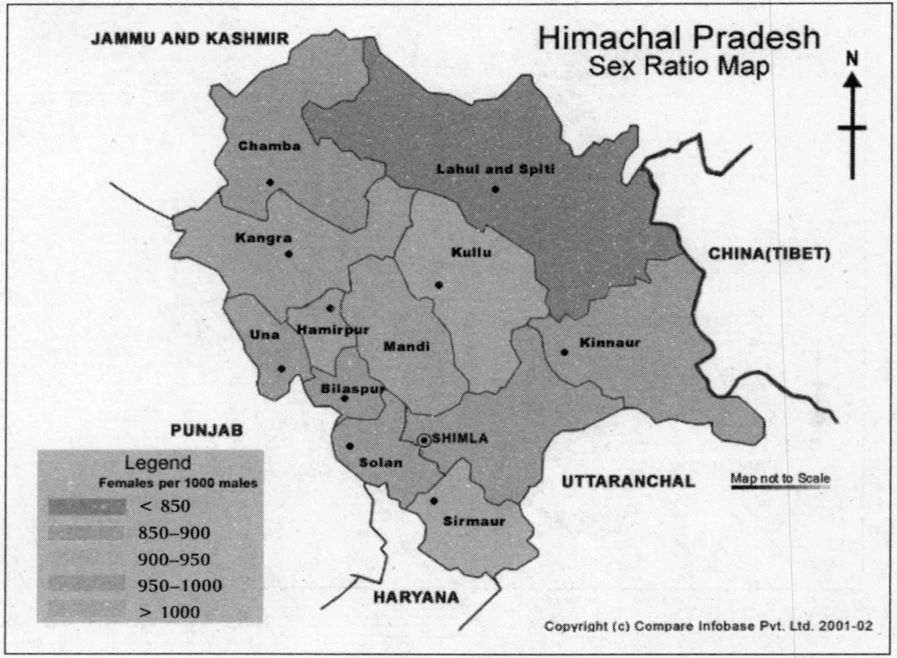

Himachal Pradesh
Sex Ratio Map

JAMMU AND KASHMIR

CHINA(TIBET)

Chamba

Lahul and Spiti

Kangra

Kullu

Kinnaur

Una

Hamirpur

Mandi

Bilaspur

SHIMLA

Solan

Sirmaur

PUNJAB

HARYANA

UTTARANCHAL

Legend
Females per 1000 males

< 850
850–900
900–950
950–1000
> 1000

Map not to Scale

Copyright (c) Compare Infobase Pvt. Ltd. 2001-02

Rethinking Female Foeticide:

Perspective and Issues

4

Rainuka Dagar

The sharp increase in the masculine sex ratios in India has drawn intense public engagement but female foeticide continues unabated. The concerns vary to include implications for demographic imbalance, increased victimisation of women, continuity of gender hierarchies and the challenge to the popular development paradigm–which in spite of the expanding infrastructure and its availment, has witnessed widespread female foeticide. A number of competing discourses attempt to confront the spread of female foeticide. These include technological determinism which identifies the proliferation of new reproductive technologies that preclude male sex selection as the bane of female foeticide. The enforcement agenda that is spearheading intervention seeks punitive measures to regulate the social norms that legitimise male child preference. The entitlements failure that views women's disadvantaged status and subsequent female foeticide as a lack of access to resources and facilities and the attainment of female reproductive rights that aims to provide women control over their lives and bodies, are some dominant endeavours to tackle female foeticide.

The pronounced concern emanated from the increased visibility acquired by missing girl children in Census reports[1]; the development paradox–whereby the developed states registered a decline in the child sex ratio (Bose 2001: 3427); and the use of life-enhancing technological innovations for life aborting purposes.[2] This paper explores the debates that surround female foeticide, and the constraints of the existing approaches to undermine female foeticide, in particular the fall-out of a form-centric approach to address the phenomenon. In doing so, it highlights the need for an alternative perspective to combating female foeticide.

I

Approaches to Female Foeticide: A Lineage

Two distinct approaches to combating female foeticide have emerged in India. These are the provision of equal opportunities and addressing technological determinism. The underlying assumption of both these approaches is that the existing development paradigm has a built-in mechanism to capacitate or incapacitate women's empowerment and has a varying impact on female foeticide. In keeping with the 'liberal-equilibrium' view spawned by the understanding of universal equality among individuals, thus both men and women, by virtue of their being humans, are equal and the uplift of society depends on ensuring that the rights of individuals are safeguarded. Such a position argues that the key problem for women is discrimination, including both unconscious and indirect discrimination (Crowley and Himmelweit 1994). This strategy is adopted to provide equal developmental benefits to women by promoting and protecting individual women and by checking discriminatory practices. The effort as analysed by Kabeer is directed at policies and mechanisms to enhance women's access and control over resources (Kabeer 1995: 7). Technological determinism, on the other hand, locates the cause of the declining sex ratio in the spread of new reproductive technologies, particularly sex determination, and targets the access of these to check female foeticide.

Under the equal opportunities approach further strands take shape. Equal value represented by the Draft National Advocacy Strategy (NAS) for pre-birth elimination of females in India. 'Ending the Practice Changing the Mindset' aims at giving equal value to a male and a female child with a seemingly ingenious use of a demand and supply model (NAS 2002: 14). Another strand is represented by the more conventional transformation of gender placements by enhancing access and participation of women to resources (Government of

India 2001). This approach manifests in gender policy prescriptions. This is also being characterised by a variant of right to entitlements–women's effective command over resources is expected to place them on an equal footing with men (Agnihotri 2000: 44). While yet another position within the equality approach is of reproductive rights for women that promote women's control over their bodies and reproductive choices to check the practice of female foeticide (United Nations Population Fund 2000).

The liberal equality approach finds widespread acceptance among governments and international conventions. According to the Planning Commission,

> The Constitution of India provides for equal rights and privileges for men and women and makes special provisions for women to help them improve their status in society. A number of social enactments have been put on the statute book for removing various constraints which hindered their progress. In spite of these measures, women have lagged behind men in different spheres. (GOI 1985: 321)

The National Commission for Women, through its objectives, functions, powers and priorities, follows the approach of providing women with equality of opportunity. It has been set up with the main objective of 'safeguarding the interest of women, gaining for them equality of status and opportunity and eliminating, as far as possible, any discrimination against them' (GOI 1992). Similarly the national policy for the empowerment of women (2001) identifies as its goals:

(i) Creating an environment through positive economic and social policies for full development of women to enable them to realise their full potential.

(ii) The *de jure* and *de facto* enjoyment of all human rights and fundamental freedoms by women on equal basis with men in all spheres–political, economic, social, cultural and civil (GOI 2001: 2).

This policy goes on to elucidate the basic needs strategy aimed at investment in humans (in this case women) through a greater emphasis on health, education and equitable distribution of wealth and resources to empower women. It further identifies masculinisation of the sex ratio, and by, implication female foeticide as a reflection of this inequality. 'Gender disparity manifests itself in various forms, the most obvious being the trend of continuously declining female ratio in the population in the last few decades' (GOI 2001: 1).

Female foeticide, stereotyping and violence are mentioned as manifestations of gender disparity and women's adverse placement is to be countered by empowerment of women, and equality with men is the dictum. Entitlement to rights through laws and international institutional mechanism such as CEDAW (Convention on the Elimination of All Forms of Discrimination Against Women) are ratified to 'eliminate unequal treatment and unequal opportunity. The convention ratified by India provides,

> the basis for realizing equality between women and men through ensuring women's equal access to, and equal opportunities in, political and public life–including the right to vote and to stand for election–as well as education, health and employment. State parties agree to take all appropriate measures, including legislation and temporary special measures, so that women can enjoy all their human rights and fundamental freedoms. (CEDAW 1979: 1)

These development measures have been promoted by policy interventions vis-à-vis women. To illustrate, the programme of action (POA) from the International Conference on Population Development (ICPD), to which India is a signatory, envisages 'empowering women and providing them with more choices through expanded access to education and health services' (United Nations 1994: 1). No doubt, women's education, a vital component of enhanced capacity, has shown positive linkages to the decline in fertility rates (Das Gupta *et al.* 1998: 38), infant and child mortality[3] and demographic frameworks in particular have pointed at the importance of female literacy, female workforce participation, and female autonomy (Miller 1981). Yet socio-economic development has been unable to stem the tide of female foeticide. Croll has argued that 'the assumed interdependence of fertility decline with socio-economic development has been such that identifying prerequisite socio-economic factors making for fertility decline become a development priority'(Croll 2000: 5). However, the author cautions that the same rationale does not show results when it comes to the phenomenon of female foeticide.

To empirically investigate the dependence of female foeticide on socio-economic development vis-à-vis the parameter of Gender Equity Index (GEI), the paper explores: the trend of child sex ratios in economically developed and underdeveloped states including, practice of female foeticide among groups with different income and education levels across rural-urban populations and the practice of female foeticide in socio-economic advantageously placed groups, i.e. NRIs/ethnic groups in western developed countries. The macro analysis is based on data from secondary sources including the Census of India, the Human Development Report, India, supported by published empirical studies. Primary data is drawn from surveys forming four reports confined to Punjab between 1995 and 2003.[4]

Development, it is assumed, has an isomorphic relationship with phenomena of a divergent sort, including women's empowerment. This assumption has been challenged by the phenomenon of foeticide as experienced by both developed and developing states. Economically developed states with a high per capita income and relatively better infrastructure have registered a decline in the sex ratio, particularly so in the 0–6 age group. Similarly, the higher income groups, urban populations and the educated have been found to practise a relatively higher extent of female foeticide.

The view that economically developed states that offer advanced infrastructure facilities are in a position to provide easy access to scientific technologies of sex determination and these states reflect a collusion of development and technology through a sharp decline in their 0–6 sex ratios is well propounded. According to Bose:

> Those familiar with the field situation in Punjab, Haryana, Himachal Pradesh, Chandigarh and Delhi know that the ready availability of doctors during the ultrasound test and consequent female foeticide, the good transportation network and the ability to pay for the services of the mobile doctors are factors responsible for the widespread recourse to ultrasound in rural areas also. (Bose 2001: 3428)

States such as Maharashtra, Gujarat, Punjab and Goa, no doubt, would affirm to the proposition that developed states have registered the highest decline in their child sex ratios (If per capita income is taken as an indicator of economic development).[5] Further explorations of data reveal female foeticide is prone to the most economically backward states also, while states with similar development indicators reflect dissimilar child sex ratios, and child sex ratios are affected by cultural neglect practised in populations in lower income groups, where female foeticide may or may not be widespread.

Table 4.1
Sex Ratio (0–6 Years) and Per Capita Income in Selected States, 1981–2001

State	1981	2001	Decline in child sex ratio	Per capita income 1999–2000 (at current price) in Rs
India	962	927	-35	15,562
Goa	926	933	7	44,613
Maharashtra	956	917	-39	22,604
Punjab	908	793	-115	22,797
Gujarat	950	878	-72	18,926
Kerala	970	963	-7	17,709
Karnataka	974	949	-25	16,654
West Bengal	1149	963	-186	14,817
Andhra Pradesh	992	964	-28	15,040
Rajasthan	954	909	-45	12,074
Bihar	981	938	-43	4,813

Source: 1. Census of India. 1991. *India: Primary Census Abstract: General Population*. Part II–B(i) Vol.1.
2. Census of India. 2001. *Punjab: Provisional Population Totals*. Paper 1 of 2001.
3. Government of Punjab. 2004. *Statistical Abstract of Punjab, 2003*.

States such as Rajasthan and Bihar, which are among the states with the lowest per capita income in the country, also reflect the same trend, and even a sharper decline in the 0–6 sex ratio than, for instance, the 'developed' state of Maharashtra[6] (Table 4.1). Again, states with a moderate per capita income (near India's average) may report a sharp or a marginal decline in their child sex ratios. West Bengal is found to have the most drastic decline in its 0–6 sex ratio of 186 points between 1981 and 2001. On the other hand, Kerela, Karnataka and Andhra Pradesh, with similar per capita incomes, show a decline of only 7, 25 and 28 points respectively in the same period. Clearly, if per capita income is an indicator of economic prosperity, it has no defining role in determining the declining child sex ratio.

According to studies on female foeticide, urban and upper income groups, who have access to medical facilities, utilise these to practise their preference for the desired sex of their child. The sharper decline in the urban birth sex ratio at the all-India level, as in many other states, is cited as evidence (Gill 2002). Estimates of sex-selective abortions calculated by a study (UNFPA 2001: 10), report that urban areas in Haryana and Punjab witnessed a five-fold and an 18 per cent increase, in contrast to the declining trends in the rural areas.

A number of micro studies have found that the particular form of gender abuse of female foeticide is reported to be higher among the upper income groups and educated groups. A study by Kulkarni in Mumbai reports that in 1986, doctors performing sex determination tests revealed that the majority of their clients were from the middle class and others from the upper class, with a very small number from the lower classes (Gupta 2000). Moreover, some of the medical procedures for sex selection are so expensive that the clientele, perforce is from the upper income groups. The Foundation for Research in Reproduction in Mumbai, while performing the Ericsson technique charged Rs 4,000 per insemination, which on an average requires 3–4 insertions for a pregnancy. Ninety-six per cent of its initial clients wanted a son and two-thirds of them were from the business community (Gupta 2000). Similar reporting is done by Ravinder regarding a doctor who had a diary of 450 'cases' of sex determination tests. According to the doctor, 'initially, only moneyed people from the middle castes came for the tests. They keep coming even now, but our main clientele has changed. Now it is the educated middle class' (Ravinder 1993). Another study in Delhi reports a substantial clientele from educated women.

Not only do developed states and groups resort to female foeticide but also people from empowered populations, with relatively better resources and rights, are its practitioners. It is a challenge to the entitlements approach to combat female foeticide in ethnic groups who resort to birth sex preference practices in developed societies (Gupta 2000). These groups enjoy secure endowments and female entitlements to resources. Yet they resort to female foeticide. In The Netherlands, the issue of ethnic minorities seeking male children by aborting female foetuses created sufficient furore to be reported in newspapers in 1994. The debate found support from some medical practitioners on grounds of a right to exercise a cultural preference, with others arguing against this choice, since these people now lived in The Netherlands and did not need sons as an old age insurance. The demand found reflection in sex selection choices being made by ethnic minorities through the facilities offered by the Gender Preselection Clinic opened in Utrecht in 1995. Gupta reports that of the 19 per cent ethnic minorities, significantly with a higher education using the clinic services, predominantly desired a son, contrary to other clients of the clinic (2000). Such instances indicate that even when the benefits of development accrue, son preference remains unabated, even manifesting in the phenomenon of female foeticide.

Further doubts about the development agenda arise when analysing data of states ranking high on the gender equality index (GEI). In fact, states improving on the GEI are simultaneously boosting the masculine sex ratio. Himachal Pradesh, for instance, was ranked 4 on the GEI in the 80s and in the 90s became the most gender equitable state. Yet it recorded one of the most dramatic declines in the child sex ratio, a fall of 74 points from 1981 to 2001 (Table 4.2). In other words, while gender enjoys increasing equality on the development parameters, female foeticide also increases. Himachal Pradesh has registered a substantial increase in its female literacy rate (from 37.7 in 1981 to 68.08 in 2001), as also a vast improvement in its female work participation rate (31.86 in 1981 to 43.7 in 2001) but during the same period it has seen masculinisation of its child sex ratio.

Himachal Pradesh is not the only state to have simultaneously enhanced female capacities, including female life expectancy, and also a deteriorating child sex ratio. Maharashtra, Orissa, Punjab, Gujarat are some of the other states that belie the popular linkage of development with gender status. Clearly, development parameters such as female education, access to facilities, particularly health facilities, do not protect women from gender abuse. Obviously then, gender equity is no criterion for gender empowerment. The analysis cautions against an isomorphic dependence on development to dis-

Table 4.2
Female Literacy Rates and Child Sex Ratio in Selected States

States	Increase in literacy rates from 1981 to 2001	Decline in child sex ratios from 1981 to 2001
Gujarat	20.14	-72
Himachal Pradesh	30.36	-74
Maharashtra	26.5	-39
Orissa	25.83	-45
Punjab	26.91	-115
India	24.41	-35

Source: 1. Census of India. 1991. *Primary Census Abstract: General Population*. Pt. II-B(i).
2. Census of India. 2001. *Punjab: Provisional Population Totals*. Paper 1 of 2001.

mantle the structure of gender dominance. Education, work participation rates, enhanced health, declining fertility have been subsumed under the existing gender hierarchies to manifest in the
phenomenon of female foeticide. Moreover, socio-cultural contexts
shape the forms of gender subjectivities, thus male child preference
may manifest as female infanticide in some areas and as female
foeticide in other populations. Blanket categorisation of 'developed
states' as the bedrock of particular phenomenon is reductionist and
also gender neutral.

Access to development has been unable to transform the gender
position and bring about a change in the power equilibrium of society. Yet gender-related policies continue to promote and even achieve
their specified targets of increased access but are unable to counter
female foeticide. For instance, the National Health Policy (2000)
targets controlling infant mortality rates and promoting the two-
child family norm (GOI 2002). The IMR rates are declining, but so
is the birth of the girl child (Registrar General of India 2001). Also,
addressing the IMR gender gap seems to be outside the scope of its
mandate. While in 1981 infant mortality rates in accordance to
biological vulnerability of male children were favourable to the girl
child with mortality rates of male 122 and female 108, increasing
penetration of health facilities bypassed the survival rate of males to
that of females in 1991 (male IMR 74 and female IMR 79). The trend
continued in 2001 (male IMR 64 and female IMR 68). In other
words, developmental benefits accrue differentially to males and
females. The two-child norm is also becoming a reality, but at the
cost of displacing the girl child (UNFPA 2000: 26). The reproductive health approach to population stabilisation and sustainable development adopted by the Department of Family Welfare and UNFPA
India, calls for increasing 'women's control over their bodies and
lives'. Is 'women's right to choice' a protection against an informed
choice to undergo female foeticide? The Women's Empowerment
Policy (2001) views women's unfavourable status as an entitlement
failure—'lack of women's access to resources, facilities and infrastructure' (GOI 2001). Yet if increasing female literacy rates, enhancing life expectancy, increasing health benefits to women,
increasing female employment, were the basis of realising equality,
then states like Punjab, Himachal Pradesh, Orissa, West Bengal,
Maharashtra should not have witnessed large numbers of missing girl
children. Clearly, the existing gender-related policies do not have an

answer to the gender-differentiating hierarchies as highlighted by the increasing female foeticide even when policy objectives are being met.

If empowerment is merely to provide access, participation and skills within the existing gender differentiating system, it will be absorbed within the gender hierarchies. 'Social activity is the ideological setting within which skills are used and power is exercised' (Allen 1975: 213). These efforts to empower women are being subsumed under the prevalent gender ideology to appropriate the value of female education to promote health of the male offspring, female income and property rights as dowry and absorption of female labour in the unorganised sector at the cost of exclusion from the formal sector. If power is a derivate of skills, then empowerment mandates transformation and reallocation of skills from gender based functions. Thus access to livelihood, increased resources or increased participation in decision-making itself may not have the capacity to change women's unfavourable social placement. Economic independence has been purchased at the cost of doing a double day and increased vulnerability to sexual harassment. In fact, participation per se of women in socio-economic processes may just lead to newer forms of violence.

Notwithstanding the contradictions that emerge from the 'entitlement failure' to arrest female foeticide, the proposed initiatives to halt female foeticide by NAS (National Advocacy Strategy) 'Ending the practice changing the mindset' and related frameworks (UNFPA 2000) is propelled by the same liberal assumption of gender equality. In this instance, for the male and female child by placing the discriminatory manifestation of female foeticide in a demand and supply framework. To quote the draft strategy 'while no scientific study has been conducted to identify and rank the reasons for Pre-Birth Elimination of Female (PBEF), it is agreed that there are many obvious demand and supply side factors' (NAS 2002: 13). The category of the demand and supply model depends upon addressing the gender power hierarchies at the level of a manifestation, in this instance, the form of female foeticide. The differentiation of genders, structural placements, cultural practices, role typing and causation of gender conditions are segregated from the phenomenon. It is the bypassing of social conditions of dominance that allows a demarcation of supply and demand factors or the supply has to be curtailed and the form will be eradicated—as the short-term strategy elucidates. Yet even without the so-called supply factors of technology, the birth of a female child was being socially determined. A host of traditional methods, ranging from religious bigotry to the Chinese calendar were practised prior to the advent of the new reproductive technology of sex selection.[7] There are no separate factors of demand or supply of the male child. The assumption behind both is the same—the practice of gender differentiation. Both 'practitioners' and 'users' of the PBEF techniques are imbued with the same thinking—it works in collusion, like dowry exchange—the givers and seekers, like fathers who do not give property rights and daughters who do not seek the rights. There are no separate factors—the small family norm does not seek to promote female foeticide, the male child preference continues to run its writ—be it large or small families and it is always at the cost of the female child, be it female foeticide or cultural neglect. Similarly, there are no socio-economic imperatives to a girl's birth–the costs of raising a son—from celebration to expenses to acquire degrees/jobs, are not perceived as costs since the perceived advantages in terms of income, status and security accrue to the 'family' not to the 'other' as in the case of the girl. Given this socio-cultural context, an enforcement approach that targets only technology, may perhaps succeed only in making the services go underground. In Maharashtra, the public campaign against inhumanity and brutality against the girl child was successful in clamping down the initial spread of PBEF technologies, but with the increasing legitimacy of pre-birth selection and sex determination technologies, a legal enforcement alone will not work unless it is pro-actively imposed.

Moreover, the strategy is behaviour-oriented rather than addressing the more structural interests and values that articulate male child preference.

> The National Strategy recommends the ways to achieve changes in the behaviour of the multiple stakeholders on account of whose acts of omission or commission the practice of the pre-birth elimination of females continues unabated and is on the rise. The strategy links in with broader efforts to progress towards the vision of gender equality. (NAS 2002: 16)

This vision of gender equality finds expression in another strand to curtail the phenomenon of female foeticide—that which is centred on the right of women to make their own choice about reproduction and sexuality; in other words to exercise control over their bodies (UNFPA 2000).

In theory, the conceptualisation of equality is conceived on grounds of universal uniformity and in operative reality, it concedes the existence of an established standard as the prescribed ordain for the human species. Spike Patterson argues that the principle of equality enshrined in human rights discourse, is imposed by taking the standpoint of men.

> Human rights are gender specific. This is established empirically by reference to gender-differentiated human rights practices, and conceptually by reference to the model of human nature underpinning the rights traditions. Both in application and in theory, human rights are based on the male as the norm. (Patterson 1990: 305)

The thesis that the dominant notion of women's rights is individual-oriented and its negation that difference between male and female may be recognised and each is given control over his/her body, is gender-perpetuating, says Patterson (1990).

The institutionalisation of discrimination is impregnated with a bias, a differentiation, and a hierarchy. And power hierarchies are expected to be transformed by a change in the mindset. Such a strategy is corrective in nature. The state is targeted as an active medium for distributing equal opportunities, and at the same time, for providing measures for the redress of violation of these efforts. No causation, only manifestations of women's existing status is addressed. By assuming that equal opportunities can be availed of by adjustments in the systemic functioning, whereby prejudices, stereotypes and sex roles can be combated by awareness programmes, provision of health, education and income, the approach ignores the underlying ideology, values and social practices that determine women's unfavourable placement and therefore restricted access to opportunity.

> Liberal solutions can only improve the access of a relatively small number of women to the prizes of existing society. However, if women as a whole are to be liberated, a fundamental transformation of the structure of society is needed, not just a different allocation of who does what. Such restructuring would involve not only liberating women from their domestic and nurturing roles, but also changing the goals of the public world of work and politics. (Crowley and Himmelweit 1994: 16–17)

Even if women are 'empowered', they would continue to take gendered decisions. Intervention is made to rectify the imbalances at the level of visible impact, namely discrimination and physical abuse. It presupposes that discrimination and abuse is directed at defined 'victims' i.e. women, by defined 'perpetrators'. The problem is thus dealt within the preview of 'radical individualism' rather than any social patterning or manifestation of structural conditions (Phillips 1994). Focus is thus on individual and segregated aspects of society for redress–'where at the micro level the "users" and "service" providers of female foeticide form the core strategy'. These acts, if seen as only individual acts and described as aberrations, result only in corrective justice being dispensed whereby the victim is provided with relief and the perpetrator is targeted for punishment. In fact the NAS strategy focuses on short and medium-term goals that revolve around an effective implementation of the law with some provision for formal equality (NAS 2002: 15). Thus, corrective methods which are individual and relief-centred are practised.

The underlying thrust of the equality of opportunities approach in particular has been to ensure that women have access to and control over resources and an increase in income and decision-making would result in greater access for women to health, education and other material resources. The availability of infrastructure and services does not ensure their utilisation by females. The availability of infrastructure is reflected in male access to health and education, yet females are discriminated in varying proportion to their socio-economic settings. Thus the opportunity to equal rights does not ensure their availment. In fact, given the increased access to development benefits witnessed by women, it would be fair to observe that, 'In spite of dramatic changes in economic and political relations, the ideology of gender hierarchy has not been eliminated but simply modernised' (Patterson 1990: 316).

The systemic discrimination against women operates through the incorporation of values and norms that are ideologically determined and based in the gender system. This prescribes differential placement and roles for males and females on the basis of biology. Empowerment, therefore, is a function of transforming the gender-based system, which is shaped by anonymous social mechanisms which provide invisibility to the deprivation, discrimination and abuse that women face. As Allen analyses, ideology, in this case the gender system, is a process by which ideas, values and purposes act to influence behaviour and is essentially a mechanism of social control (Allen 1975: 224). It is these gender values that are socially codified, anonymously institutionalised and practised as cultural capital that manifest as systemic discrimination.

The normative acceptance of power hierarchies renders the systemic deprivation and discrimination as decrees of nature, unchangeable, and outside the purview of decision-making. This institutionalised power has its basis in gender equation, and provides visibility only to brutal acts. Built-in prejudices and biases promote the gender system and even shape the interests of disenfranchised groups to present conflicts as invisible. It is here that the function of ideology is defined wherein interests and ideas are shaped to determine not only the areas of decision-making and prescribing an agenda for decision-making but also to determine the 'socially structured and culturally patterned behaviour of groups and practices of institutions' (Lukes 1974: 22) that prevail to determine people's perceived interests. This level of power has been presented as the strategic gender needs by Moleneux who concedes that 'the relationship between what we have called strategic gender interests and women's recognition of them and their desire to realise them cannot be assumed,... even the lowest common denominator of interest such as equality with men, control over reproduction and greater personal autonomy and independence from men are not readily accepted by all women' (Molenuex 1995: 234).

II

Form-centric Initiatives: The Punjab Study

To empirically investigate the validity of the proposition of deploying development as a defining variable to overcome institutional bias to uplift women's status and tackle manifestations such as female foeticide, a disaggregate analysis of the situation in Punjab is being undertaken. Also examined is the import of a form-centric inquiry and initiatives to undermine the phenomenon of female foeticide. The empirical study draws on data from four surveys conducted between 1994 to 2002, extends to nearly 12,000 respondents that include male-female respondents from households, government functionaries, support structures such as local bodies' members and opinion-making sections. The paper uses this data to describe the patterns of practices and government initiatives to combat female foeticide.

Examining efforts in Punjab to address the issue of female foeticide, which are largely spurned by governmental initiative, this section analyses the historical context and the issues that are left unattended in the war against declining child sex ratios. While the national policy on advancing women's status finds continuity in the state through schemes, programmes and positive discrimination, the defined approach to combat female foeticide is ingenious to the state, given that 21 per cent of female foetuses go missing in Punjab as against the national average of 1.4 per cent (calculated from Census, 2001). Punjab which has the lowest child sex ratio (793) in the country directed its efforts 'to stop the menace of pre-selection techniques'.[8] An analysis of the departmental measures to promote a healthy sex balance, reveals preponderance of an enforcement perspective within the gamut of technological determinism.

According to health and social welfare functionaries, 68.5 and 72 per cent of the respective initiatives were enforcement oriented (Table 4.3). This included organisation of public camps, meetings, including self-help groups, plays, door-to-door campaigns to spread the legal ramifications of the PNDT Act and checks of pregnant women and raids on clinics which offer ultrasound technology. All IEC material circulated by the Health Department pertains to the criminality of female foeticide with an emphasis on spreading aware-

Table 4.3
Government Initiatives Reported by the Punjab Line Functionaries

Department	Awareness against female foeticide	Enforcement oriented	Generate importance of girl child for family
Social welfare (ICDS)	36	48	24
%	51.4	68.5	34.2
Health Deptt.	38	69	11
%	39.5	72.0	11.4

Source: IDC Field Survey 2003. 70 functionaries of ICDS and 96 of health department.

ness regarding the ban on pre-sex-selection techniques. The Social Welfare Department did lay stress on spreading awareness against the practice of female foeticide and this centred around appeals to the public to refrain from the brutal act of female foeticide. Some activities also pertained to giving importance to the girl child such as celebrating *Lohri* of girls and the UNICEF programme of Meena Day. A number of notifications to this effect have been issued by the Social Welfare Department.[9] Investigations reveal a wide gap between the identified problem of female foeticide and the method for its resolution. The assumptions of the state health department being that it is lack of legal literacy among backward populations, which an approach of fear can combat. The department for women's issues extends its understanding to include a cultural fallacy of male child relevance which, in the 21st century, is misplaced since girls have no biological barriers to achievement. Therefore, the view that awareness and facilities for enhancing women's capacities can bring about the requisite behavioural change. The policy approach to combat female foeticide through spread of legal literacy seems ill-conceived given that the groups which were found to practise female foeticide were predominantly aware that sex determination was illegal and they belonged to the upper income groups as well as the educated sections of society. Table 4.4 reveals that more than 77 per cent of those who undertook foeticide were aware that it was a crime. Also, this awareness was to the extent of 91 per cent among the upper income groups. Similarly among the educated groups 87 per cent were versed with the legal ramifications (see Tables 4.4 and 4.5).

Yet they resorted to female foeticide—clearly informing the informed will not be effective in checking female foeticide. Moreover, the awareness campaigns led by the government departments and some NGOs[10] in the state promote the idea that there is no difference

Table 4.4
Respondents Used Sex Determination and Knew the Laws by Income

Strata of the respondents who used sex determination test	Awareness of SDT law (%)	Awareness of property law (%)
Upper	91.7	100.0
Middle	77.0	92.0
Lower	58.0	56.0
All Respondents	77.0	82.0

Source: IDC Field Survey 2002.

Table 4.5
Respondents Used Sex Determination and Knew the Laws by Education

Educational qualification	Awareness on sex determination test (%)	Awareness of property law (%)
Illiterate	86.0	67.0
Primary	63.0	58.0
Matric	0.0	–
Graduate	87.0	96.0
All Respondents	77.0	82.0

Source: IDC Field Survey 2002.

between male and female children and thus discrimination against the female should not take place. However, a glance at the popular perception regarding the worth accorded to the male and the female child reveals a vast difference. Table 4.6 shows that the male child is a prospective earner and source of dependence (according to 43 per cent and 58 per cent respectively) while the girl child has to be provided with protection (45 per cent) and represents the burden of dowry collection (55 per cent).

Table 4.6
Respondents' Perception on the Value of Son and Daughter

	Male	Female	Total
Male child as valuable earner	39	38	77
	41.94	43.68	42.78
Parents dependent on male child	51	54	105
	54.84	62.07	58.33
Female needs protection	50	32	82
	53.76	36.78	45.56
Female child is expensive to give dowry	48	51	99
	51.61	58.62	55.00

Source: Dagar 2002.

And interestingly, this experience of differential value of the male and female child is a perceived reason of female foeticide by the very functionaries who are imploring people to refrain from female foeticide. Most accord female as a liability (60 and 36.4 per cent respectively) and male as a symbol of status and preferred child (44 and 61.4 per cent as in Table 4.7).

No effort is, however, forthcoming to change the factors for perceived male child as a provider, protector or procreator. In fact, the

Table 4.7
Government Line Functionaries' Views on Reasons for Female Foeticide

Department	Male child preference/ status	Girl a liability	Illiteracy	Small family norm
Social welfare (ICDS)	31	42	5	3
%	44.2	60.0	7.1	4.3
Health Department	59	35	11	1
%	61.4	36.4	11.5	1.0

Source: IDC Field Survey 2003.

functionaries' own bias for the male child's importance can be gauged by the overwhelming number (80 and 63 per cent) stating that by seeking God's grace, the boon of a male child can be acquired. In other words, physical annihilation should not occur, but the justifications and the legitimacy of the importance of the male child remain unaddressed and condoned (19 per cent and 25 per cent) by even traditional methods of begetting a male child (Table 4.8).

It is not only utilitarianism that spurns these groups for a male child but even the emergence of a normative concern where they feel the male child enhances their status as is predominant in the case of landowning families. Another factor that plays an important role in family politics is the small family norm. The emergence of the two-child family and even one-child family, in many cases, has ensured the birth of only male children. So not only middle income families, who cannot support large numbers, but also the rural, landed families are found to have only one offspring—a male. It is common for the landed respondents to say that landholdings are shrinking and even if they have 22 acres, this would not support two male children and that they are planning to have only one male child. Forty per cent

Table 4.8
Per cent Government Functionaries on Religious Bigotry for Male Child

Department	Condone female foeticide	No opinion	No harm in seeking God's grace for a male child
Social Welfare (ICDS)	18.6	1.4	80.0
Health Department	25.0	11.4	63.5

Source: IDC Field Survey 2003.

Table 4.9
Peasants Chose to Have a Single Son in Malwa, Punjab, by Age

Age of the respondent	Per cent peasants with a single male child
18–25	35.0
25–35	15.0
35+	40.0

Source: Dagar, Rainuka 2002.

of the couples over 35 years, in landed households, were found to have only one offspring, a male (Table 4.9).

These perceptions of both respondents and functionaries are rooted in social structures and are reflected in the historically unfavourable condition of women in the state. In fact the disaggregate analysis reveals that rather than technological determinism, held responsible for the present sex imbalance, it is social placement and the cultural context that direct the use of sex-selective techniques and that the form of gender abuse changes in the changing context. Thus if Punjab had to deal with female infanticide during the early 20th century, it is female foeticide that has become the bane of social development in the early 21st century.

III

Technological Determinism: An Analysis of Sex Ratios in Punjab

While the predominant programmes in Punjab target the spread of technology in checking female foeticide, sex ratios have been highly imbalanced prior to the invention of technologies of pre-birth sex selection. Sex ratios register a further decline after birth when these technologies are inapplicable. Moreover, within defined locales, social groups resort to female foeticide differentially in accordance with historically defined male child preference.

Historically, Punjab has had the dubious distinction of having a highly masculine sex ratio. In fact with the advance towards the 21st century, the adverse sex ratio in Punjab has improved. At the turn of the century, the Punjab sex ratio stood at 832, improved to 882 in 1991 and fell comparatively to 874 in 2001. The historically adverse sex ratio testifies to the unfavourable condition of women in Punjab. The lack of technology has not been a hindrance to the disposal of unwanted females. Yet misappropriation of 'technology' is indicated in the adverse sex ratio at birth, as well as, in the sharp decline in the sex ratio in subsequent years. In Punjab the child sex ratio at birth was 946 in 1981 and it fell to 854 in 1991. In both the decades the sex ratio at birth was higher and it declined for the one-year age group. In 1981, the sex ratio at birth was 946, while for infants it fell to 921. Similarly in 1991, the sex ratio at birth was higher at 854 and for one year of birth, it fell to 845. The fall in the infant sex ratio and also in the other age groups, reflects factors that operate after birth, such as cultural neglect to replace technology. To state an example of neglect–a premature girl child needed to be kept in an incubator that would have cost Rs 25,000. The family decided that this amount could be better utilised as a fixed deposit for her dowry, if she survived without medical care. The baby was not provided the needed medical attention and died.

Higher female child mortality has affected the decline in age-specific sex ratios. Miller found that the proportion of female mortality increased after the fifth month (Miller 1981). She attributed girl child mortality to the quest for a male child. In Punjab, infant and child mortality in 1991 was higher in all age groups and even decreased for female infants in 1981 and 1991 (Tables A4.1, A4.2 and A4.3 in the annexure). Female child mortality increases in the one to four age group when social factors continue to intervene to affect survival (Chatterjee 1990: 3). In fact in Punjab, the sex ratio in the 10–14 years age group in 1991 was the most adverse at 876 (Table A4.4).

The systematic and consistent adverse sex ratio at birth, declining child sex ratios, higher female infant and child mortality rate and the increasingly adverse sex ratio with increasing age, reflect the importance and negative impact of social factors that continue to intervene to negate life chances for females. In rural Khanna, Monica Das Gupta found clear evidence in 1984 of the role of behavioural factors in raising the mortality rate of girls. She reported that after the first month of life, environmental and care-related factors, that are susceptible to societal manipulations, come into play (Das Gupta 1987: 81). Cultural negation of the female sex is a historical reality. Importantly, the continued decline in sex ratios from birth to infant to child, points to the need for an agenda that addresses the female's right to life and survival rather than to only assert for the right to birth. Birth right is no protection against cultural neglect, dowry deaths, wife beating or female infanticide.

Technology Differentially Appropriated Irrespective of Access

Besides the variations in the sex ratio among child age groups, regional variations in the sex ratio reflect social impediments to the natural sex ratio. While the 2001 sex ratio of Punjab is among the lowest in the country, large variations within its districts exist. Ludhiana, with 824, has the lowest female representation while Hoshiarpur with 935 has the most favourable sex ratio. A look at the pattern of sex ratio over the century (Figure 4.1) reveals that there has been a historical consistency among the regions with regard to sex ratio.

Malwa, which is characterised as a feudal region with late agricultural development, has the poorest sex ratio. In fact, historically, the districts of Ropar, Fatehgarh Sahib and Ludhiana share the lowest sex ratio. In contrast, the prosperous Doaba region, which in-

Figure 4.1
Region-wise Sex Ratio of Punjab from 1901 to 2001

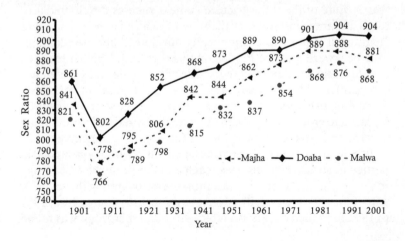

cludes Jallandhar and Kapurthala, has had the most favourable sex ratio, always above the state average. The Majha region bordering Pakistan, with districts of Amritsar and Gurdaspur, had sex ratios hovering around the state average.

An analysis of the sex ratio and child sex ratio reveals a distinct pattern based on the cultural zones of Punjab. Districts comprising the backward area of Malwa, namely Bathinda, Mansa, Sangrur, Fatehgarh Sahib, Patiala and Ropar, and pockets of the Majha region had the most adverse sex ratio as well as an adverse child sex ratio in 2001. Interestingly, in most of these districts (Fatehgarh Sahib, Patiala, Mansa, Sangrur and Ropar) the decline is far greater in the rural child sex ratio (Table A4.5 in annexure). The rural areas seem to have surmounted the distance and accessibility factors to reduce female births.

What is revealing is that districts with the lowest sex ratio and the lowest child sex ratio are also those which have witnessed the largest decline in the child sex ratio since 1991. These areas represent the most hostile conditions for women. It is perhaps here that pre-natal diagnostic techniques have been misused the most.

Differential Use of Technology and Socio-cultural Predispositions

Regional disparity in the misappropriation of technology reveals that in spite of the infrastructure context such as development of roads and transport links, availability of health facilities and other facilities, it is not the 'economically developed' but the economically backward areas of Punjab that have recorded higher levels of female foeticide. Cultural predispositions of male child preference can be inferred from the sex ratio in the rural and urban areas also. Rural Punjab has registered a higher decline in the sex ratio in the 0–6 years age group even though the overall sex ratio of rural Punjab is better than that of urban Punjab (Table A4.5 in annexure).

Besides these regional disparities, population groups grounded in particular social relations have reacted to this pre-birth technology in a differential manner. For instance, sex ratios among the Jat peasantry have been historically adverse as the Census figures, from 1901 to 1931 for which data is available, show and this group was found to have the highest incidence of female foeticide (Table 4.10). An analysis of the qualitative data clearly indicates the importance of the male child to the Jats who comprise the peasantry, and their socio-cultural and economic linkages with land. As one young Jat father explained,

The birth of a son enhances my status while that of a girl lowers my head. Land is the mother for Jats and looking after it is akin to caring for your mother. If boys are there the land will be looked after, but if there are only girls then the land will be sold. Boys are the owners of land, they are the tree of the house that flowers and fruits. (Dagar undated)

While sex ratio Census data by community is not available, micro studies in the field reveal that female foeticide is most practised in

Table 4.10
Sex Ratios for Jats, Gujjars and the State of Punjab

Year	Punjab total	Gujjar	Jats
1901	858	841	805
1911	818	805	764
1921	829	821	781
1931	831	821	802

Source: Census of India. 1931. India: Imperial Tables. Part II. Vol. I.

Table 4.11
Per cent Reported Female Foeticide by Household Head's Occupation

Occupation	2001–2002	2002–2003
Peasantry	26.7	15.5
Business class	15.4	12.4
Service	18.5	6.2
Labour	7.0	9.2

Source: IDC Field Survey 2003.

Table 4.12
Per cent Respondents Reported Female Foeticide by Caste

Caste group	Extent of female foeticide
Jat	13.2
Non-SC	9.9
SC	9.5
Total	10.9

Source: IDC Field Survey 2003.

the peasantry constituting Jats (Table 4.11). Female foeticide was reported to be the highest among the landed groups. These caste and occupational differences are found among groups located in the same area, across income and locale (Table 4.12).

'Empowered Population' and Foeticide

'Empowerment' in terms of higher access to education, health, income, decision-making, available more in the urban areas, has been the said panacea for discrimination against women. If access to development indicators were to uplift women's status, female foeticide should not be found in the upper income groups, among women professionals, women who are decision-makers or among non-resident Indian (NRI) Punjabi populations that are relatively better placed in developed countries.

As for the various 'advantages' of sex determination tests, it was the better educated groups who found these tests more advantageous than the lower educated groups. Similarly the upper income groups were found to practice female foeticide more widely than the lower income populations (Table 4.13).

In a study of the women respondents who used modern methods (ultrasounds, in-vitro fertilization techniques) to determine the sex of their foetus, 83 per cent were 'decision-makers' (Dagar 2001). Of the total women 'decision-makers', 78 per cent mentioned having consciously resorted to methods to determine the male sex of the foetus. Male child preference is not only bound by physical territory, cultural setting, economic and educational access. It also derives its relevance from the urge to establish one's cultural identity.[11]

Table 4.13
Per cent Respondents Reported Practice of Female Foeticide by Income[12]

Strata	2001	2002
Upper	18.3	15.7
Middle	23.2	12.6
Lower	15.5	6.2
Total	19.4	10.9

Source: Dagar, Rainuka 2002.

The development and application of medical technologies in particular, have raised a number of sociological debates. Do these offer reproductive rights and choices to women or is the development of technologies itself ideologically laden? According to Pursell,

As the material manifestations of social relations, tools are concrete commitments to certain ways of doing things and therefore certain ways of dividing power. It is the same technology from which labour is saved or jobs destroyed. (Pursell 1994: 218)

As argued, new reproductive technologies have been appropriated to perpetuate the retrograde social set-up. Moreover, utilisation or misappropriation of technology is embedded in historical social relations and even debates on technology are shaped around cultural predispositions. In the context of reproductive technologies, for instance, the pre-birth technology of ultrasound, amniocentesis, in-vitro fertilization etc. have given rise to debates centred on genetic screening, a search for the perfect child (Gupta 2000 and Rothman 1989) and the related debate on eugenics among native populations in western Europe. Gender counselling is a vital component in the practice of these technologies with issues centred around the ethical, legal and philosophical questions that arise in the use of particular qualities in a child (Gupta 2000). Yet in the Asian context, it is the same technologies that have given rise to the issue of endangered daughters and sex-selective births. The utilisation of technology is, no doubt, centred around socio-cultural preferences and the values that emanate from them. In other words, technologies are not supra social, but bias is built into the technology itself (Mies 1987). The usage and spread of technologies reflect a prior hierarchy of gender, social placement, religion and cultural specificities.

IV

Masculinisation of Sex Ratios: Emerging Debates _____

The treatment of symptomatic manifestations as autonomous phenomena, addresses social conditions as fragmented. Masculine sex ratios, female foeticide, dowry, *sati* and wife beating are all forms of gender violence emanating from the practice of gendered differentiation. Isolating a form of violence from its causal linkages, confines the analysis to being only descriptive. If the gender hierarchies are not addressed, then the system of dominance flourishes unhindered. To exemplify, if the concern is only for the declining sex ratio then the issues being addressed would be of demographic imbalance, lack of girls for boys to marry etc. The social message that is conveyed is that girls are necessary for reproduction and population stability.

These sentiments in fact find favour with the dominant 'gender-imbued' population. According to one middle-aged rural, landed woman, 'If girls keep disappearing at this rate then boys will be in difficulty. Whom will they marry? Three-four brothers will have to make do with one woman—like the Pandavs.' Another concern voiced was that 'now girls will have to be brought from Bengal and Orissa—earlier girls used to take dowry, now they will have to be bought' (Dagar 2002).

Such an approach views the female identity only vis-à-vis her existing typed role, re-emphasising the existing gender norms that may be promoting the imbalance in the first place. The point being that forms of violence cannot be corrected if disassociated from their historical, socio-cultural, economic and political context. Delineating from determining and supportive factors denies the existence of power hierarchies that systematically disadvantage on the basis of gender; changing the phenomenon in the changed contexts, yet the hierarchies remain unchanged.

The urgency to control the use of sex determination tests with a view to checking the declining sex ratio has thrown up the following issues:

Practice versus Norm

The concern for female foeticide emerging from the declining sex ratio has made controlling the practice of female foeticide central to the strategy and even assumptions regarding the emergence of imbalanced sex ratios. The Sikh clergy proclaimed a social boycott of those Sikhs who practised female foeticide.[13] This resolution was hailed as a frontal opposition to female foeticide. There is no opposing the positive initiative of the clergy to undermine this form of gender violence. However, this resolution on its own may not translate into desired results. The issue of male child preference that fuels the practice of female foeticide remains unattended. While the misuse of technology has been denounced, religious bigotry and blessings for a male child are routinely supported by Sikh institutions such as Gurudwaras. *Deras* continue to proliferate the boon of the birth of a male child, as is the situation with other religions and sects (Dagar 2001). In fact, the unfavourable status of women needs to be confronted in its entirety rather than addressing the practice and expecting it to change the value accorded to the male child. This concern is better represented by people to whom the worth of the male child accrues, with the girl child as the 'other' who stands as a drain on family resources.

Another example of demarcation of the practice from its material and historical context can be drawn from the content analysis of support structures and line functionaries' interventions to combat female foeticide.[14] While the idea of female child as the 'other', displaced through lineage, inheritance and patriarchal role identities is to be undermined, female foeticide is located in the higher worth of the male child (97 and 90 per cent), considering the female a liability.

Yet at the level of problem resolution, the majority of the government line functionaries relied on legal enforcement (68.5 and 72.0 per cent; see Table 4.3). Female liability was to be underscored by educating women and telling the community that there is no difference between male and female children when the community experiences the male to be God's gift and the female to be a burden. In other words, while female foeticide is perceived to be practised due to both discrepant worth of the male-female and the undisputed value of the male child, at the level of resolution, only the practice is targeted. Training on female foeticide has been imparted to line functionaries with a verdict to abolish the use of pre-birth sex determining technologies. The strategy hinges on providing awareness of the illegality of these technologies and urging people to see reason in the comparative worth of the male and female child. Interestingly, two practices of dowry harassment and *Lohri* have been focused on— one as a cause (dowry exchange) and the other as a display (*Lohri*) of male-female discrimination. These practices are being targeted for bringing about a change but only at the level of arousing the people's sense of morality, without arousing the gamut of interlayered processes that intermesh to proclaim male hegemony and associated cultural values.

Gender versus Reproduction Rights

The debate for female control over their bodies as a measure to counter female foeticide may be far stretched. The issue of abortion rights has a different meaning in the western world from that in India. The question here is not of control over sexuality to escape repeated pregnancies but to escape sex-selective abortions. In India the concern of individual women may not just be the issue of abortion rights, but repeated birth of girl child, to gain freedom from repeated pregnancies. Without the aid of pre-birth sex-selective technologies, women may decide to continue with births until they arrive at the desired number of male children (Dagar 2002). In fact, the desired number of male children and sex defined family configuration has been an accepted factor in demographic studies. Voices from the field are worried, according to one woman, if the tests are no longer available then it will be girl after girl taking birth and reproduction halted only at the birth of a son (Dagar). Unsuccessful attempts to bear a male child have led to women hiring the womb (Vinayak 1997) and even supporting bigamy (Dagar 2001) to allow for a male child. What is the guarantee that if women have control over their bodies, they will not resort to female foeticide?

Excessive Dependence on Legal Apparatus

If female foeticide as a form of gender abuse is analysed as an autonomous phenomenon causing a sharp decline in child sex ratios, then this reductionism perforce depends on the PNDT law and its enforcement to counter the expression of people's preference. In Punjab, 84.2 per cent of the local body, i.e. *panchayat* members were of the same view and demanded stringent enforcement of the law to tackle the problem. Yet 12 per cent found the impact of the law to be dismal (Dagar 2002). Reliance is on fear to bring about a behaviour change since the problem is identified in the realm of attitudes and mindset rather than the realm of values and social structures. The law is control-oriented rather than an instrument for the protection of freedom or the promotion of rights. According to Brenner when the '...ability to win the material and political conditions of power for women diminishes, reliance on the coercive arm of the state comes to play more central part' (Brenner 1996: 55). Can laws and punitive measures be expected to rectify social attitudes and norms which actually have their origin in social structures? Legal measures can be effective when a behaviour is perceived as socially unjust. The law can intervene to regulate that which is socially desirable. It would perhaps be pertinent to understand the conditions under which corrective measures can contribute to the protection of rights. Law centric intervention, even if safeguarded against bias or gaps in legislation, will face biased application and adjudication in accordance with dominant norms. To overhaul a preference rooted in generations, interest groups need to emerge, take shape and assert. If interest articulation is restricted to a selective practice, the channels of communication that articulate these interests, normative rules and social values through anonymous mechanisms, will distort, reshape and dilute the implementation.

Principles and Assumptions : Pro-life and Parental Choice

Liberty and value for human life are integral principles within the context of human rights. In the domain of female foeticide these principles conflict. While pro-life supporters condemn as immoral the practice of female foeticide, the parents assert their right to have a family of a particular sex composition (Wertz and Fletcher 1993). Legal support to discriminatory elimination of life is stated in the PNDT Act. Yet the principal of liberty, voiced as a parental choice to desire a small and sex-defined constituent family, falls in the gambit of a criminal choice. Can one human rights principle be privileged over the other when all human rights are inalienable? However, if this debate transcends to the assumption that guides the contextualising of the principle then both the pro-life and parental choice supporters may be seen to be guided by the same logic of male child preference. These perceptions were empirically captured to reveal that as many as 37 per cent of the pro-life asserters, had practised (Pramod and Dagar 1995: 30–31) their preference for male child, albeit through religious bigotry—visits to quacks, pilgrimages and pandits for evoking God's blessings for a male child. While one was visible and life eliminating, the other was shrouded in customary practice. Again, when the gamut of patriarchal structures are addressed, the rights debate is contextualised with both the right to life and the right to choice expressing different forms of gender discrimination, highlighting the power hierarchies that dictate the approach.

Agent and Site of Violence Targeted

The acts of commission are visible, and easily discernible as life depriving, while the acts of omission remain outside the very frame of reference when the act of female foeticide is the focus for the redress of the declining sex ratio. The clinics, practitioners and individuals stating their preference for a male child are most visible and targeted for criminal proceedings. The pilot project of Punjab identifies 'high risk' women—those who have had two or more girl children without a male child (Nagpal 2003). Follow-up and enforcement teams are acts of omission of cultural neglect, discriminatory medical, maternal and life-enhancing entitlements and God's favour for the male child blessings remain outside the ambit of perceived social violence and are left unattended, without a causal connectivity to patriarchy. It is easier to target a defined practice such as female foeticide rather than the diffused linkages bound by anonymous social mechanisms which are more difficult to grapple with, and capture the people's imagination to target themselves. Thus it is the urban, upper income and educated population that is found to practice female foeticide, while the lower income population may be guilty of cultural neglect. Both are contributing to the declining female population.

Professional Ethics or Social Collusion: Demand and Supply Strategy

The market mechanics of female foeticide obliterate the fact that social reality is not segmented but a conglomeration of vying interests and values. Neither is social reality demarcated to define demand or supply factors. Profit may not be the only reason that new reproductive technologies proliferate. While male child preference can be priced, and profit accrued, doctors may also believe in the necessity of a male child and may perform foeticide as a social service in case of second or third birth order girls. Responding to the decline in sex ratio in Punjab, the medical association of doctors in Amritsar decided not to perform sex determination tests. Giving this logic, a doctor informed patients that only for the third pregnancy in case of two prior girls would they now perform these tests. Doctors are part of society and imbued with similar norms and value systems. Therefore, medical ethics may justify, protecting a woman from repeated births after a number of girls have been born. The analysis does veer away from form-centric initiatives and the inability of developmental goals to challenge the phenomenon of female foeticide.

V

Policy Initiatives _____

1. From Birth Right to Life Rights

To attribute primacy to right to birth rather than to the all-encompassing right to life is a reductionist approach. It is evident that cultural predispositions could not deny the right to birth, but could distort the natural life cycle (e.g. female infanticide).

To focus strategy to check and regulate application of sex-selection technology without questioning the values and norms dictating individual choice and social practice, may detract from addressing the core issues. To label enforcement as a short/medium term intervention in the absence of a correct gender framework, may prove counter productive. In other words, single locus, linear milestones may not be adequate for an intermeshed complex social phenomenon like male child preference.

2. Targeting the Norm rather than the Practice

Male child *per se* is a value and 'male child preference' a sociocultural norm. Gendered practices derive their sustenance and justifications from superordinate-subordinate gender hierarchical system. The concern for female foeticide emerging from the declining child sex ratio brought the visible distortions to the forefront of the interventionist framework. Rather than addressing the practice and expecting it to change the value accorded to the male child, the need is to confront the norms and their representation beyond the gender identities such as caste, ethnic and religious.

3. From Women's Empowerment to Gender Justice

The visible face of powerlessness in the gender system are women. Instead of empowering women with male support, it is the social context that disempowers them, which has to be addressed. The exercise of bias is ideologically rooted in institutions, gender norms, roles, practices and beliefs and exercised through 'anonymous social mechanisms'. Social processes and the web of structural and cultural institutions have to be dismantled to allow the empowerment project to root out gender hierarchies. So it is not women or men that have to be 'sensitised' but practices such as dowry, manifestation of masculinities–femininities, transforming sexual division of labour and women's rights to inheritance that have to be targeted.

4. From Control Over Resources to Redistribution of Hierarchies

The entitlements approach envisages women's control over resources as the ambit of empowerment. Institutional gender power hierarchies would shape the agenda for resource management. Developmental access and decision-making themselves may not be sufficient to undermine the 'socially structured and culturally patterned behaviour of groups and practices of institutions' that prevail to undermine people's (women's) perceived interests. The unequal gender power balance rather than resource shall have to be transformed and—located. Thus it is not the number of male nurturers or women breadwinners that have to be increased, but the roles of nurturing, procreation and that of a provider, that have to be detached from a gender value.

5. From Form-Centred to a Holistic View

The answer to life-enhancing mechanisms resulting in life-depriving outcomes, lies in the understanding that pre-natal diagnostic techniques do not exist in a vacuum but function in accordance with social conditions of patriarchy. The appropriation of medial technology to diagnose the sex of a child is part of the systemic gender discrimination, since scientific intervention is not exempt from social predispositions. Addressing only technological practices, a form of social differentiation would not undermine the differential per se. In other words, female foeticide occurs because there is male child preference in society. The male child preference emanates from the perceived higher relative worth of the male over the female. Not only does the male have more developed capacities but has culturally-accumulated, normative hegemony. It is ingrained that the male has more developed capacities than the female. Therefore, addressing 'reversal of flows of inter-generational wealth' is unable to capture the symbolic value of a male child. In order to combat this male child preference, not only has the female productive worth in society got to be enhanced, but her identity as the 'other' has also to be abolished.

Annexure

Table A4.1
Infant Mortality Rate in Punjab

Year	Male	Female
1983–87	81.93	85.05
1984–88	78.97	84.64
1985–89	77.90	80.27
1986–90	66.42	71.10
1987–91	64.27	65.73
1988–92	62.50	63.57
1989–93	60.31	62.41

Source: SRS Mortality Differentials by Age and Sex in India 1983–93.

Table A4.2
Child (1–4 Years) Death Rate in Punjab

Year	Male	Female
1983–87	6.23	12.80
1984–88	7.14	12.99
1985–89	7.13	12.41
1986–90	5.24	9.81
1987–91	4.62	8.89
1988–92	4.53	8.57
1989–93	4.17	7.56

Source: SRS Mortality Differentials by Age and Sex in India 1983–93.

Table A4.3
Infant Mortality Rate in Punjab, 1981, 1991 and 2001

Year	Male	Female	Persons
1981	138	114	127
1991	81	53	74
2001	43	63	52

Source: National Human Development Report 2001.

Table A4.4
Sex Ratio by Age in Punjab, 1981–2001

Age group	1981	1991	2001
0–4	925	878	794
5–9	877	887	821
10–14	872	876	859

Source: 1. Statistics on children in India 1993, 1998.
2. Census of India 2001, 2004. Report and Tables on Age.

Table A4.5
Sex Ratio and Child Sex Ratio in Districts of Punjab, 1991 and 2001

State/Districts	Sex ratio 1991			Sex ratio 2001			Sex ratio 0–6 age group 1991			Sex ratio 0–6 age group 2001		
	T	R	U	T	R	U	T	R	U	T	R	U
Punjab	882	888	868	874	887	848	875	878	866	793	795	789
Gurdaspur	903	905	895	888	895	868	878	881	868	775	789	729
Amritsar	873	871	876	874	885	859	861	864	856	783	789	772
Kapurthala	896	910	857	886	907	843	879	875	891	775	773	779
Jalandhar	897	907	883	882	904	859	886	891	879	797	806	786
Hoshiarpur	924	932	890	935	947	888	884	887	873	810	813	800
Nawanshahr	900	898	914	913	914	911	900	898	913	810	811	805
Rupnagar	870	870	870	870	869	871	884	883	886	791	787	800
FG Sahib*	871	870	873	851	859	832	874	872	881	754	747	774
Ludhiana	844	880	812	824	877	784	877	886	869	814	812	816
Moga	884	883	889	883	885	873	867	867	866	819	820	811
Firozpur	895	898	887	883	893	857	887	894	864	819	824	804
Muktsar	880	877	888	886	888	883	858	864	839	807	810	798
Faridkot	883	882	884	881	876	892	865	867	861	805	805	806
Bathinda	884	888	873	865	868	860	860	866	844	779	789	756
Mansa	873	871	881	875	875	878	873	883	814	779	780	775
Sangrur	870	866	881	868	869	864	873	877	863	784	779	798
Patiala	882	875	899	864	862	868	871	870	872	770	764	786

Source: Census of India, 2001. Provisional Population Totals: Supplement District Total. Paper 1´ of 2001.

Table A4.6
Districts of Punjab in their Placement by Child Sex Ratio in India, 2001

	State	District	Sex ratio	Percentile Rank
1	Punjab	Fatehgarh Sahib	754	0.00
2	Haryana	Kurukshetra	770	0.00
3	Punjab	Patiala	770	0.00
4	Punjab	Kapurthala	775	0.01
5	Punjab	Gurdaspur	775	0.01
6	Punjab	Mansa	779	0.01
7	Punjab	Bathinda	779	0.01
8	Punjab	Amritsar	783	0.01
9	Haryana	Sonipat	783	0.01
10	Haryana	Ambala	784	0.02
11	Punjab	Sangru	784	0.02
12	Haryana	Kaithal	789	0.02
13	Punjab	Rupnagar	791	0.02
14	Haryana	Rohtak	796	0.02
15	Punjab	Jalandhar	797	0.02
16	Gujarat	Mahesana	798	0.03
17	Haryana	Jhajjar	805	0.03
18	Punjab	Faridkot	805	0.03
19	Haryana	Karnal	806	0.03
20	Punjab	Muktsar	807	0.03
21	Haryana	Panipat	807	0.03
22	Haryana	Yamunanagar	807	0.04
23	Punjab	Nawanshahr	810	0.04
24	Punjab	Hoshiarpur	810	0.04
25	Gujarat	Ahmadabad	814	0.04
26	Punjab	Ludhiana	814	0.04
27	Haryana	Mahendragarh	814	0.04
28	Haryana	Rewari	814	0.05
29	Jammu & Kashmir	Jammu & Kashmir	816	0.05
30	Gujarat	Gandhinagar	816	0.05
31	Haryana	Jind	818	0.05
32	Haryana	Sirsa	818	0.05
33	Punjab	Moga	819	0.05
34	Punjab	Firozpur	819	0.06

Source: 1. Census of India, 2001.
2. Provisional Population Totals: Supplement District Totals Paper 1 of 2001.

Notes

1. The data that have galvanised this social concern are indeed alarming. While child sex ratios declined from 945 in 1991 to 927 in 2001, this fall was as high as 82 points in Punjab with Haryana, Himachal Pradesh and Gujarat reporting a fall of 59, 54 and 50 respectively.

2. Not only did sex ratios at birth become more masculine (For all India, these ratios fell from 967 to 939, between 1981 and 1991, and to 915 by 2001) but the number of sex determination clinics and subsequent female foeticide were becoming rampant. (Sharma 2000, Sooch 2000).

3. In fact, a number of studies have also shown the diametrical impact of education on delaying marriage age, decreasing fertility rate, lowering child mortality etc., among other, the NHFS data. According to NHFS data infant mortality declines with increase in female literacy (Table 4.1), as do the child mortality rate (Table 4.2) and the total fertility rate (Table 4.3), (International Institute for Population Sciences; Das Gupta 1987).

4. In all the reports data is drawn from a sample of three cultural zones of Punjab namely Majha, Malwa and Doaba and representative of urban and rural population. Atrocities Against Women in Punjab (1995) by Pramod Kumar and Rainuka Dagar. The data was collected in 1994 from interviews (including a neighbourhood analysis and incident of case studies) in which 4,656 people were interviewed.

   Combating Violence Against Women in Punjab (2001): A total of 2,874 respondents were part of the sample base (this included household survey, case incidents, narratives, opinion making sections and focus group discussions).

   Identifying and Controlling Female Foeticide and Infanticide in Punjab (2002a). The sample of this study was 1,483 (this included households, narratives, case studies and focus groups discussions). Combating Gender Differentiation and Female Foeticide in Punjab (2002b). The number of respondents who were part of the sample was 2,933 (this included interviews with respondents from households, government functionaries and narratives).

5. The per capita income in these states is better than India's average and they have also declining 0–6 sex ratios. Punjab, with a per capita income of Rs 23,254, has registered the sharpest decline in the 0–6 years sex ratio from 908 to 875 and 793 in 1981, 1991 and 2001 respectively.

   Gujarat's 0–6 sex ratio falls from a relatively better 950 in 1981 to a perceptively low of 878 in 2001, while boasting of a per capita income of Rs 18,625 in 2001.

6. Bihar 0–6 sex ratio was 981 in 1981 and declined by 43 points to 938 in 2001, and Rajasthan figure dropped by 45 during the same period, whereas in Maharashtra, a developed state, it dropped by 39 points.

7. The legitimacy to male child preference can be gauged from the existence of local traditional practices to acquire a male child and include places of worship designed specifically to acquire a male child (Baba Buddaji Gurdwara), the presence of *hakims/dais* specialising in potions and quackery, the presence of local places of pilgrimage and '*pirs*' that grant a male child to the seeker (Chintpurni Jwalaji, *Dargah* of Lakkhon da Pir) (Dagar 2001).

8. Crowley and Himmelweit forwarding a radical feminist critique to this extent mention that: 'They were sceptical of the extent to which legislation could improve the position of women, since discrimination was only a symptom of the underlying problem. Further, their structural view of women's subordination meant that all aspects of society were to be viewed as part of the same system and could not be seen as neutral instruments to be used by feminism. Thus, for example, the state, as part of the same system of oppression, was unlikely to produce legislation which really benefited women.' (Crowley and Himmelweit 1994)

9. Government of Punjab, Directorate of Social Security and Women and Child Development Notification No. S 109 (I.C.D.S.)– 2002(38635–43 dated 18/12/02.

10. For instance see *The Tribune* 2002.

11. Doctors with established practices in cities of Punjab mentioned in interviews that a tangible clientele for sex selection comes from NRIs. In one 45 minutes interview with a renowned gynaecologist in Amritsar, the researcher recorded three calls from UK seeking appointments for sex determination and one for a sex-selective procedure. According to an *Amritdhari* (baptised Sikh) female respondent settled and working in a ticketing agency in Canada, but visiting her in-laws in Ropar was undergoing female foeticide in Ropar after the birth of three daughters. 'When the first daughter was born, it didn't matter much but we were upset when the second child was also a girl and felt doomed when the third was also a girl. Then the family supported me to use a doctor's services to ensure the fourth child was a son.' (Dagar 2003)

12. The income groups categories for the IDC studies are:

Lower – Annual household income below Rs 25,000
Lower middle – Annual household income Rs 25,000 – 75,000

Upper – Annual household income Rs 75,000 – 1,50,000
middle
Upper – Annual household income Rs 1,50,000 and above
13. For details see *The Tribune 2001*
14. This IDC study was conducted on health and social welfare functionaries and panchayat women in the year 2002–2003.

References

Agnihotri, S. B. 2000. *Sex Ratio Patterns in the Indian Population: A Fresh Exploration*. New Delhi: Sage Publications.

Allen, V.L. 1975. *Social Analysis: A Marxist Critique and Alternative*. London: Longman.

Arditti, Dueli Klein and Shelly Minden (eds.). 1984. *Test Tube Women: What Future for Motherhood?* London: Pandora Press.

Bose, Ashish. 2001. 'Fighting Female Foeticide: Growing Greed and Shrinking Child Sex ratio', *Economic and Political Weekly*, 36 (36): 3427–29.

Brenner, Johanna. 1996. 'The Best of Times, the Worst of Times: Feminism in the United States' in Monica Threlfall (ed.), *Mapping the Women's Movement: Feminist Politics and Social Transformation in the North*. London: Verso.

CEDAW. 1979. *The Convention on the Elimination of All Forms of Discrimination Against Women*. www.un.org/womenwatch/daw/cedaw

Chatterjee, M. 1990. *Indian Women: Their Health and Economic Productivity*. World Bank Discussion Paper No. 109. Washington: The World Bank.

Croll, Elisabeth. 2000. *Endangered Daughters: Discrimination and Development in Asia*. London: Routledge.

Crowley, Helen and Susan, Himmelweit (eds.). 1994. *Knowing Women: Feminism and Knowledge*. Cambridge: Polity Press.

Dagar, Rainuka. 2001a. *Combating Violence Against Women in Punjab*. Chandigarh: Institute for Development and Communication.

———. 2001b. *Life Enhancing Mechanisms—Life Depriving Outcomes: A Case of Female Foeticide*. Chandigarh: Institute for Development and Communication.

———. 2002. *Identifying and Controlling Female Foeticide and Infanticide in Punjab*. Chandigarh: Institute for Development and Communication.

Das Gupta, Monica. 1987. 'Selective Discrimination Against Female Children in Rural Punjab, India', *Population and Development Review*, 13 (1): 77–100.

Gill, P.P.S. 2002. 'Abortions More Prevalent in Urban Punjab', *The Tribune*, Chandigarh; 4 July.

Government of India. 1985. *Seventh Five Year Plan 1985–90*. New Delhi: Planning Commission.

———. 192. *National Commission for Women: The Mandate of the Commission*. www.ncw.nic.in.

———. 2001. *National Policy for the Empowerment of Women* www.wcd.nic.in/empowerment.htm.

Government of India 2002a. *National Human Development Report 2001*. New Delhi: Oxford University Press.

———. 2002b. *National Health Policy 2002*. New Delhi: Ministry of Health and Family Welfare.

Gupta, Jyotsna Agnihotri. 2000. *New Reproductive Technologies, Women's Health and Autonomy*. New Delhi: Sage Publications.

International Institute for Population Sciences. 2000. *National Family Health Survey (NFHS–2): Punjab 1998–99*. Mumbai: International Institute for Population Sciences.

Kabeer, Naila. 1995. *Reversed Realities: Gender Hierarchies in Development Thought*. New Delhi: Kali for Women.

Kulkarni, S. 1986. *Prenatal Sex Determination Tests and Female Foeticide in Bombay City—A Study*. Bombay: Foundation for Research in Community Health (FRCH).

Lukes, S. 1974. *Power: A Radical View*. Macmillan: London.

Mies, M. 1987. 'Sexiest and Racist Implications of New Reproductive Technologies', *Alternatives*, 12: 323–42.

Miller, Barbara D. 1981. *The Endangered Sex: Neglect of Female Children in Rural North India*. Ithaca: Cornell University Press.

Molenuex, M. 1995. 'Mobilization without Emancipation? Women's Interests, State and Revolution in Nicaragua', *Feminist Studies*, 11(2): 234.

Nagpal, Arvinder. 2003. *'Pilot Project to Launch PNDT Ac'*, Paper presented in the workshop on 'Rethinking on Perspectives, Approaches and Methodologies for Combating Female Foeticide' held on 11–12 April, Institute for Development and Communication, Chandigarh.

National Advocacy Strategy. 2002. *Pre-birth Elimination of Female in India: Ending the Practice, Changing the Mindset*. www.indiafemalefoeticide.org/draft.doc. 17 June.

Patterson, V.S. 1990. 'Whose Rights? A Critique of the "Givens" in Human Rights Discourse', *Alternatives*, 15: 305.

Phillips, A. 1994. 'Feminism, Equality and Difference' in L. McDowell and R. Pringle (eds.), *Defining Women: Social Institutions and Gender Division*, pp. 205–22. Cambridge: Polity Press.

Pramod Kumar and Dagar, Rainuka. 1995. *Atrocities Against Women in Punjab*. Chandigarh: Institute for Development and Communication.

Pursell, Carroll. 1994. *White Heat*. London: BBC.

Ravinder, R.P. 1993. 'The Campaign Against Sex Determination Tests', in Chhaya Datar (ed.), *The Struggle Against Violence*, pp. 51–99. Calcutta: Shree Publications.

Registrar General of India. 2001. *SRS Bulletin*. 35 (1). New Delhi: Registrar General.

Rothman, Barbara Katz. 1989. *Recreating Motherhood*. New York: W.W. Norton.

Sharma, Vibha. 2000. '9 Out of 10 Clinics in City are Abortion Centres', *The Tribune*, Chandigarh; 13 July.

Sooch, Pawandeep. 2000. 'Female Foeticide Rampant', *The Indian Express*, Chandigarh; 10 August.

The Tribune (Chandigarh). 2001. 'Takhat Bans Female Foeticide: Offenders to be Excommunicated', 19 April.

The Tribune 2002. 'Education Can Help Curb Female Foeticide', 4 January.
———. 2002. 'Daire can Create Awareness: Bhatt', 31 January.
———. 2002. 'Steps to Check Female Foeticide', 20 October.
United Nations. 1994. *Summary of the Programme of Action of the International Conference on Population and Development.* Cairo, 5–13 September.
United Nations Population Fund. 2000. *Population Stabilisation and Sustainable Development.* New Delhi: United Nations Population Fund.
———. 2001. *Sex-Selective Abortions and Fertility Declining: The Case of Haryana and Punjab.* New Delhi: United Nations Population Fund.
Vinayak, Ramesh. 1997. 'Surrogate Mothers: A Womb for Rent', *India Today,* June 23.
Wertz, D.C. and J.C. Fletcher. 1993. 'Prenatal Diagnosis and Sex Selection in 19 Nations', *Social Science and Medicine,* 37(11): 1359–66.

PART 2

Meaning and Social Context of the Depleting Number of Girls

The Mindset behind Eliminating the Female Foetus*

5

Tulsi Patel

The late twentieth century advances in new reproductive technologies (NRTs) have generated a great deal of interest in social anthropological literature. These have given rise to new socio-cultural dilemmas around the women's and feminists' desire to overcome gender exploitation derived from biological reproduction (Firestone 1971 and O'Brien's 1981). Having control over one's body and deciding about one's reproductive contours mediated through reproductive technological advance and intervention, has not been uniform for women in all societies and parts of the world. Varying feminist positions on biological reproduction in the wake of new reproductive technologies (NRTs) have come about (See Franklin 1995) and so have meanings of biology and kinship, often mediated through different states' legal codes.

Introduced in the 1960s to monitor high-risk pregnancies, foetal-ultrasonography had become by early 1980s, a routine aspect of pre-natal care in most of the industrially advanced countries, and gradually also in many others. Among the scientific advances in pre-natal diagnostic screening techniques, ultra-sonogram, in particular is taken up for discussion in this essay. Ultrasound scan has almost become synonymous with the sex determination test in India by 1990s. What has sonography come to mean to people, and what makes people access it? Based on a multi-sited fieldwork, this paper analyses the

*An earlier version of this paper was presented at the workshop, 'Missing Girls in India: Political Economy of Emotions', in Department of Sociology, Delhi University on 30–31 October, 2003. I am thankful to all participants who commented on it.

experience of 'those/other' people (women and couples) who feel it fine to use the pre-natal diagnostic technology for producing 'the optimum sex composition' of their children. With the help of case accounts picked since the early 1980s from various field sites in Rajasthan and Delhi, and focus group discussions (FGDs) and interviews conducted in Delhi during 2002–2004, the paper focuses on the discourses and considerations in the use of sonography. The trajectory in the diffusion of pre-natal diagnostic screening with the intent to abort female foetuses into the Indian society is followed.

The paper has two parts. The first part begins with a section providing a context of the use of new reproductive technologies (NRTs) in their place of birth, and their transnational migration, i.e. their use in India. It follows the section on methodology in collecting data on the thriving secret practice engulfing a large number of Indians, a practice which is publicly seen as unethical and is officially illegal. The narratives provide the third section. The second part of the paper discusses how daughters in everyday life come to be considered a 'burden' for parents, their families, including both sets of grandparents. It discusses how the birth of grandchildren brings together the affinal relatives' and consanguineal kin's common views about the sex of children born.

What are the considerations in the minds of people (their mindsets) that enable and perpetrate the elimination of the female foetus? Mindset is most commonly brought up in discussions in seminars and conferences in different parts of India alongside culture with regard to sex determination tests accessed with the intention of sex selective abortion. By mindset I mean here the cultural and intersubjective experience and field of understanding. Mindset seems to me to approximate Bourdieu's concept of habitus. Mindset is postulated not simply as an abstract entity of the conscious mind. It is to be seen as both conscious and reflexive activity as well as influenced by shared and embedded predispositions.[1] While infanticide and/or foeticide is an individual activity, it is also a socially adaptive activity. The question thus raised is how does the mindset relay the patriarchal structuring of the family with the aid of science? The serious impact of the foetal-ultrasound technology is evident through the public debates around the ethics of the practice and the worrisome adverse sex ratio of the children in India, confirmed officially by the decennial Census of 2001. The paper tries to understand what all constitutes the making and working of the mindset at the micro level, aggregating at the macro level into highly-skewed sex ratios, in the range of 927 to 750 girls for 1,000 boys (Sehgal 2006). And what is it that still makes it a commonly held view that girls are not in short supply, if any thing, rather boys are valuable as well as scarce? What is so overbearing that goes into raising daughters as against sons and sustains the general feeling that girls are 'not ours' but someone else's property (*paraya dhan*), they are a burden, and are held in trust to be duly handed over to their lawful owners?

I

New Reproductive Technology and Elimination of Defective Babies _____

Parents' and pregnant women's expectations have, in the last five decades of the 20th century, clearly changed with advances in knowledge and technology regarding delivery of health care during childbirth, especially in the West. Medical technology, such as ultrasound and amniocentesis offer much more reliable antenatal screening and diagnosis than was previously possible. This has enabled people to know the unknown aspects of a foetus. Ultra-sonography is medically considered a harmless test in the sense that it has no radiation, and no pricking is involved. No fluid is taken in a routine sonography. It involves just a probe on the abdomen where sound waves are sent, they reflect back and are picked up by the probe again. It is indeed a technological feat and empowers man over nature. It is common to have three sonography tests, one in each trimester of pregnancy, in the West.

The technology for foetal testing has brought down to a great extent, high risk births, such as babies born with neural tube defects or Down's syndrome, known to be the main contributing factor for mentally retarded babies in the world. The main diagnostic test for Down's syndrome is amniocentesis. It provides opportunities for women to have late babies without being interrupted, in their studies for professional advancement early in life. It is only done and warranted in high risk pregnancies where the mother is: 1) more than 35–40 years old, to rule out Down's syndrome as it is known to happen in mothers who are first time pregnant at an advanced age, and 2) where there is a family history of a genetic disease. If the foetus tests positive, the parents have a choice to keep or terminate the pregnancy. The results of the test take up to one month to obtain, by which time the pregnancy will be advanced. Since the desirable time for the test is between 16–20 weeks, it is risky and painful to abort at the advanced stage of pregnancy. The test is diagnostic and usually provides definite confirmation of Down's syndrome and other chromosomal anomalies of the foetus, except in some cases of ambiguous results because of laboratory errors (Harpwood 1996). With an increasing number of women coming under the fold of antenatal screening since the medicalisation of birth began in the early 20th century, foetal testing has attracted a greater involvement of women in decisions about their treatment and that of their unborn babies in the West.

Since the mid-1980s, the most common test in India is ultrasound, colloquially known as sonography and in some areas as *janch* (literally, inquiry or test). Usually sex of a child can be determined at 16–20 weeks of pregnancy by sonography and at a similar time or even earlier by amniocentesis. It is for knowing the sex of the foetus that ultrasonography is mostly used in India, though officially speaking it is a routine ritual in state and private hospitals and maternity homes to diagnose foetal congenital anomalies. Sonography is done routinely in all hospitals in India, wherever it is available (therefore officially, it is largely though mistakenly, understood as non-available in rural areas in India).

Even before entering into the hospital, pregnancy has never been an absolutely private affair for a woman. Anthropological studies (Douglas 1960, Levi-Strauss 1966, Jordan 1980) have shown that biological phenomena are culturally organised; pregnancy and childbirth are socially and culturally immersed activities (See Jeffery et al. 1989, Jordan 1980, Shostak 1983, Patel 1994). Pregnancy, childbirth, abortion and infanticide have been in the political arena for quite some time in the western world. These matters have not remained limited to the familial domain. They have also moved out of the domestic and entered the larger political arena.[2] The evolution of the discursive shift of pregnancy from the micro and the private to the macro and public political domain is traceable most directly to the emerging consumer movement of the 1960s and 70s, notwithstanding the early 20th century birth control movement. This was coupled with the second wave of the women's movement that reiterated with force some of the earlier issues it had on its agenda. Unwanted pregnancies and legalising of abortion were brought under the purview of rights. In India, abortion was legalised in 1971 to encourage population control and is called Medical Termination of Pregnancy (MTP) Act of 1971. Termination of pregnancy is permissible until 20 weeks in India. Economic, social and health considerations, including reasons, such as not wanting another baby so early and failed contraception are good enough for getting an abortion.

Methodology

Besides a conscious and long-drawn follow up of chance cases that I came across with regard to the use of sonography since the early 1990s, interviews with medical doctors and staff of NGOs working with women in Delhi were also conducted for a period spanning over two years in 2002–2004. The chance cases collected from Rajasthan in north-west India were those I happened to overhear during social gatherings where an oblique reference to someone was overheard. I pursued the matter further without causing the unease of being too intrusive. In one of the several subsequent meetings with the person who had in the first instance given away the clue, I managed to find more information. The lady herself does not know that I know about her having used ultrasound screening to test the sex of her foetus. Yet, I think that I have fairly reliable information. The women reporting the events to me have no ulterior motives to malign or speak behind the concerned lady's back. In one of the vignettes in Delhi, I was present on the scene and witnessed it while I attended a delivery case in a reputed government hospital. The data was also collected through focus group discussions (FGDs) and unstructured interviews with doctors and college teachers in Delhi for about two years. On the whole, the data for this paper thus pertains to urban north India. Pockets of north India are notorious for violence against women, especially for female infanticide in the past until the early decades of the 20th century (Clark 1993, Panigrahi 1972, Vishwanath 2000, and in this volume). The region is also infamous for female child neglect, especially of the second and later birth orders (Das Gupta 1987). It was with Visaria's (1971) important study showing excess female mortality as the main contributor to adverse sex ratio in India that several other hypotheses including higher altitudes, maternal anaemia and obesity as factors for adverse female male ratios were laid to rest.

Unfortunately, though not unexpectedly, data from individual interview-schedule administration was not forthcoming on the topics, be it ultrasound scan, amniocentesis or female foetus abortion. This was perhaps for ethical and legal reasons. Since 1994, law in India prohibits the use of pre-natal diagnostic techniques (PNDTs) to test the sex of the foetus. The Act provides for the regulation of the use of PNDTs for the purpose of detecting genetic or metabolic disorders or chromosomal abnormalities or certain congenital malformations or sex-linked disorders. It provides this for the prevention of the misuse of such techniques for the purpose of sex determination leading to female foeticide. PNDTs include all gynaecological, obstetrical or medical procedures and techniques such as ultra-sonography, foetoscopy, taking or removing samples of amniotic fluids, chorionic villi, blood or any tissue of a pregnant woman for being sent to a genetic laboratory or genetic clinic. All genetic laboratories and clinics are to be registered, even advertising of these facilities is an offence. A violator of the law is liable to imprisonment up to three years and/or a fine up to rupees 10,000. The PNDT Act 1994 (and its amendment in 2002 has been an achievement for Indian feminists and civil society groups, see appendixes for details). The ban was achieved through the introduction of two private members' bills, one in Maharashtra (state) assembly and another at the centre (Indian parliament) in 1986. In 1986 itself, the bill was passed in Maharashtra state (Vibhuti Patel in this volume for more on this). Government hospitals are supposed to refuse to declare the sex of the foetus even if people are often curious to find it out. People both in urban and rural areas are aware of the ban. Unlike the openness about foetal tests prior to the ban, they are shrouded in secrecy presently. It must be pointed out that even the cases picked up before the promulgation of PNDT Act, 1994 were not discussed openly, they were a family secret, known to only close friends or well-wishers. It was not easy to collect data on ultra-sonography for abortion in the pre-PNDT period, though conversation was possible if well pursued. But since 1994 it has become more difficult. FGDs proved the most successful means of getting information on this matter as these allowed an open discussion about the practice in existence without identifying an individual with the act. This is similar to Favret-Saada's (1980) experiences with finding out about witchcraft practice in Bocage (France), where everyone knew of someone who engaged in it or encountered it but not the informer himself or herself.

The 'public secret' kind of sense with which the issue is infused is enough to generate a sense that something is the matter about these tests, a feature not totally absent in the pre-1994 period. Information about the sex of a foetus is possible to obtain through tests in private clinics/hospitals but at a very high cost. On the ethical front, sex identification tests are culturally understood to mean that they are conducted for having 'desirable sex composition' of children in families or simply put, elimination of female babies. There is little open encouragement or acceptance of the practice. Son preference is intensive as it is extensive in India and also south Asia as a whole. It does mean that the less preferred sex is eliminated, whether through infanticide, neglect or foeticide. Despite its widespread prevalence there is something that is encircled with a great deal of hesitation in discussing about the practice. It is an act having a mixed meaning associated with it, it is both good and bad at the same time, bad enough to keep it shrouded and good enough to continue the practice. When there is a sense of conspiracy felt by people, they do not want others, especially researchers to know about those activities. The challenge was to collect data about a practice people are not willing to talk about and least wish to be associated with. What emerged by way of a constant side conversation around this issue, the stress to provide reasons that make it a lesser evil if not justify it, gave away some of the clues to the mindset behind the popularity of the practice.

Birth as a Power Game: A Rite of Passage for the Mother

As mentioned above, reproduction is at the heart of feminists' (of various hues) explanations for subordination of women. It is also seen by demographers as being so, especially revealed through the theory of demographic transition. Birth of a child has been regarded as a critical event, considered with substantial social and individual significance. Moreover, the birth of the first child is of special importance since it signifies the transition of the parents into a new social status. It marks the sexual and social maturity of the mother, the visible significance and cementing of the marital tie. Births are empowering for parents, especially for mothers in a number of cultures (Handwerker 1990). The absence of being able to give birth makes it clear how critical birth is for couples, especially women. Societies where women's basic identity is primarily through motherhood, the pressure to perform and conform is enormous. The failure stigmatises the woman. It spells a doom and amounts to social ostracism of sorts. The fear is of dissolution of marriage and the consequent evaporation of all a childless woman has by way of status. The harrowing experiences of childlessness, faced particularly by childless women in rural India (Patel 1994), in Delhi (Widge 2001), in Egypt (Inhorn 1996) and in many parts of the world (Inhorn and Balen 2002) are palpable. The ideology of motherhood is pervasive in these societies. The desire for pregnancy and childbirth is a recurrent theme.

It is not only that motherhood brings status to a woman but also it is an attribute without which she is useless. A woman in patrilineal society gains status and position through motherhood, especially through producing sons for the family and the lineage (Patel 1994, 2004). She justifies her existence and is privileged only as a mother of son/s. The cases cited Patel (1994) describe how disconcerting and disheartening births of 'daughters only' can be. The fact of being born male or female carries different behavioural expectations permeating most spheres of life. While a son's birth is much desired, a daughter's (if she happens to begin her mother's fertility career) is acceptable and tolerated. 'Every one knows that it is better to spend a hefty amount now than to raise another daughter, who is in any case going to be someone else's property and drain the family resources all her life', said Kamni, a young mother when I asked her during one of our several chatting sessions as to what people think when they go for ultrasound and abort if it is a female foetus. By the phrase, drain on resources all her life, she meant the constant flow of gifts that will continue not only from parents to her and her affinal family members, but also from her mother's brother to her and to her children, their male spouses and her conjugal family members, at least until her children's wedding if not later on too. Similar comments have been recurrently made by people when probed with reference to the hoarding that boldly announced this perception. The common advertisement in Punjab and Delhi as in many parts of north India in the late 1970s and early 1980s, before the success of the feminist pressure to ban amniocentesis for sex detection, had struck the right chord with people. It stressed on the economic sense and lured people thus: 'Spend rupees 500 now rather than spend 50,000 or even 500,000 twenty years later' (in marrying off a daughter). This advertisement did not make a distinction between the first and subsequent daughters, and signifies the attitude towards the daughter as a category.

Daughter as a Burden: A Heavy Responsibility on Parents' Shoulders

At the outset, I want to make it clear that female foeticide is not approved and/or practised for the first female foetus. As majority of the births in India still take place at home, ultrasound is rarely conducted as part of the antenatal routine examination. The first baby is accepted with joy. It is a relief for the families, both conjugal and natal, that the mother and baby are fine. Of course, if the first-born were to be a son, the families are overjoyed. Fifty years ago when a daughter came first, there was joy and relief, except perhaps among the castes notorious for female infanticide. Like at present, it was even then accompanied with earnest hope that the second baby would be a boy. Mothers and families with successive daughters were sympathised with as they had to continue to have babies until at least one son was born. My research in rural Rajasthan (Patel 1994) shows that while it is important for women not to be pregnant when their children's fertility career begins, most of the few women who did have a baby after they became grandmothers were the ones who had no son. It was not very comfortable for these women to produce babies while their grandchildren were born. There was a sense of awkwardness and shame associated with childbirth at that late stage in life. But their dilemma was understood by many, even though their childbirth was not openly approved. Family strategies were actively planned and executed until the social optimum number and sex composition of children was obtained.

What has changed in the past fifty years is the ability of parents to modulate the composition of one's children, especially with the introduction of foetal-sonography. Parents now do not consider it worthwhile to have daughters until a son happens to arrive. Presently, they usually want only two children and wish that at least one among them is a son. Thus, this paper should not give the impression that young parents in modernising India, like to have only sons and no daughters. I take the risk of repetition that one daughter a couple is not seen as undesirable, it is more than one daughter that makes the latter ones undesirable. There is a large body of research available on neglect of daughters, higher mortality of daughters than of sons, strikingly low sex ratios by parity and birth order mentioned in this volume (in essays by Visaria, Dagar, Kapoor, Bose and Vibhuti Patel, and earlier by Das Gupta 1987 and Kishor 1993).

I had followed up on one couple who went for two ultrasound tests after having a son as their first baby because they wanted to have a daughter. Unfortunately for them, even after being assured twice by radiologists that the foetus was a girl, they had a boy. If the first child happens to be a boy, most parents do not go for the ultrasound test as it does not matter what sex the second baby is. There are a few couples I have met in Delhi who have not had more than one child, a daughter, while there are many others who have had three or four daughters and finally gave up without resorting to sex selective abortions even if the last or the last two daughters were born after 1980, when ultrasound had become available in Indian hospitals. The latter themselves feel as losers in the game of family strategising and so do their relatives and neighbours. Most young couples who set out on their fertility careers around the late 1990s desire only two or at the most three children. They do not wish to have more than one daughter. It is this desirable family composition they manage to achieve that needs to be kept in mind in the ensuing discussion about the daughter, i.e. the second and subsequent daughters, being considered as an avoidable burden in the following sections of the paper.

The importance of a daughter for the parents, who find her emotionally more close and who is more concerned about the parents than a married son, is also commonly heard. If there is only one daughter parents try their best to amass whatever they can to raise her and marry her off, keeping with the prevailing expectations of their caste, class and such circumstances in mind which also contribute towards setting of standards for raising daughters in the group. One may recall Krishna, who in the *Gita*, exhorts Arjuna to glow by making sacrifice. A daughter's parents glow in the sacrifice of making the gift of the virgin to the suitable recipient. Giving additional gifts to a daughter and her conjugal family at all life cycle ceremonies and festive occasions is also a means of earning *punya* (religious merit) for the parents and the brother. *Huani/huasni* (a generic term in Rajasthan for a married daughter of the household/family) brings *punya* to the natal kin by receiving gifts from them. Those who have no daughters do so for daughters of the male agnates. Marrying off a *jethuti* (daughter of the husband's elder brother) earns more *punya* and glow, i.e. symbolic capital than marrying off one's biological daughter, was often stated by people in the village studied by Patel (1994). Sisters do have a ritual and social significance in their brother's life in north India, i.e. even among those communities that do not practise cross-cousin marriage. A married sister's ceremonial and ritual significance in North India is vividly described by Jamous (1992). Daughters are adopted and/or brought in to be raised and their marriages arranged in mythological and scriptural texts in India. Mahabharata mentions Pritha, the daughter of Sura adopted by Kuntibhoja; Santa, the daughter of King Dasratha was adopted by King Lomapada (Kane 1946). Such an act was not a ritual requirement, nor did it economically strengthen the adoptive family. Nevertheless, it helped the family attain *punya* through giving the daughter as gift in marriage. The other aim was to strengthen friendship between families. As a goodwill gesture, girls were adopted (Karve 1953). The reasons for which daughters were adopted were different from those mentioned for adopting sons. As long as there is only one daughter, the ceremonial, ritual and religious, as well as the everyday life's mundane aspects are not seen as enormously burdensome.

In many ways it neutralises the expenses as the son's wife brings in dowry and the subsequent flow of gifts. Having only one daughter is not an all out loss, but having more daughters than sons is a relative loss. The glow from sacrifice is attained through one daughter and each of the subsequent daughters adds only a little more, if at all, to the parents' and the family's glow, i. e. symbolic and social capital. With more than one daughter, parents get apprehensive about being able to find a suitable match which comes at a considerable cost. The burden of the single daughter nevertheless remains until the suitable recipient of the virgin gift is handed over the gift. She is considered a burden more in the ritual, religious and sexual sense rather than predominantly an economic one. It is in this light that the category of the daughter comes to be considered a burden on the shoulders of the parents and the family. The cautionary note is not to see each of a couple's daughters as unwanted but several daughters are surely unwanted.

Rugji, works as a support staff in a school in a large city in Rajasthan. He is a Jat, was married in his early twenties to a girl in her late teens. She stayed in the village while Rugji worked in the city. He went to his village house three to four times a month. His parents and wife lived jointly with two of his older brothers, their wives and the latter's small children. In the first few years after marriage, Rugji begot two daughters one after the other. The first daughter was born in his wife's natal home as is customary. As she enunciated the onset of the mother's fertility career, she was welcome. There was joy but with an undercurrent of the feeling that after all she is only a girl. Like in most first daughter's birth events, there were no celebratory songs that accompany a son's birth, also noted for a village in U.P. by Wadley (1993).

The second daughter's arrival had led to innuendoes and insult for his wife from her conjugal relatives. Even her natal family members were clearly sad. This daughter was born in the conjugal home. The mother had not faced such a dislike after her first daughter's birth. She was not happy about living with the larger family in the village, especially as she had the option of moving to the city with her husband. By this time, he also wanted his wife to join him in the city. They moved to a small, one bedroom house as tenants with their two daughters. Soon his wife discovered that she had missed her periods (*kapada*) for two months. She was not close to any of the neighbours, though she had taken a liking for one lady a few houses away, the family her husband was in touch with for long.

Over the next few weeks Mrs Rugji became friends with the lady and gathered courage to discuss her pregnancy with her friend. She wanted to find out some place where sonography could be obtained to test the sex of the baby she was carrying. Her friend was willing to help her. It took a few more weeks before they found a clinic and got the details about the amount required for sonography. She took rupees 500 with her and went to the clinic with her friend. Though she carried a female foetus, she was denied termination of pregnancy as she was too late, which could lead to complications. She could only pray that next time she got a son. No one from her in-laws' family came to help her when she had a third daughter. The neighbours were consoling the couple for their misfortune in having three daughters in a row.

Next time she was pregnant, her husband, father of three daughters knew what his pregnant wife was up to and had given her more than 500 rupees to cover the expenses of the test. The course of action was repeated with the help of the same friend. The test showed that this time too it was a girl, but also advised her to come for another test in a week's time as the staff at the clinic she had earlier approached, after four months of her previous pregnancy, wanted to be fully sure about it. Again the same exercise had to be repeated and the expenses arranged. On second attempt it was confirmed that the foetus was a girl. There was not much time wasted in deciding to abort the foetus. The only hesitation was the money required for it. Mrs Rugji had to consult her husband, arrange for another 1,000 rupees and return to the clinic. What is the worth of 1,000 rupees if the expense can avoid an enormous and long drawn, social stigma and one's economic disaster later? Mrs Rugji was escorted home by her friend after the abortion. She was listless and weak for a few days. Her friend helped her with the cooking and the girls. She was up and about in a few days, and life was normal again.

They wanted their daughters to be educated, unlike the mother. All girls in the neighbourhood went to school and so would their daughters. It means expenses on education, better clothing and care in grooming of the girls. Mrs Rugji was also aware of the fact that once educated, parents would prefer the girls to marry educated and preferably salaried boys. In one of the meetings at another wedding, she told me:

> A suitable match is not easy to come by. The girl's beauty and health are important, but so is her schooling and the dowry that urban boys usually get at weddings. It all means expenses. Where will the money come from if there are more daughters. One is more than enough. In the past it was not so bad. Girls were precious. Boys' people kept a watch for girls and approached her people for her hand. Now it is just the opposite in our community too, it is now like Rajputs and Brahmins. Things are changing with education and city life.

She had put the abortion behind her, relieved of another unwanted daughter coming into the family. Mrs Rugji repeated the test at the same clinic when she was pregnant again. Both she and her friend had gone to the clinic and she was overjoyed to hear that it was a boy this time. She had finally conceived a son. The stigma of sonlessness and the gloom of having her head constantly bowed down before all relatives and family members was to disappear soon. She could hold her head high having produced an heir to the family, an armour against being insalutory had she been a failure in this regard. Though the conjugal family was overjoyed, they did not all rush to greet her, though she expected it to happen. She revealed it in her complaining tone when she recalled it for me later. Her friend and other neighbours managed to look after the girls and the house while Rugji shuttled between the home and the hospital. The mother-in-law and one of her husband's brothers came two days later to look after her and the household. She treated herself well through the pregnancy and was looking forward to the celebrations after a boy was born to her. And as expected, she was full of joy to have given birth to a boy and the joy spread in the neighbourhood with the news. Mayo's (1927) description about young meek women assuming a sense of pride and moving about the house with an air of confidence, which she gave nearly a century ago, continues to hold good in India even today. There were smiles and congratulatory greetings received by the Rugji family. Much congratulatory mood prevailed for several days and Rugji was happy to share his blessed state with friends, neighbours and relatives. Both his family and his wife's family members were excited with the birth of their son. Continuity of Rugji's family line is not just the concern of his parents and siblings, but also of his wife's parents and siblings. Rugji's children were a matter for concern for both the families, even if not in identical ways. She said, 'I managed all the household chores and arranged for a feast for the larger family, relatives and friends two months after the boy was born.' There was no feast organised after any of the girls' birth.

Most neighbours were unaware of the fact that Mrs Rugji had been through a sex test and aborted a female foetus. Later, Mrs Rugji's friend related the whole case and expressed her dilemma and justified helping her out in this manner. She was able to absolve herself of any serious moral issues by saying that she did not do it for any money, and would not have done it had there been no daughter already born in the family.

'Mrs Rugji was illiterate and had come from a village. If she was not helped and escorted she would have landed herself in greater trouble and might have been cheated or even maltreated by the ultrasound clinic in the private medical care system. Worse, still, she might have got a fourth daughter. It is rewarding to see how jubilant she is after her son's birth. If you have to settle for someone who is not your own match (i. e. give the gift of a virgin daughter to one who is lesser in education, and social, economic and cultural capital), is it a happy feeling for parents all their life?', asked her friend.

Hypogamy is proscribed. It is a ready recipe for downward social mobility of a family even among the lower and untouchable castes.

And endogamous marriage is also usually strategised with the intention of upward social mobility within the caste. Parents with several daughters, do not get identically placed sons-in-law. Often their kin as well as affinal relatives help them to locate suitable boys. Such help is not only sought but highly appreciated, but it means investing resources, which the family may not be able to spare, having spent on more than one daughters' education and upbringing. Additional daughters to a couple are an uneasy feeling and appear more burdensome than having only one daughter.

A Son Meaning Space
Under the Sun

A son's birth is a means of privileging the mother. Thus the dilemma of being the second sex and yet craving for the first is resolved through the practice of patriarchy. Majority of the Indian women would be shattered to only have successive daughters. The birth of a son is perceived as an opportunity for upward mobility while the birth of a daughter is believed to result in downward economic mobility of the household and the family.

Mrs Rugji was as keen as was her husband and perhaps her mother-in-law to have a son after having had three daughters in a row. Most women would be if they were in Mrs Rugji's position. I met her after her son was over a year old and found her a different person, she was more sure of herself. Confident in her mannerism, she said, 'Now I don't care if my in-laws say anything. I just ignore it if it is unpleasant. Earlier, it would unnerve me, I was worried all the time.' Very often, meek women assume an air of confidence in dealing with their conjugal relatives after they have a son. A man commented about his wife, 'Something is different about her. I feel she is happy on her own and busy with herself. It is different from when we had the first child, a daughter three years ago.' 'A mother's height increases by two-finger-width when a son is born to her', was a common phrase in the town and in the adjoining rural areas in Rajasthan. It is not just women who feel elated upon bearing a son. The case of Rajuji who married thrice, one after another woman to have a son, but never managed to have one, is a telling one. Though he had two daughters, his status in the village as an old man was not the same compared to others of his age cohort. Most of his contemporaries had one or more able-bodied sons, their wives and grandchildren living together. It was not a usual sight for an old man of his age to carry water, or take cattle for watering, done usually by younger household members. But Rajuji did it as he had no one else to relieve him from such menial chores when it was his time to be in *hatai* (meeting) taking place frequently at some public spot/joint or someone's house in the village (Patel 1994).

A son's birth immediately means the reverse of that of a daughter's. An old man in a Rajasthan town was known in his neighbourhood for his popular address for new-born babies in the locality. Employed with the Indian Railways, his family occupation was tailoring, in which he joined after returning from work and on weekly holidays. Tailoring brought him in touch with many more people in the locality. Every time he heard of someone having got a son, he said, 'Oh, so *Muffat Lal* (a free lad) had arrived'. If it was a daughter, he would say, 'Oh, so came the *Ayee Chuki* (enough of coming)'. Because a son's upbringing and education cost is evened out through the dowry he commands at his wedding, he is almost free for his parents as it were, thus *Muffat Lal* for a son.[3] On the other hand, expenses in raising a daughter have not only to be incurred, she has to be paid dowry on top of it all, in order to marry her off, the prime responsibility of the parents, thus one is enough of a coming (*Ayee Chuki*).

The stigma of sonlessness is not an abstract one, but rests on very hard ground, it is very palpable. The misery of not being able to produce a son is not limited to the household or the mother-in-law daughter-in-law dyad but spills rather quickly beyond the family. It is a failure to perform. As mentioned earlier, infertility is a curse, next is inability to bear a son. It is nearly as stigmatising, lesser so in large cities in Delhi in fleeting conversational acquaintances among neighbours. But among the family and relatives, it is a major debility for parents. It soon brings to fore the blame game within the family. Despite what science of reproduction might say about the sex of the baby being dependent on the Y chromosome, people blame the woman for her inability to provide a son to the family. Often, it is not even blame. It comes as a serious worry for the woman's natal kin that she is unable to bear a son for the conjugal family. The fear that a co-wife might be fated, lingers. Ways and means of conceiving a son are mentioned in Indian folklore, traditional medical systems and in *Kama Sutra*. Sonless women and couples try various medical, religious and shamanic means to have a son. The idea of all relatives forming a sort of panoptican as it were in Balinese society (Wikan 1990) is close to what goes on in Indian families too. People's affective commitments and fears are mediated through the family and community. Let us see how stigma and disadvantage operates in everyday life for daughters and their parents (and other family members often included).

While attending on a labouring friend in a two-bedded waiting room outside the labour room of a hospital in Delhi in 1982, I witnessed a Punjabi nurse working in the same hospital brought in just after giving birth to her second child, also a daughter. Crestfallen, she wept inconsolably for several hours, oblivious of the physical state she was in and the cultural prescriptions for a nearly motionless quietude towards quicker recovery. She would sob and curse herself softly but every now and then break into a mournful wail wishing away her reality. She did not wish to accept the fact that she had given birth to a second daughter. She was a working woman and the fact that her daughters could take up jobs when they grew up, was nowhere a consideration through her plight. On the next bed lay my friend who had a five year old son at home with her parents-in-law and knew no one would mind whatever the sex of her new baby was. The suffering nurse on the other hand, was totally beside herself. I did not see her take even one look at her daughter throughout the day. In normal circumstances she would have been monitoring the lady lying on the next bed. All through the day, several of her doctor and nurse colleagues came to console her, to have heart, but she cursed herself and her ill luck for producing two daughters in a row. No amount of aural and touch (holding her hand, palming her forehead) convincing from her colleagues calmed her. They tried to pacify her and said,

> She has come to you but has brought her own *bhag* (fate/share) with her. *Rab bauhath deooga*, God will give you a lot, (resources and strength—the words are unstated but implied) for her care and upbringing.

Her state was so miserable that her colleagues made efforts to convince her husband not to be harsh to her when he came to visit her. The unhappy husband could not empathise more with his wife. Whatever happened to the newborn girl did not invite anyone's attention. She spent the whole day and the night in that room before being moved elsewhere. As an attendant, I was on the side sofa used as a bed at night. Still suffering from the trauma, the new mother had not slept until I fell asleep at night, nor had she eaten anything. Next morning, her colleagues shifted her to another room. Apparently, she was not so upset when the first daughter was born. Often such a frenzied state is witnessed by others around and older girls in the family come to accept the importance of a son for a woman. But in one case in 1993 all three daughters in a family committed suicide the day the mother delivered a boy in a hospital in Chandigarh after several years of numberless efforts by the mother through ultrasound tests and abortions. The eldest was 19 years at that time. The father returned home after visiting his wife and the new-born son and found all three daughters had hung themselves in a suicide pact (Baligar 1999).

The micro politics of the family disadvantages its women, especially younger ones. It is with the birth of sons that mothers get a stronghold into the family. Whether the husband and in-laws approve or not, women find producing girl babies, especially after one, to their detriment. They have a vested interest in avoiding a daughter's birth, especially after one has been born. Bumiller (1990) recounts the killing of daughters by low caste women in south India. Mothers justified killing of daughters so that the girls could avoid repeating the same miserable life (Shiva 2002, also mentioned in Bose in this volume). It is in the light of a plethora of considerations such as the above that the *Rig Veda* prayer asking, 'birth of girl be granted elsewhere and here grant a son', becomes meaningful.

II

The Everyday and the Occasional: Practice of Raising the Burdensome Daughter

The saying, 'may even my enemy not have a daughter' and '*jako maar rayo kartar*' (one whom the maker [God] is slow-poisoning) comes from the pain and suffering a daughter's birth and upbringing can cause to her parents, and her paternal and even the maternal grandparents. For the next descending generation, the grandparents on both sides find their interests merging with respect to their grand-children. They are consanguines for their grandchildren, even if they are affines to each other in their own generation and in many respects until their children's generation. The shift from being affinal rela-tives in one generation to becoming consanguineous relatives to the next descending generation has been discussed by Dumont (1966, 1975) and Vatuk (1975) both through kinship terminology and flow of prestations. The two sets of grandparents and grandchildren are clearly differently referred terminologically for those through the son, compared to those through the daughter and vice-versa in Rajasthan. Yet like Vatuk and Dumont, I find both the terminological and generational shift in turning affines into consanguines relevant for understanding the gentle prodding and advice a woman's natal kin give her on several matters pertaining to her life, including her reproductive experience. After having had one daughter, having another daughter is a cause for concern to a woman's parents and brothers as much as it is to her husband's parents and siblings. The convergence of interests between what were two affinal families is mediated through the marriage tie furthered through procreation. The two affinal families are ideally interested in enhancing their social, cultural and economic capital. Marriage ties of children are preferably arranged between households of comparable status and position which in turn support conditions, circumstances and per-petuates all forms of capital accumulation.

A hypergamous marriage for a daughter is not just an expensive economic proposition but it makes good common sense for status maintenance and enhancement for the two affinal families. Marriage strategies (Bourdieu 1976) are also family strategies, which include reproduction of the social optimum kind. Kin and close relatives are thus mutually interested in each other and their procreation. There is a semblance of a sort of panoptican formed by the relatives through exchanging notes and frequently evaluating actions of relatives. People are polite and inquire about the activities and well-being of family members and relatives when they meet others. Daughters' relatively shorter honourable domiciliary right in their parental home is ex-pressed in different ways. Often girl children are not included in reporting the number of children one has.[4] They are *paraya dhan* and will be gone soon, is so very often said in many contexts in daughters' faces and about them in referring to them in conversations. 'She is grown up now', 'it is time to think about her match (marriage)', and 'you have some major expenses ahead of you, now that your daughter is grown up', are commonly made statements among friends and relatives. Among the Delhi's middle class, friends of a grown-up girls' mother ask her, 'is she thinking of settling down?', 'you might be worrying about her settling down these days', 'it'll be good if you find some one nice for her'. So the overbearing sense of responsibility to find an unmarried girl a house she can call her own is shared by the well-wishing relatives both on her father's and mother's sides. A mother in Delhi after visiting her 28 year old daughter's house a few months after her marriage said,

> I was so happy to see her run her own household, minding the maid, paying to the newspaper man, the guard, buying little things for the house and having tea when her husband got back from work; I came back so relieved to see her happy in her house. She is also thinking of taking up some job soon.

Her daughter had resigned from her job in Delhi to join her husband in another city, as is common for women to do. She enjoyed sharing her experiences about her daughter with friends, neighbours and families of her siblings and her husband's siblings with a sense of pride and satisfaction.

What makes the daughter a dispreferred, i.e., undesirable offspring, whose birth brings displeasure if not mourning, and a son a preferred child? Is the low social value assigned to the female a cultural figment expressed through emotions? Or does the low value work out its details at the ground level to synchronise with the distress in raising a daughter? The solemn or gloom at a daughter's birth in most parts of north India, is symbolic of what awaits the family where a daughter is born. I witnessed, in a town in Punjab in 1976, a group of women from the neighbourhood visited the Gupta (Baniya) household where a second daughter was born to sympathise with the parents and the grandparents. The grandmother of the new baby sat with the visiting ladies, and they were mournfully quiet, muttering under their breath once every now and then and sat for about an hour and left quietly. No gifts or money was given to the new-born, no tea or soft drinks were offered to the visitors, not certainly because the house was in a state of pollution. They had come to express *afsos* (sympathy) with the unfortunate family, I was told. The visit signified that the visitors' shared the helplessness and gloom of the Gupta family. (In Delhi in 2003 when a professional couple had their second daughter, the neighbours sympathised differently. They said, 'Lakshmi, i.e. the goddess of wealth has come, it is okay', implying that though highly expensive she will prove to be, she might bring wealth to the family by her presence, through her *karma* and her parents' *karma*. Coming of females is often symbolically consoled through terms such as arrival of Lakshmi. Note the change in the form of expression of *afsos* between 1976 and 2003).

The expression of *afsos* of the former kind may not be openly appreciated in the Indian middle class in urban Delhi, but it exists in subtler forms and within the inner core of the household. At arrival, second and a subsequent daughter is unwelcome/tolerated in relative terms. Cormack (1953) reproduces a girl's lament upon her birth through a folk song where her birth was announced through beating a brass plate while a boy's is announced through beating of drums (see also Shiva 2002 for the continuity of the folk song even today). It is not the difference in instruments used to announce (in Rajasthan beating a bronze or brass plate is a signifier of a male birth and beating a chaff that of a female), but the meaning the community assigns to the beating of these instruments makes all the difference. Whatever, the means of announcement, the emotions felt and shared with others around and with relatives convey the difference in meanings between a son and a daughter's birth. Even in middle class professional families in Delhi, I have seen sweets distributed to close neighbours and friends upon a son's birth, while sweets are offered to them if they visit the family upon a daughter's birth. Among the lower classes, the sweets are absent if a daughter is born.

A university professor of Indian origin based in Europe told me in 2006 that he continued to get suggestions and even recipes and medicines, from friends and relatives who wished him well, to have a son until his eldest of the three daughters was to have a baby. One of his friends even sent a bottle of medicine for his wife, to enable her conceive a son. The friend had not even met her. A Muslim professional couple with multinational consultancy jobs felt so pressured after two daughters were born to them that in 2000 they again decided to take one more chance in the hope of getting a son. When the nurse came out of the labour room to give the news, she broke into a sob to have to declare that it was again a daughter. Family members tell doctors in hospitals, 'Doctor, you should have given something better' (*koi changee cheeze deni see*). The celebration and joy at a son's birth, and its reverse at a daughter's, travels from hospital to home and the neighbourhood. Boxes of sweets turn up in hospital labour rooms soon after the family waiting outside learns of a son's birth, but rarely after learning of a daughter's birth. The hospital staff don't expect sweets or cash gifts (for lower level support staff) in the latter case. In Delhi, eunuchs come to take their share of gifts/cash upon marriage and childbirth and make a good collection at a son's birth in contrast to a daughter's as they bless the baby and sing and dance around. Though there is a great deal of evidence of neglect of daughters, the open dislike and disapproval is far less once a daughter is born. From the open and aural, the attitude of daughter dislike shifts to muted and physical, i.e. medical, education and nutrition expenses may be incurred somewhat lesser on a daughter than on a son. But such selective discrimination against daughters, as discussed by Das Gupta (1987) for Punjab in mid-1980s, also varies by birth order and socio-economic contexts.

When Demand is Gift: More than Low Value or High Dowry

The excessive care and caution in raising a daughter, once born, begins early. Dowry and the subsequent flow of gifts goes on much longer, often beyond the lifetime of her parents. It is important to point out here that even among castes practising bride wealth, the flow of gifts after the wedding is usually from the bride's kin to the groom's. As an infant and toddler, a girl is like fine china, parents take care that she turns out fair and beautiful. The 'fragile' and 'handle with care' item in a china shop is to remain a desirable bride for prospective patrons. She belongs to another family and not where she is born. By corollary, any mishandling by the trustees (parents/stewards) is likely to reduce the chances for her making it big in the marriage market. Marriage being central to life for women in most parts of India, parents are seized with a daughter's marriage. Her home, her identity and her prestige come through her marriage and in turn permeate the prestige for her natal family and the conjugal one. In being raised as a preferable bride, things are easier for her and her folks. De Beauvoir (1983) was apt when she stated that for women demand is a gift. It is in the cautious and careful vigil over a daughter, her sexuality and the training given to her to be affectionate, caring and responsible for her conjugal household members, while being efficient and dexterous in household work, and if need be in taking up paid employment, that she is considered as having been raised with love and care.

In order that a daughter is desired as a marriage partner, her upbringing is accordingly fine tuned by the parents who then feel greatly relieved. Conversely, all hell is let loose. People often said a daughter has to be carefully looked after because she has to go to another house. If she has any physical deficiency, her chances of marriage, the route into another (conjugal) house, the ultimate destination, shrinks.

A boy remains at home so he could have any deficiency and no one will say anything, but a girl has to go elsewhere. Who will accept her if she is deficient. She is constantly assessed in the initial years of her married life and all blame is put on her parents for any physical deficiency.

That is why often girls with serious illness are neglected with an unstated intention, i.e. let her die rather than be a problem later on when a match for her in marriage is to be looked for. This statement was an eye opener for me into the mindset that emboldens sex differentials in medical care that all public health data speaks so eloquently about.[5] People's reason dawned on me and helped me to revise the reason from the symptom as merely a practice of the female child's neglect owing to her low social value or high cost of dowry. The consideration is to eliminate her poor chances of marriage and greater humility and social sliding down of the family, in case she survived with a physical or mental deformity after a serious illness. Marriage has a bearing on the practice of differential care in preventing a daughter from injuries or letting her die if sickly or gravely injured. Nevertheless, even girls who are normal by general standards are viewed in common discourse as economic and social burden for the family. This feeling is commonly prevalent not only in most parts of north India but also in Haryana where there is of late a shortage of marriageable brides (see Hudson and Den Boer 2004 for China).

At a training programme for medical doctors in Haryana, two contrary statements were put forth, both of which when put together convey the centrality of marriage. The most immediate concern is the humbling sense an unmarried daughters' parents feel at her birth.

All the doctors were unanimous that the common view repeated often about daughters is, 'where will we go, before whom will we bow low' (*kahan jayenge, kiske aage gidgidayenge*) for offering a girl in marriage? The stress remains on how crucial a girl's marriage is. It is a humbling experience to arrange a match for her, let alone the economic drain the marriage can be for her family. At the same meeting they also said that if a widower or a divorcee male doctor in his late thirties or early forties wished to remarry it would be tough for him to get a match in Haryana. It is certainly not the case if a young bachelor doctor wanted a match.

The sexuality of girls is closely guarded. She is likened to an earthen pot that should neither be dropped nor chipped. Unlike boys, girls are to be kept under a constant vigil. Wild girls are not good girls. They have to be escorted (if not physically at least in terms of knowing their movements, and of late by giving them a mobile phone to trace their movements) whenever they move out of the vicinity of the household. An older family member or a male sibling are the usual escorts. This is an additional task to be performed with more resources and enhanced sense of responsibility. It is a resource the family has to provide for until a girl is married off. Fathers or brothers drop and pick up the small and teenage girls of the family when they visit friends, relatives, go for movies, to restaurants, etc. Once they are college going, they are on their own for college purposes, but are escorted by a family male, mother or old servant when they go elsewhere. Such a vigil is necessitated more in urban areas and is increasingly needed in some rural areas and big towns as well.[6]

Sexual assault on unescorted girls and female children is on the rise, and is frequently reported in the media. It increases the worries of working mothers, who cannot leave their infants and/or children unescorted, especially daughters while they are away at work. Urban areas are particularly notorious in this respect. Unlike most rural areas where women can take their children with them to their work sites or leave them with kin or relatives, working women in urban areas cannot do so. An old parent-in-law in the house is good enough to keep an eye on the older child who can mind his/her younger sibling while the parents are away at work. In villages, open spaces in the residential quarters and the space in the street is rather protected and less open to strangers than in cities. Strangers are dangerous for toddlers and older children. In towns and cities children cannot even be left on their own in parks or open areas around the houses while parents are inside the house/flat to play on their own. In Delhi, it is a common sight to have a parent, grandparent or servant to watch while the toddler plays around the house.[7] It is a common site in Delhi for parent/s to see their school-going children onto the school bus or drop them at school and pick them up from school or wait for them at the bus stop when the bus brings them back from school. Among the lower income groups, children are seen to go and come, usually from the neighbouring government school in groups without being escorted by parents. But as toddlers, they have to be looked after, and it is not easy if the mother happens to be working outside the house.

For poorer women working as domestic help, their patrons do not prefer their children to accompany the mothers. Many such working women cannot afford to keep children in crèches or have other full-time female babysitters or child minders. They do not have space enough in the house to get their parents or parents-in-law to the city for the purpose. However much they might like this to be the case, they are often unable to spare enough resources for having their elders in the city. They have to leave toddlers behind with older children. But this is easier if they happen to be boys not if they are girls. It interferes with poor women's work and wages. They have to look for wage work that allows them to carry their children with them. Aneeta, a domestic maid left her two children with her mother in the village while she worked in Delhi. Later she brought her son but did not think it fit to get her daughter. Soon her son would run away from school and she had managed to get him admitted with great difficulty. Ladies in homes she worked, did not want her son to join her. She brought her daughter and her ailing mother for treatment-cum-babysitting for her daughter. She could do this as her husband had left her and had disappeared from her life. For upper and middle class as well as for the poor, more monetary and human resources and caution are required in raising a female than a male child right from early on. The cultural mindset tilts in favour of sons on the basis of everyday worries that beset daughters' parents. Among the poor, girls need to be draped more than boys, an expense that parents might much prefer not to incur. 'The boy can go naked, but the girl's body needs to be covered, it is not good to keep her naked. It is a matter of shame and may invite undue attention', said a poor grandmother in Delhi.

Raising Children: Increasingly Decreasing Gender Disparity

Over the past two decades, there has been a trend in spending money on children's education, including that of girls, especially in the lower-middle and middle classes, a trend that makes girls nearly as expensive to raise as boys. The middle class provides both boys and girls the same education, often also professional education. This is in the hope of finding for a daughter a better groom. The trend was not the same thirty years ago in Delhi. Many women and men in their thirties said they were sent to different schools than their opposite sex siblings. Girls were sent to public (government) schools, while boys to private schools. If parents could cut corners and spend higher on sons' education as English schooling meant better job prospects, it was an investment towards a betterment of the household. The parents now do not like to follow the same practice into the next generation, they send both their children to private schools. They know that this is important for making a daughter attractive in the marriage market, which is easier to manage if she is working. And they know jobs are easier to get if one has had English-medium education, possible through private schooling.

Professional girls have better chances of finding professional grooms, a medium for upward mobility. Similar expenses on schooling for sons and daughters signifies that younger parents are less discriminatory towards their children. It is also seen as an investment towards social mobility of the family as a whole first through jobs and then through search for a marriage partner. A bride needs to be beautiful, educated and good at work in the home and in her professional field. Neither such a bride nor such a groom are produced without heavy expenses for the parents. Even if a daughter has to leave her natal home to go elsewhere and it means watering another's garden, the investment is worth it and she is educated primarily to fetch a suitable boy. After a good marriage she may continue her profession if he and/or his family like her to work. Her professional life is only of secondary priority both to her parents and her husband, even though her profession might have been one of the important considerations for marrying her. It is seen as an insurance and potential for extra income. If they have only one daughter, the expenses could be near equally distributed between her and a son, but if there were more daughters, priorities might have to be altered.

Though it is commonsense to obviate expenses on daughters because spending on her is like watering another's garden, parents prefer to spend money on her education, food, clothing etc. almost as they would for a son. Thus, sons and daughters are equally expensive in upper and middle class groups. Some discrimination is likely to appear when it comes to giving higher education to girls. Heavier expenses on private education of sons may be more easily and willingly incurred than for a girl. If there is an alternative, she may be encouraged to pursue less expensive courses to enable parents to assemble towards her marriage than would be the case for a son. As for his health care, his educational expenses could mean borrowing money with an understanding that he has to be equipped with the capacity to earn to support a family. And, the cost of education is an investment, which through a good job would attract an educated bride with larger dowry. Nevertheless, this should not mean that middle class parents shy away from spending on daughters' education. They spend enough on her education to make her an attractive bride to carry herself in the prospective groom's circle, and take up a professional job too. Spending on her education enhances the parents' status through forging hypergamous affinal ties with other families. Once they have a daughter, they like to invest the household resources in her. They have disposable resources and can often give higher dowries than they might actually do. Similarly, those in the middle class, receive a large dowry, mutually honorific for givers and the receivers, though they are not usually in need of it. Efforts of status summation by individual households in competition for betterment go on through bearing, rearing and settling down one's children in socially and smybolically honourable ways.

Raising Status through Dowry: Sanskritisation of Marriage Practices

The daughter's groom does not come cheap. Matters of marriage are also matters of money and status. He has to be at least equal if not somewhat better (in education, income, social standing of his family, family's wealth, etc.) than her; and dowry can catch this match. Both the Rugji family and that of the nurse's in the Delhi hospital know this very well. Hypergamous marriages have been historically known to exist among the higher castes, who are usually, and have been mostly, also higher class. Those not already of high caste can enhance their caste status as a corporate group through hefty dowries hypergamously as discussed by Pocock (1971) in his monograph on the Patidars of Gujarat (See Vishwanath in this volume). And the caste groups' status got enhanced through the judicious balancing of resources with population control (Clark 1993).

Individual households, even while they operate through caste endogamy, are class stratified. Individual households and families try to raise their status through hypergamous marital alliances, which in turn are based on large dowries and high education and/or official/political connections. Providing a hefty dowry and arranging an exorbitantly expensive wedding, after educating a daughter, even if the marriage is not apparently hypergamous is on the rise. Both giving and receiving dowry is an honourable act for both the families concerned. Thus the popularity of dowry, though illegal in the state's eyes, is viewed as status enhancing by the society, both within the family and the community.

The customary and ritual status of the wife givers is slightly lower than that of wife receivers in the generalised exchange marriages, especially in India. This is not true of other societies like the Kachin studied by Leach (1964). Leach shows how Levi-Strauss's generalised exchange presupposes an expansion of trust and credit and the Kachin system has endless sequences of dyadic exchanges which are in the long run balanced *quid pro quo*. The notion of *kanyadan* (gift of a virgin) in Hindu scriptures expects gift giver to find a worthy receiver of the gift before whom the self-abnegating gift giver is relatively lower. It is in the sacrifice of the gift that the two come closer and yet not entirely as Parry (1986) discusses for the gift in general and also the Indian gift in particular. The feeling of such a differential status between bride givers and receivers is catching on among the lower castes, and among the scheduled castes as well among whom exchange marriage and bride wealth marriage existed (my observations in Rajasthan villages and towns over the past four decades). So is dowry on the rise, especially among those who have risen higher taking advantage through the constitutional provision of reservations in education and jobs.

Many of the agricultural and service castes and the lower castes in rural Rajasthan that practised bride price until three decades ago are shifting towards dowry, as a mark of raising their caste's status in the caste hierarchy and their household's status within their caste group (personal communication and frequent observation over this period). Berreman (1993) describes a similar trend among the hill people in Garhwal in Uttaranchal. He finds shrinking female autonomy, dowry marriages, and education without outside employment as means and consequences of sanskritisation. The feeling of the groom's family being ritually higher is symbolic of the hypergamous preference. This posture is to be maintained for almost all the time, and carried on by the bride's brother after her parents' death (See Vatuk 1975 for more on this in Uttar Pradesh). The customary claim of a daughter on parental property may be absent but her claim on her parental and eventually on her brother's property, especially by way of customary gifts to her, members of her conjugal family and her children, is highly significant and often substantial. Similar is the claim of her offspring on her brother for his presence and for customary gifts, at least until his sister is alive. The importance of the son is thus not just for the mother and the power that comes to her through his birth, but it is important for the sister throughout her life to have a brother to carry on the supply of customary gifts to her and her conjugal family. A son's father's confidence is enhanced in dealing with dowry and the ensuing gifts if they have sons who provide social and economic support as male members of the bride giving family. Besides, a brother is the emotional shield for a sister and also her husband, in case of any untoward eventuality or misfortune.

It is odd that daughter dispreference is on the rise among the wealthy and the middle class in India, and by emulation among the lower ones too. Among the very poor from lower middle and lower castes, the conditions of marriage may differ. But for those who can afford even among the lowest castes try to emulate higher caste marriage customs. Many low caste domestic service providers in Delhi borrow money from their employers and take loans from friends, and family to spend on marriages and incur larger expenses, like their richer caste counterparts and neighbours, more on daughters' marriages than that of sons. This paper does not cover those poor who have no money and for whom amassing food itself is a daily struggle.

Clearly, sons are raised and educated to be earning members who can shoulder the responsibility of looking after parents and fulfilling customary obligations towards sisters. On the other hand, daughters are raised as a means to forge alliances for upward social mobility, through which parents earn the highest social prestige and religious merit. One might argue that daughters are not customarily given rights in parental/family property. But it is through the discourse woven around raising them well for others and gaining indirectly in the process, that the son-daughter differential is made sense of. This sense of the differential is emboldened through the inability to have any right over one's daughter after her marriage, which is constantly mentioned every now and then. Besides, there are statements, such as how expensive raising of daughters and marrying them off, usually is. The burdensome daughter is increasingly proving to be a resource guzzler. She frequently gnaws at the parental assets. Parents want her to remain happy for which both human and material resources are needed. The presence of a brother for a girl is viewed in the light of not only for the performance of mortuary rituals, but also for other family rituals, including those for one's sister.

Fear of violence in married life—bride burning, wife bashing, divorce and the ensuing stigma is an emotional cost in having a daughter. It is this social discourse that charts out a daughter as a social and economic burden, whose upbringing is enormously pains-taking and uncertain until she has children, at least a son. The fewer daughters one has, the lesser the occasions of standing in attendance for a daughters' conjugal family and drain on one's material re-sources. Thus, it is thought ideal to have not more than one daughter, especially when not more than two children is seen as an ideal for a couple to have.

Models for Wedding and Other Rituals: The Role of Culture Industry

In the present times when money and wealth are accorded supreme importance, dowry and gifts at life-cycle rituals are always welcome. It is easy money and glitzy gizmos are status symbols, and more so when they come as dowry or customary gifts. These symbolise the higher status of wife receivers, and their recurrent honouring through customary gifts from wife givers. It works as a spiral. Gift receivers enhance their social standing before neighbours and kin through receiving gifts. This in turn enhances the social standing of gift givers and that of their daughter/sister in her conjugal family. Those castes that practised bride wealth justify the practice as it brings honour to their daughter in her conjugal family. A well-oiled warmth in ties between the two sets of families is expected to continue. The im-proved economic standing happens on the side.

The seductive attraction of the culture industry facilitated through media and advertisements has skyrocketed Indian, especially middle class wedding expenses. Expert statements through mass media are described as examples by Foucault as falling in the category of relevant 'surfaces of emergence' to which people gain access and identify them as relevant. Films like *Ham Aap Ke Hain Kaun*, and many TV soaps define for audiences the 'surfaces of emergence'. They as it were, provide them the meaning of happiness and satisfaction in family life. Such media provide social settings in which a discourse's facts are materialised or situated within the fields of statements. The discourse that follows the soaps and such films in parks, on morning and evening walks, in buses, trains and cars in and around Delhi deploy the media reorientation as models for real life situations, especially in matters of marriage. What it means to have a daughter is both reproduced and destabilised through a reiteration of norms, rituals and discourse of media representations as well as of actual everyday practice over time. Human bodies and the cultures in which they grow come to be blended, so that conceptually separating them is not so easy.

Maximisation of advantages in life are seen to come through managing and manipulating resources. If dowry is a resource for one party, it is a loss of resource for another, especially if unequally tilted. It makes sound social and economic sense to be in a position of receiving rather than giving dowry. There is a style of negotiating dowry among middle-class Punjabis in Delhi and Punjab. It is commonly said, 'We want only the girl in barely three clothes'(*teen kapron mein ladki chaahiye*). But this is only a manner of speaking and never to be taken literally. A huge dowry following such statements is welcome. In fact, parents prefer to give more to enable their daughter a comfortable time in her conjugal home. Northern India, especially Delhi is notorious for enhanced dowries. Not only large dowries, demanding even larger dowries is what has twisted the desirable ideal of giving and receiving dowry. Dowry communicates love, affection, respect, and honour. Of course, giving dowry is not merely economic cost and/or loss because it enhances status and honour of both dowry givers and receivers. But when honour is positively correlated and measured through the monetary extent of the dowry gifts, collectively evaluated by the concerned families and other relatives, the economic burdensomeness of the daughter heightens.

In Delhi there are several event management companies run professionally that specialise in organising expensive weddings, besides those seen through Bollywood films and TV soaps. There are boutiques and designers for bridal and wedding wear. Their exquisite pieces are very expensive but set standards to strive for. They set off a competitive spree among those families or households planning weddings to have their event marked by arrangements that outdo others to be remembered for long even after the event. This recount of arrangements, dresses, invitees, venue, menu, music, dance, etc. are all items that can be arranged by event managers, a new profession, to add to family honour. Unlike many women professionals in Delhi who got married around or soon after India's independence in a rather simple style, many of them in a *khadi saree* with no dowry, to reasonably good matches told me,

> Young college going girls these days want very stylish and lavish weddings. They want designer dresses, fashionable jewellery, and accessories. They often say that this is a once in a lifetime occasion, and also expect to receive a substantial dowry. It is justified as girls say this is the time when they receive something in bulk from their parents. The thinking is very different from our times. We did not want to be burdens on our parents during those days and also shunned the institution of dowry. Now girls think very differently. They think about having all comforts in their conjugal home soon after their wedding and want their parents to contribute towards their smooth married life. (Narang, a college teacher)

Young women in smaller towns in north India also held similar views and openly stated so when asked. Dowry is meant to bring happiness and comfort to the married daughter. Punjabis commonly express that a daughter takes/receives all the time in the proverb, '*Kuanri khaaye rotiyan te byayi khaaye botiyan*', literally, an unmarried one eats bread and a married one eats you up. She takes even after death; a married daughter's cremation expenses come from her natal home for her last rites to be duly performed. This signifies that the wedding and dowry are not the end of a series of expenses incurred on a daughter. A Punjabi upper-middle class mother in her sixties used this proverb if a daughter is not given enough gifts, *Ghar ki deewaren roti hain*, literally, walls of the house weep. This explains the importance of keeping a daughter and her conjugal family happy to keep one's own house happy, including its material structure (the walls). Raheja's (1988) poison in the gift and the necessity to give gifts for one's own well-being is resonating here. Gift giving begins soon after the betrothal is fixed. The flow of gifts to a daughter's conjugal family begins from the point of *thaka*, (booking the boy for the girl in marriage). For a couple of rituals before the wedding, when the two families visit each other, gifts and/or cash in envelopes (*lifafa*) is presented to the groom's relatives. Some of the rituals are new and are adopted from TV soaps and Bollywood films. A colleague in her fifties, teaching in the university in a town, was surprised when she was asked to join other relatives in taking henna (*mehndi*) to the bride's house two days before the wedding of her cousin's son that she had come to attend in Delhi. When she said that it was a new ritual and she was not aware of it, the reply was, 'Don't you want the *lifafa*? We'll all be given *lifafe* (plural) there.' Such gifts are handed over while bidding good bye to visitors from a daughter's conjugal family. Gifts and cash for members of her fiancé's household, family and relatives and often for most of the relatives who come for the wedding are provided. The proverb goes,

'The groom is happy with the bride, the *barati* (the party of people accompanying the groom) for wedding are happy with the feast' (the honour given in all humility by the brides' family, and/or the accompanying gifts).

The first year of marriage of their son, who is a banker posted abroad, the car load of gifts came to the middle class Agarwal house every now and then. Their son and daughter-in-law were not in Delhi. But the son's in-laws brought gifts on the first *Diwali, Holi, Lohri, Karwa Chauth*, and the birthdays of their daughter, son-in-law, latter's parents and sister. The first year of their daughter's marriage, they came to pick up the son-in-law's sister several times for a meal at a restaurant, to a film show, etc. Such courtesies with humility are extended to generate goodwill for one's newly married daughter. Such gift-giving wanes in frequency and amount with time, especially after grandchildren are born. The first *Lohri* of a grandchild is very significant, maternal grandparents are expected to give large amounts of gifts. Some of the sweets and gifts are distributed among friends, neighbours and mostly among relatives later on. I have received gifts and sweets on several occasions from many families in Delhi, including the Agarwals, when a married son's mother proudly announced that the sweets and gifts came from her son's in-laws. After the grandchildren arrive, the flow of gifts is then diverted to grandchildren. That is expressed in the often emphasised phrase for a mother at a daughter's birth. The mother is told by many of the women who meet her after a daughter is born to her, 'Now the days for you to dress up gorgeously are over' and 'a daughter's mother, you now have to start accumulating for her'. These sayings are common even among communities irrespective of whether they have been practising dowry or not. Usha, a Punjabi academic in Delhi, recounted how her husband's brother's family receives expensive gifts for their grandchildren from their maternal uncles and grand-parents.

> 'The three sons' six children receive gifts on their birthdays, at ear piercing ceremonies, on ritual and festive occasions.' Each one's mother's natal kin try to give gifts which are the latest items on the market and are a craze with children. 'Birthday gifts are becoming a newly-introduced expense. We did not have such gift giving during our childhood. Each affinal relative tries to outdo the other through expensive gifts at birthdays, marriage anniversaries, and other festivals and ritual occasions.'

A woman's natal family owes her even until her death. Obviously her parents are usually dead when she is old herself. It is her brother/s who are expected to provide for the expenses for her last rites upon her death.

Bringing the Threads Together

With a decline in infant and child mortality along with a myriad associated developments, younger couples are more confident of taking the risk of putting a stop to their fertility after having fewer children (See Patel 1999 for how this logic worked in rural India). The other risk they take in arresting fertility earlier than their parents did, is owing to a sense that life is getting harder. Both material cost and human cost of raising children is rapidly rising. The demands children make on parents is on the rise. They live off their parents until they begin to earn a steady income for which parents are expected to spend on them and provide opportunities. Parents aspire for a better life for themselves and even better for their children. For fruition of aspirations, the number of children one has, is to be curtailed. What is critical is the control of the sex composition of a possible number of children, which can now be fine tuned more carefully with sonography. Female foeticide is being substituted for female infanticide for who ever can scrounge the finances to avoid having many daughters. Beside the emotional dilemmas, the low cultural value a daughter has in the context of uncertainty around her rearing, and eventually in settling her down in marriage are major considerations right from the time she is born. Kin and other networks support this perception. A silent approval to the subsequent course of action is a sign of social sanction. Nevertheless, female foeticide is not seen as an act appreciable in others' eyes, but committed for the welfare of the family, which includes gendered structures with the male in authority. In the micro politics of the family and the household, sonography has turned more stringent and instrumental in supporting the culture of son preference and dislike of daughters. To have a place under the sun, son(s) is required. One daughter is acceptable but not a string of them. The sex of a foetus is assumed to be created biologically but technologically detectable, and thus considered terminable.

Accumulation of privileges has always remained of special advantage in social relationships. By having male babies a woman and her family gains social prestige and are more often than not, treated as more privileged than in the absence of male offspring. The desire to have male babies is expressed frequently in blessings showered on the respectfully bowing new bride till she has borne sons. May you be the mother of a hundred sons (Bumiller 1990) and 'may you continue to have sons and bathe in milk' (*dudhon nahao pooton phalo*), and flower and prosper (*phulo phalo*) are commonly heard blessings for a young bride. The cultural construction of motherhood and the problem of failure to achieve at least one son, assumed interest in medical anthropology. Involuntary childlessness was medicalised as the disease of infertility (Becker and Nachtigall 1992). The converse of it all is in having sons preferably with at the most one daughter. A sonless woman's future is dark but not that of a daughterless one. Daughterlessness has not been a social or a sociological concern. There is the commonly held notion of the desirable sex composition of children, discussed in Patel (1994) as the social optimum sex and number of children. What better way to achieve the ideal sex composition of one's children than to use amniocentesis and ultrasound technologies? The neglect and part rejection of parturient women with female babies is common as is the prioritised attendance on them if they deliver a baby boy.

Both the emotional and micro-political considerations in the everyday and the occasional over the gendered life course are exacting for parents. Mediated through institutions such as sexuality, marriage, procreation, family and modern education for daughters, parents find daughters a burden. Bride wealth practising castes are increasingly adopting dowry often influenced by the culture industry and more rapidly as they come to urban areas. Among those with high economic aspirations, sonography provides avenues. It is an odd fact that the upwardly mobile and those with better economic resources adopt sonography in favour of sons to avoid having more than one daughter. It is supported by the constant generation of discourse around two issues, which assumes a facticity of sorts. First, the demographic composition of households. Second, around marriage and gift-giving practices that make daughters seem as sexual, social and economic burdens. The usual humble posture maintained by a daughter's parents as wife givers also provides a continuous fuel to this discourse. In the power relations between the bride's and groom's families, the former always have to give in and put up with any humiliation, indignity, and oblique or direct insults on the part of the latter. The uncertainty regarding tracing the right match and subsequently the cordiality between affinal families is enhanced in urban areas as not many families know each other over generations, a factor adding to the feeling that a daughter is one too many.

Where honour comes through material acquisition, it is reasonable to avoid dispensable costs. People do not mind accepting dowry for their sons. Dowry is easy money, 'get rich quick' formula spreading throughout the society. By the late 1980s, dowry has ceased to be delimited only to certain upper castes. The middle and lower castes considered emulating upper castes through dowry as a means of upward mobility in the caste hierarchy. Sanskritisation, to use Srinivas' concept and its resurgence in recent times in Indian society (Shah 2005) includes imitation of higher castes in marriage alliances, customs, such as dowry, and other rituals. The custom of dowry, also seen as a means to enhance the family's and caste's status, has not only remained limited to the Hindus but has spread among all communities in India irrespective of their class, community and religious background. Its extreme manifestation was seen in the increasing state of dowry-related murders. The registered cases are on the rise but unregistered cases are estimated to be several times more. Berreman (1993) compares the autonomy of Garhwali women in the hills with those in the plains and finds the loss of women's agency through their envy and emulation of high caste plains customary practices in the process of sanskritisation. Proscription of hypogamy and the gift of a virgin to a deserving and rightful man is socially constructed. Marriage strategies are also family strategies. Both religious injunctions and the socio-economic are imbricated in the plethora of supporting mechanisms and thought structures. Dowry marriages, disrespecting of widow remarriage and women's freedom to initiate divorce, and spending equally on sons and daughters' nutrition, education, etc. combine to make fewer daughters an attractive option in times of a small family norm. Conditions of gender hierarchy seldom mystify conditions of production for parents in general.

Cultural politics has surrounded the occurrence or non-occurrence of biological events, such as conception, pregnancy, miscarriage, induced abortion and childbirth, operating routinely at the micro political level in the household and the family. The ability or inability to reproduce has cultural meanings. Sonography enables to achieve or at least have the potential for desirable biological outcomes having culturally coloured meanings and they have a potential to reduce the separation between 'desirable' and 'actual' outcomes. And, especially during ruptures of time-honoured social arrangements people get secretive among themselves too.

Notes

1. I am thankful to Dr Roland Hardenberg to help me tease out this notion of the mindset.
2. In India, for instance, the localised and caste specific practice of female infanticide, and its recording during the colonial period that ensued a discourse pan-Indianising infanticide has been questioned and debated from a feminist cultural history perspective by Bhatnagar, Dube and Dube (2005).
3. It is not uncommon to come across statements justifying dowry by saying that it eases if not evens out for the parents of a son, the cost of raising and educating him. His wife would reap the benefits of his upbringing and income more than the parents (personal communication with Prof. Gita Dharampal Fricke).

4. Kalaivani in personal communication mentioned this happening in Andhra Pradesh in south India, where the term for 'insignificant', or 'some one who'll not be there in any case' is invoked in response to a query about girl children. Arima Mishra mentioned about how the term for involuntary childlessness and sonlessnesss is often the same in Oriya language spoken in Orissa, personal communication.

5. A father lost no time in deciding that it was better that his gangrene-afflicted daughter died rather than her leg be amputated when a doctor suggested so. He instantly said, 'It is better that she died, who'll look after her after I am dead?' Reported in Minocha, A. A. in a paper on informed consent in medical practice in an edited volume in the honour of A.M. Shah (forthcoming).

6. Saraswati Raju reported that in villages in Haryana parents now fear sending their teenage girls to school on their own and withdraw them from school if they cannot escort them while commenting on my paper on 'Science Gender and Social Networks: The Missing Girl Child in India' at the Institute of Social Sciences, Vasant Kunj, New Delhi, on 26th September, 2003.

7. Chritsa Fricke, a school teacher in Heidelberg said she played in the forest close to her house in the village and wandered around alone and came home whenever she wanted to. Her grandparents and parents had nothing to worry about. All in the small village she grew up in, around the WWII, knew who she was. That was safe enough. 'None of my three daughters had that kind of carefree childhood even if Heidelberg was also smaller than what it is now'.

References

Agnihotri, S. B. 2000. *Sex Ratio: Patterns in the Indian Population, A Fresh Exploration.* Sage: New Delhi.

Arditti, R., Duelli-Klein, R. and Minden, S. (eds.). 1984. *Test-Tube Women: What Future for Motherhood?* London: Pandora Press.

Baligar, V. P. V. 1999. *Mother and Child.* New Delhi: Rawat.

Becker, Gay. and Robert D. Nachtigall. 1992. 'Eager for Medicalisation: The Social Production of Infertility as a Disease', *Sociology of Health and Illness,* 14 (2): 456–71.

Berreman, G. D. 1993. 'Sanskritization as Female Oppression in India', in B. Miller (ed.), *Sex and Gender Heirarchies,* pp. 366–93. Cambridge: Cambridge university Press.

Bhatnagar, R. D., R. Dube, and R. Dube. 2005. *Female Infanticide in India: A Feminist Cultural History.* New York: State University of New York Press.

Bourdieu, P. 1976. 'Marriage Strategies as Strategies of Social Reproduction', in R. Forster and O. Ranum (eds.), *Family and Society: Selections from the Annales,* pp. 117–44. Baltimore: The Johns Hopkins University Press.

Bumiller, E. 1990. *May You Be a Mother of Hundred Sons*. New York: Fawcett Columbine.

Clark, A. W. 1993. 'Analysing Reproduction of Human Beings and Social Formations, with Indian Regional Examples Over the Last Century', in A. W. Clark (ed.), *Gender and Political Economy: Explorations of South Asian Systems*, pp.115–45. Delhi: Oxford University Press.

Cormack, M. 1953. *The Hindu Woman*. Westport: Greenwood Press.

Das Gupta, M. 1987. 'Selective Discrimination Against Female Children in Rural Punjab, India', *Population and Development Review*, 13 (1): 77–100.

De Beauviour, S. 1983. *The Second Sex*. London: Jonathan Cape.

Douglas, M. 1960. *Purity and Danger*. London: Routledge and Kegan Paul.

Dumont, L. 1966. 'Marriage in India: The Present State of the Question III. North India in Relation to South'. *Contributions to Indian Sociology*, 9 (December): 90–114.

———. 1975. 'Terminology and Prestation Revisited', *Contributions to Indian Sociology* (NS), 9: 197–215.

Favret-Saada, J. 1980. *Deadly Words: Witchcraft in Bocage*. Cambridge: Cambridge University Press.

Firestone, S. 1971. *The Dialectic of Sex: The Case for Feminist Revolution*. London: Cape.

Franklin, S. 1995. 'The Anthropology of Science', in J. MacClancy (ed.), *Exotic No More: Anthropology on the Frontline*, pp. 351–58. Chicago: University of Chicago Press.

Handwerker, W. P. (ed.). 1990. *Births and Power: Social Change and the Politics of Reproduction*. Boulder, Co: Westview Press.

Harpwood, Vivienne. 1996. *Legal Issues in Obstetrics*. Aldershot: Dartmouth.

Hudson, V. M. and A. M. Den Boer. 2004. *Bare Branches: The Security Implications of Asia's Surplus Male Population*. Cambridge: MIT Press.

Inhorn, M. and V. Balen. (eds.). 2002. *Infertility Around the Globe: New Thinking on Childlessness, Gender and Reproductive Technologies*. California: University of California Press.

Inhorn, M. 1996. *Infertility and Patriarchy*. Philadelphia: University of Pennsylvania Press.

Jamous, R. 1992. 'The Brother–Married Sister Relationship and Marriage Ceremonies as Sacrificial Rites: A Case Study from Northern India', in D, de Coppet (ed.), *Understanding Rituals*, pp. 52–73. London: Routledge.

Jeffrey, P. R. Jeffrey, and A. Lyon. 1989. *Labour Pains and Labour Power*. London: Zed Press.

Jordan, B. 1980. *Birth in Four Cultures: A Cross-Cultural Study of Childbirth in Yucatan, Holland, Sweden and The U.S.* Shelborne, VT: Eden Press.

Kane, P.V. 1946. *History of Dharmasastras*. Vol.3, 2nd Edn. Pune: Bhandarkar Oriental Research Institute.

Karve, I. 1953. *Kinship Organisation in India*. Bombay: Asia Publishing House.

Kishor, S. 1993. 'May God Give Sons to All: Gender and Child Mortality in India', *American Sociological Review*, 58: 246–65.

Leach, E. R. 1964. *Political Systems of Highland Burma*. London: Bell.

Levi-Strauss, C. 1966. *The Savage Mind*. Chicago: University of Chicago Press.

Mayo, K. 1927. *Mother India*. New York: Harcourt Brace and Co.

Miller, B. 1981. [1991]. *The Endangered Sex. Neglect of Female Children in Rural North India*. Ithaca, NY: Cornell University Press.

O'Brien, M. 1981. *The Politics of Reproduction*. Boston, Mass.: Routledge and Kegan Paul.

Panigrahi, L. 1972. *British Social Policy and Female Infanticide in India*. New Delhi: Munshiram Manoharlal.

Parry. J. 1986. 'The Gift, the Gift and the "Indian Gift"', *Man*, 21 (3): 453–73.

Patel, T. 1994. [2006]. *Fertility Behaviour: Population and Society in a Rajasthan Village*. Delhi: Oxford University Press.

———. 2004. 'Women's Status in Fertility Studies and *in situ*', in M. Unnithan-Kumar (ed.), *Women's Agency, Medicine and the State*, pp. 203–22. Oxford: Berghahn.

Petchesky, R. P. 1985. *Abortion and Woman's choice: The State, Sexuality and Reproductive Freedom*. Boston: Northeastern University Press.

Pocock, D. F. 1971. *Kanbi and Patidar: A Study of the Patidar Community of Gujarat*. London: Oxford University Press.

Raheja, G.G. 1988. *The Poison in the Gift: Ritual, Prestation, and the Dominant Caste in a North Indian Village*. Chicago: University of Chicago Press.

Rapp, Rayna. 1995. 'Accounting for Amniocentesis', in S. Lindenbaum and M. Lock (eds.), *Knowledge, Power and Practice: The Anthropology of Medicine in Everyday Life*, pp. 55–76. Berkeley: University of California Press.

Sehgal, R. 2006. 'Delhi's Skewed Sex Ratio: 24000 Girls Go Missing Every Year'. Available online at http://www.infochangeindia.org/features290.jsp (downloaded on 2006.01.31).

Shah, A.M. 2005. 'Sanskritisation Revisited', *Sociological Bulletin*, 54 (2): 238–49.

Shiva, M. 2002. *Skirting the Issue: The Girl Child, Seen but Not Heard*. New Delhi: VHAI.

Shostak, M. 1983. *Nisa: The Life and Words of a !Kung Woman*. New York: Vintage Books.

Vatuk, S. 1975. 'Gifts and Affines in North India'. *Contributions to Indian Sociology* (NS), 9(2): 155–96.

Visaria, P. 1971. *The Sex Ratio of the Population of India*, Census of India 1961, Monograph No. 10. New Delhi: Office of the Registrar General, India.

Vishwanath, L.S. 2000. *Social Structure and Female Infanticide in India*. Delhi: Hindustan.

Wadley, S. S. 1993. 'Family Composition Strategies in Rural North India', *Social Science and Medicine*, 37 (11): 1367–76.

Widge, A. 2001. *Beyond Natural Conception: A Sociological Investigation of Assisted Reproduction with special reference to India*. Ph.D. Thesis, Jawaharlal Nehru University, New Delhi.

Wikan, V. U. 1990. *Managing Turbulent Hearts: A Balinese Formula for Living*. Chicago: University of Chicago Press.

Between a Rock and a Hard Place: The Social Context of the Missing Girl Child

6

Alpana D. Sagar

The female-male ratio (FMR) in India, which had been showing an overall decline from 1901 onwards, revealed a marginal increase in the 2001 Census. Paradoxically, this improvement in the overall sex ratio was accompanied by a decrease in the sex ratio of the 0–6 years age group. The implications of this are disturbing, to say the least, as it means that discrimination against the female child has increased in India over the last decade. This has increased the concern about, and brought centrestage, the need to tackle the issues of female foeticide and infanticide.

In this article, I not only examine the present situation, but also argue that this problem needs to be located in its social context for any solutions to be found. I do this over three sections. In the first section I look at some of the changes in the overall as well as in the 0–6 years sex ratio over time, and explore some of the reasons for these changes. In the second section I unveil the complexity of this issue by using primary data[1] to reveal the helplessness of many of those caught in this trap, as well as to demonstrate the multiple levels at which this phenomenon operates. In the subsequent section I consider some of the solutions being offered today to improve the sex ratio. Finally, I conclude by iterating that if we truly want to improve the sex ratio in our country we need to work at the macro as well as at the micro level.

I

Vulnerabilities of Girls Reflected in Facets of Female Discrimination in India _____

This section introduces the complexities leading to the low 0–6 years sex ratio in India. I begin by examining time trends in the overall and 0–6 years age sex ratio at an all-India level, as well as for a few selected states. This data demonstrates that while the problem of female infanticide/foeticide may be greater in some states than in others, on the whole an anti-female bias seems to be pervasive throughout our country. I then present work that has utilised NSSO (National Sample Survey Organisation, several rounds) data and reveals that while sex ratios are below unity in poor families, they are even lower in the well-off families. Subsequently, I examine all-India trends in gender differentials in infant and child mortality. This reveals that in addition to infanticide, communicable diseases, as well as malnutrition, are a cause of increased mortality of girls below 6 years of age, thus contributing to the low 0–6 years sex ratios.

Time Trends of Sex Ratio in India

The sex ratio is known to be a manifestation of the interplay between biological and social factors. *Ceteris paribus* the female male ratio (FMR) should be about 1020–1070:1000 and in fact in many developed as well as in developing countries, the sex ratios are in favour of the female. For example in the USA it is 1058, Japan 1034, Burma 1016 and Ethiopia 1066 (Banerjee and Jain 2001). In India however, there has been a decline in the FMR till 1991, though female life expectancy has been increasing over time. However, the FMR was marginally higher in the 2001 Census than in 1991 (Table 6.1) though it continues to be on the lower side. Unfortunately, the census data also reveals a decreasing sex ratio in the age group 0–4 years and 0–6 years.

One of the causes of low sex ratio in childhood i.e. infanticide, has been widely documented over the years (Athreya and Chukatha 2000; George *et al.* 1992; Viswanath 1973). However, the recent phenomenon of the increasingly sharp decrease in 0–4/0–6 years age sex ratios is believed to be the result of the increased use of ultra-

Table 6.1
Trends in Sex Ratio in India, 1901–2001

Year	1901	1921	1931	1941	1951	1961	1971	1981	1991	2001
FMR	971	955	950	945	946	941	931	935	927	933
0–6 years	–	–	–	–	–	976	964	962	945	927
0–4 years	–	–	–	–	–	–	–	990	980	972

Source: Banerjee and Jain 2001, Premi 2001: Female-Male Ratio.

sound and amniocentesis for sex determination followed by sex-selective abortion (Krishnaji 2000). An important question is whether this falling sex ratio in the 0–4/0–6 year group is ubiquitous through-out India or restricted to those states known to have a high anti-female bias.

Till recently it was believed that states in the north and west–Punjab, Haryana, Gujarat, Madhya Pradesh, Rajasthan, Uttar Pradesh and Bihar, showed clear anti-female intervention, while those in the east and south like Kerala, Andhra Pradesh, Assam, Orissa and Karnataka, did not show this anti-female bias. These differences in demographic structures had been identified in literature, with an economic, social and cultural divide between the north and the south of India (Krishnaji 2001). It was believed that this divide was respon-sible for the difference in status amongst the women of these areas. However, as we see in Table 6.2, the present evidence seems to indicate that regardless of the North South divide, the phenomenon of selective female elimination has spread across much of the coun-try, though its intensity varies across states. Thus, while previously, as a general rule of thumb, states in the east and south tended to have 0–6 FMRs more than 960–980, today a phenomenon termed 'northernisation of sex ratio' (Agnihotri 2003) is prevalent. In fact, Ilina Sen has shown that from 1901 onwards, there has been a general shift of districts with higher sex ratios to the lower decile groups (Sen 2001). Additionally, Sudha and Rajan (1999) have used reverse sur-vival methods to estimate sex ratio at birth and they find increasing masculinisation in this ratio in several parts of India. According to them the disappearance of endogamy in the South and the universalisation of dowry are to a large extent responsible for this shift.

Table 6.2 also reveals that the prevalence of decreasing 0–6 years age sex ratio is not necessarily linked to the overall economic devel-opment of the state. Except for Kerala[2] where both the FMR and the

Table 6.2
Trends in FMR and 0–6 Year Sex Ratios in Selected States of India

Zone	State	1971 FMR	1981 FMR	1991 FMR	2001 FMR	1971 0–6 yr	1981 0–6 yr	1991 0–6 yr	2001 0–6 yr
North	Punjab			882	874	892	908	875	793
	Rajasthan	911	919	910	922	931	954	916	909
	Uttar Pradesh	876	862	876	898	899	935	928	916
South	Andhra Pradesh	977	975	972	978	986	992	974	964
	Karnataka	957	963	960	964	968	975	960	950
	Tamil Nadu	978	977	974	986	964	967	974	939
	Kerala	1,016	1,032	1,036	1,058	972	970	958	962
West	Gujarat	934	942	934	919	956	947	928	878
	Madhya Pradesh	920	921	912	920	944	978	952	931
East	Bihar	957	948	907	921	958	981	959	938
	Orissa	988	981	971	972	984	995	967	950
	West Bengal	891	911	917	934	1,007	981	967	963
	India	931	935	927	933	954	962	945	927

Source: Census 2001 Paper I, Banerjee and Jain 2001.

0-6 sex ratio have increased in the 2001 Census, and for Gujarat and Punjab, where both have fallen, for all other states, while FMR has increased, the 0–6 ratios are seen to have fallen. There is in fact, mounting evidence from across the country that with increasing affluence, female infanticide is being transformed into female foeticide! (Swaminathan, M et al. 1998). For example, data from the 2001 Census also reveals that the overall urban 0–6 CSR (child sex ratio) is 903 while the overall rural 0–6 CSR is 934 (Agnihotri 2003). This seems to indicate a greater discrimination in the urban/richer areas. We also know that while the 0–6 CSR has been below 900 for all districts of Delhi, it is the lowest– 845 in south-west Delhi which is one of the most prosperous districts of Delhi (Times of India 2003). Since urban health, especially amongst better-off sections, is known to be better than rural health across sexes, this fall in CSR in the more affluent areas, cannot be taken to mean a higher mortality in the rich. In fact, in view of the concentration of medical services in the urban as compared to the rural areas, it is most probable that this decreasing CSR is indicative of increasing sex-selective abortion. Similarly, data from the 55 round of NSSO-1999-2000 (Agnihotri 2003), very clearly reveal that overall female male sex ratio is most favourable for women in the poorest families and most unfavourable for the richest households in both urban and rural areas (Table 6.3). This once again is indicative of increasing sex-selective abortions in the richer families. Further work done using the 43, 50, 52, and 55 rounds of NSSO (Siddhanta, Nandy and Agnihotri 2003) reveals a more consistent trend of declining sex ratios with prosperity especially with later rounds.

It is important that we further examine and investigate such information. It is imperative for us to understand why better-off families that do not seem to have the economic compulsions of the poor, have

Table 6.3
Sex Ratio and MPCE* Class by Rural and Urban Area

Area	MPCE	0–14 years	FMR
Rural	0–225	946	1004
	>950	804	858
Urban	0–330	903	949
	>1925	819	836

Source: Agnihotri 2003, July 1999–June 2000 NSSO Rural and Urban Survey.
Note: *MPCE: Monthly Per Capita Expenditure.

poorer female-male ratios than the latter. It seems that women's secondary status has significant implications for their health, well-being and survival.

Time Trends in Gender Differentials in Mortality in India

The present worsening in 0–4/0–6 years sex ratio includes not only an increase in female foeticide but also an increase in female mortality during infancy as well as in childhood as compared to male mortality. Table 6.4 reveals that the increase in female infant mortality as compared to male infant mortality began from the 1970s. It is noteworthy that not only is infant mortality in females greater than that of males, death rates are also higher in females as compared to males in the 0–4 years age group. An examination of the percentage contribution of deaths during 0–1 years, as well as 1–4 years of age by sex, over time reveals differences in trends of male and female mortality (Table 6.5). There is for the 0–1 years age group, a slow though sustained decline in male mortality. On the other hand infant female mortality reveals an initial fall followed by a marginal increase. Similarly, there is an increase in proportion of female deaths in the age group from 1–4 years, while male mortality for the same age has decreased over time.

This is significant since if all other things remain equal, the greater biological vulnerability of the male as compared to the female should lead to an excess male mortality during infancy as well as during childhood. It is only during the reproductive period, where repro-

Table 6.4
Infant and Child Death Rates (0-4 Years) by Gender

Year	Infant mortality rate		0–4 years death rate	
	Male	Female	Male	Female
1905	231	218	–	–
1936	170	153	–	–
1955	99	91	–	–
1964	76	72	–	–
1972	132	148	–	–
1984	104	104	39.6	43.1
1993	73	75	22.7	24.8
1999	71	73	22.2	25.6

Source: Premi 2001, Agnihotri 2000.

Table 6.5
Per cent of Total Infant and Child Mortality (1–4 Years), 1970–1998

Age	0–1 years		1–4 years	
Year	Male	Female	Male	Female
1970	54	46	49	51
1980	55	45	46	54
1990	55	45	46	54
1998	53	47	46	54

Source: GOI 1970, 1980, 1990 and 1998.

duction is an additional risk factor, that female mortality may be expected to increase over male mortality. Thus this higher mortality of girls as compared to boys, during infancy as well as in the first four years of life is indicative of social discrimination in the neo-natal as well as in the post neo-natal period. This would imply situations of not only infanticide but also neglect leading to higher mortality of the female child. Another question that comes to mind is–what are these girls dying of? Table 6.6 shows that mortality due to many of the communicable diseases is higher among girls than boys despite their greater biological strength, and in fact the gap seems to be widening with time. Additionally, there are more deaths among girls due to anaemia—an indicator of malnutrition amongst girls in this age group. This seems to indicate that a lower social status of girls— especially in a situation of poverty—is reflected in discriminatory nutritional and health care practices. This could lead to an increased mortality. We see therefore that along with foeticide and infanticide,

Table 6.6
Per cent of Total Mortality in 1–4 Years by Selected Diseases

Disease	1980		1990		1998	
	Male	Female	Male	Female	Male	Female
Respiratory	11.6	12.3	12.1	14.5	11.3	12.0
Gastrointestinal	9.5	10.4	11.6	11.6	7.3	10.1
TB	0.4	0.31	0.8	0.4	0.9	0.6
Malaria	0.9	0.9	0.9	1.3	1.2	1.4
Measles	0.9	1.3	0.5	1.2	0.7	1.0
Anaemia	1.5	3.4	3.3	6.3	3.8	5.1
Total	22.4	25.21	25.9	29.0	21.4	25.2

Source: GOI 1980,1990,1998.
Notes: 1. *Respiratory includes:* Influenza, Pneumonia Whooping Cough.
   2. *Gastrointestinal includes:* Cholera, Typhoid, Acute Abdomen Dysentery and Gastroenteritis.

Table 6.7
FMR and 0–6 Year Sex Ratios in Selected States, 2001

State	FMR	0–6 Years
Madhya Pradesh	920	931
West Bengal	934	963
Jharkhand	941	966
Uttar Pradesh	899	916
Bihar	921	938

Source: GOI 2001. Census of India, 2001. Report I.

it is social discrimination—often in the presence of poverty—against females in the 0–4 years age group, that is contributing to the decreasing child sex ratio. Therefore, while we need to tackle the issues of foeticide and infanticide we also need to consider all the other causes for child mortality while planning strategies for improving the under-six sex ratios.

However, it is also worth noting that while all India FMR is better than the 0–6 years sex ratio, some states as dissimilar as Madhya Pradesh, West Bengal, Jharkhand, Uttar Pradesh, and Bihar—to name a few—have better sex ratios for the group in the age 0–6 years than overall sex ratios (Table 6.7). These higher 0–6 sex ratios with lower FMR are indicative of the fact that having survived till the age of six years, these girls die at an older age. This is worth noting as it reveals the fact that while female foeticide and infanticide are no doubt extremely important, the bias against older women is no less significant (Table 6.8). In fact Table 6.9 reveals how little progress

Table 6.8
Per cent of Reported Deaths (excluding Senility) by Age and Sex, 1998

Age group in years	1998	
	Male	Female
Below 1 year	14.1	16.3
1–4	3.8	5.8
5–14	4.2	5.3
Total	22.1	27.4
15–24	4.9	6.6
25–34	6.6	7.1
35–44	8.2	6.4
Total	19.8	20.1
45–59	16.5	11.1
60+	41.6	41.4
Total	58.1	52.5

Source: GOI 1998.

Table 6.9
Per cent of Mortality for Age 5–14 Years by Sex, 1984 and 1998

Selected Communicable Diseases	1984		1998	
	Male	Female	Male	Female
Respiratory	11.0	15.3	8.6	9.6
Gastrointestinal	21.5	19.2	12.5	16.8
Anaemia	2.3	2.1	3.3	4.7

Source: GOI. 1984, 1998.
Notes: 1. Respiratory includes: Influenza, Pneumonia, Whooping Cough.
   2. Gastrointestinal includes: Cholera, Typhoid, Acute Abdomen Dysentery, and Gastroenteritis.

(or even regress), we have made in eliminating communicable diseases as a cause of death from 1984 to 1998 (for girls 5–14 years in this case).[3] Thus, while sex-selective abortion may be increasing among the well-off, in poorer families, a number of older girls would be bound to be continuing to die due to poor nutrition as well as decreased access to health care.

In this context it is worthwhile pointing out that the overall percentage of mortality among girls in the 5–14 years of age vs. overall mortality among females has increased from 48 per cent to 50 per cent, although the percentage of female mortality by total mortality in other age groups has decreased. Also, overall female mortality as a percentage of total mortality has decreased from 46 per cent to 43 per cent while male mortality has increased commensurately (GOI 1973, GOI 1982, GOI 1992, GOI 2002). In other words, mortality has increased for girls in the age group till 14 years as compared to boys. Thus the girls who are not eliminated in childhood have to pay a heavy price as we have seen in Tables 6.6, 6.7, 6.8 and 6.9. Higher female morbidity and mortality (despite higher male biological vulnerability), discrimination in allocation of food, in education and subjection to gender violence are the lot of women (GOI 1998, Malobika 1993). While there is no doubt that female foeticide/infanticide is a crime, we cannot ignore the question of higher female mortality in childhood, that is again due to the twin demons of poverty and discrimination against the girl child. We have already seen through mortality data by age (Table 6.8) that not only is mortality for girls more than for boys at ages 1–4 years, mortality is more for females till the age of 35 years as compared to that for males! This clearly indicates that girls who survive foeticide and infanticide may still succumb due to inequitable access to food or medical care. The end result for them thus stays the same, and it is there too that we need to focus our energies.

Therefore, while the decrease in the 0–6 years sex ratio is generating a lot of discussion today, the issue of higher female mortality in later life that is also due to gender bias likewise needs to receive special attention. The quality of life of these girls till they die as juveniles or in womanhood is linked to the same issue that is responsible for the low sex ratios viz. their low social status. A question we therefore need to ask ourselves is, whether attempting to prevent female foeticide and female infanticide is sufficient, or would we need to improve women's overall status in order to improve sex ratios?

We thus see the following issues thrown up by this data:

i) While the sex ratio has been decreasing for almost a century, it is only recently that the FMR has shown a marginal improvement. However this has been accompanied by a fall in the 0–6 and 0–4-age child sex ratio. This is indicative of a high probability of increasing female foeticide and female infanticide.

ii) Interestingly while there is a 'northernisation' of the southern states in this phenomenon, another observation is that this bias also seems to be more among the rich urban groups as compared to the poorer rural population.

iii) While mortality rates are higher for girls than boys during infancy, this higher mortality is seen to persist till the girl is fifteen years of age. Finally, even if girls survive beyond the age of fifteen years, they often still continue to be socially vulnerable and have a higher mortality than boys and men.

II

The Social Context of Female Elimination[4] _____

We have seen in the preceding section that the low FMR (especially in the 0–6 year age group) is only the tip of the iceberg of the pervasive discrimination faced by females. In fact, sex-selective abortion and infanticide are only the latest manifestations of a long history of anti-female bias that is evident in the historically declining sex ratio of the population in India. The central issue is social subordination and oppression of women cutting across age, class, caste as well as time and space. Therefore, if we wish to question and tackle the pervasiveness of this phenomenon we need to understand the conditions that create such a world. In order to do this we would need to place this phenomenon against the larger backdrop of historical, social, cultural, economic and ideological factors.

In this section, we explore some historical, political, social and cultural reasons for this anti-female bias in India in order to understand the conditions that create such a world. The experiences of poor women from a slum in Delhi are used to demonstrate women's position today, as well as to bring forth the dilemmas of many women (and often their families), who may be pushed into accepting female foeticide and infanticide. The experiences of these poor women also demonstrate the multiple levels at which these phenomena operate.[5] Through the issues raised we further elucidate how these biases continue to operate throughout women's lives. It is also pointed out that richer women may be in similar traps.

Anti-female Bias in Colonial India

It was in 1789 that Jonathan Duncan of the Bengal Civil Service first 'discovered' female infanticide.[6] The British claimed that it was the high caste Khatris, Bedis and Rajputs who were primarily responsible for female infanticide in India, and believed that the cause of such a practice was caste pride/hypergamy/dowry. The British Government attempted to suppress infanticide through ban and regulation, and finally through the Act of 1870. However they did not seem to note that female infanticide was also being practised by families from other Hindu castes and Sikhs who received bride price, as well as by Muslims who did not follow the practice of dowry (Snehi 2003), which would indicate that daughters were, *per se*, for multiple reasons, not desired as much as sons. Snehi (*ibid*) has also pointed out that according to Oldenberg who explored marriage, gender and property rights in Punjab it was the 'masculinisation' of the economy under the British that increased the desirability of the male child. The forms of agrarian development and revenue policies

of Punjab under the British led to the establishment of private property, the reinforcement of class differentiation among the rural people,
the monetisation of revenue and the compulsion of cultivation of
indigo and opium. This transformed the society of Punjab. The high
revenues pushed peasants into indebtedness and from there to jobs
in the army, with its cash wages as well as awards of land and
pensions. Since only men could own property, this led further to
greater son preference in the family. Thus British policies helped to
strengthen a practice that already existed and was rooted in an anti-
female bias. In the present time, an escalating dowry system, increasing landlessness and poverty, with high gender differentials in wages
and decreasing economic opportunities as well as marginalisation of
women have been suggested as reasons for increasing son preference
(Sudha and Rajan 1999).

The Present Social Context in the Delhi Slum

Most of today's societies are patriarchal, and consider women the
physically and cerebrally weaker sex. Understandably, women living in these patriarchal societies are conditioned into accepting this
social valuation of themselves as undistorted and authentic. They
therefore live out their lives such that their secondary social status
is reaffirmed.[7]

Socialisation of girls

It is important to realise that these women in the slum do not voluntarily carve out subordinate lives for themselves. Social pressures
assist in moulding the forms of their lives. For most women, there
is a creation of a poor self-image from childhood onwards, with
socialisation into duties and responsibilities. Girls grow up believ-
ing that being selfless, putting the interests of all and sundry before
their own, and being caretakers for their families, is one of the most
important facets of their lives. From childhood itself, female children see the special emphasis that is laid on the role of women in
bearing children, particularly sons, to carry on the husband's family
name and traditions. The importance shown to their brothers further
accentuates their understanding of the significance and desirability
of males. Most women realise that they are being given a subordinate
status that is reflected in all aspects of their lives. Many of them

accept it, for they have been told time and again, that their aim in life is to be good daughters, and later good wives and mothers and good housewives. Women in fact tend to feel worthless unless they prove themselves by realising these aims. The fact that these women need to consider their own selves as important, or believe that they by themselves have any intrinsic value, has always been negated. For most women consequently, there is no sense of self-esteem or recognition of self worth, and no structure that gives them an identity away from their family. Hence they believe themselves and their lives *per se* to be worthless, and their feeling of hopelessness is reflected in a statement by one of them–'What is there in a woman's life?'

Social pressures have, over time, hammered in the realisation for women that they must learn to be submissive, and that accepting neglect and abuse without rebelling is part of being exemplary women. This is typified with the role models of Sita, Sati and Savitri being held up before them. Women learn to defer to their men folk in all decisions pertaining to the household, themselves or otherwise, as a mark of respectful submission. Of all those who are aware of this subordinate status as an injustice, almost none are able to fight and overcome this social circumstance. Their acceptance (no matter how unwilling), of their low status is reflected in their statements: 'no man gives his wife as much value as he gives even his stomach' or 'if the man is alright, it is good for the woman, otherwise her life is of no use', and even 'in-laws treat you well only if your husband cares for you.' In fact, one woman went as far as to say 'God should not create one as a woman. It is good if one has no daughter. At least she won't suffer.'

Social pressures have also conditioned women into accepting that a family is needed for them to fulfil their aim in life-all these pressures manage to annihilate their feelings of self and autonomy, converting them into passive, quiescent models of ideal womanhood. Patriarchal societies stress, not only their need for these 'womanly' qualities, but also the women's need to have sons—indeed, married women gain in stature if their first-born is a son. Accordingly, women grow up with the knowledge that their function in life is to selflessly serve their families, to be passive, humble and obedient, and to carry on the family name by bearing strong and healthy sons; by being a 'mother machine'.

Female devaluation through work

Historically, 'the woman's place is in her home' and women's housework has always been in the category of unrecognised work. This is true for all women, regardless of whether they are housewives or wage earners, Hindus, Muslims or Christians, those with husbands in secure jobs, or irregular work or chronically unemployed. For all these women the bottom line is that the house *per se* is their responsibility, and they are the ones who usually have to manage most aspects of managing it—a full-time job, though an unpaid and an unsung one. Social norms in most societies ensure that women's labour in housework is either devalued or invisible. Such a situation strengthens the understanding that women are non-productive members of a household. Non-inheritance patterns intensify this situation.

In addition, employment patterns as seen in the Gautam Nagar slum reveal that women's work is always considered less skilled than that of men, and the sexual division of labour ensures that they have always been relegated to the poorer paying 'feminine' marginalised jobs (Table 6.10). This table reveals that about 42 per cent of the women out of 1,312 in Gautam Nagar slum, were working for wages.[8] Of these, a large number–almost 63 per cent –were working as domestic help (*kothi*). About 13 per cent of the employed women worked either as daily wage unskilled or semi-skilled labourers (DW), and another 12 per cent were rag pickers (SES, Self-Employed Small). The remaining 11 per cent of employed women worked in various jobs—cleaning women in shops (Private), alms seekers, small '*parchun*' (minor groceries) shop owners (SEM, Self-Employed Medium), and very rarely sweepers (1 per cent) in Class IV government jobs.

The men seemed to have slightly better options. About 10 per cent had succeeded in obtaining permanent Class IV government jobs. About 25 per cent were working in small shops as helpers, or as cooks in small *dhabas* (roadside eateries), etc. Two per cent were in permanent private jobs—jobs that bring with them security, a regular income and retirement benefits. About 18 per cent were working as construction workers on daily wages, and about 12 per cent were plumbers, masons, carpenters, electricians, etc., who though working seasonally, earned better daily wages (DW). Another 2 per cent were Class IV employees working on daily wages. In terms of wages and regularity, however, they were akin to those in daily wage jobs.

Table 6.10
Occupational Distribution in the Delhi Slum by Gender

Gender	Perm/Govt	Pvt.	DW	SES	SEM	SEL	Kothi	Houses	Not Working	Mas	Total
							Occupation distribution in slum*				
Women	0.5% (6)	2.3% (30)	5.5% (72)	5% (66)	1.1% (15)	0.4% (5)	26.3% (345)	58.3% (765)	–	0.6% (8)	100 (1312)
Men	10.2% (144)	27% (378)	32% (444)	9% (131)	8.5% (119)	9% (128)	0.5% (7)	3.5% –	0.3% (51)	(4)	100 (1406)

Source: Data from 1,480 households with 1,312 women and 1,406 men
Note: DW–Daily Wages, SES–Self-Employed Small, SEM–Self-Employed Medium, SEL–Self-Employed Large.

Nine per cent were self-employed, small-time workers like *pheriwallas* (hawkers), cobblers, etc., and their earnings were similar to those of daily wage-unskilled workers, and almost as irregular (SES). There was another 9 per cent ('large' self-employed), who owned *kabari* (recyclable household refuse) shops or *dhabas* in the slum or outside or plied their own auto rickshaws (SEL). About 8 per cent were 'medium' self-employed, *kabariwallahs*, vegetable and fruit-sellers, pan or teashop vendors etc (SEM). Less than 1 per cent were working as domestic help. Only about 4 per cent were unemployed (not working), some chronically unemployed, but most had either lost a job due to illness or were in between jobs.

We see thus that the urban employment markets push women into their traditional work, that of housework, and their employment usually tends to be for routine domestic activities of women such as preparing food, cleaning, washing, childcare, etc.—work that is stated to need no skills and hence is poorly paid. Men on the other hand have more as well as better options for employment. This employment profile reflects the existing views on women's work capabilities, and in turn affects their social standing.

Dowry and devaluation of women

Norms of dowry further devalue women and the female child is considered an economic drain on her family in the slum. This devaluation and commodification of women leads to an increase in violence towards them at all levels. Fathers often can only visualise the dowry they will have to pay to marry off their daughters. They say, 'who can afford to marry off two daughters in these expensive days! Even one daughter is one too many!' Interestingly mothers see in their daughters future helpers in household tasks, and maybe potential wage earners when somewhat older. Women say, 'a son to carry on the father's name, and a daughter for the mother—to help her and make her life bearable', and yet they also socialise their daughters into accepting their inferior status.

Female devaluation and health care

While most parents do care about their daughters, and term them the Lakshmi of the house, yet girls are rarely given the love or respect they deserve. In a situation where choices often have to be made between advantages for the daughter or the son, the daughter usually loses out. Therefore, in comparison to her brothers who will carry on the bloodline, and presumably support the parents in their old age, the girl child tends to be neglected. While the final difference in care may be only marginal, in situations where health of members of families is already borderline, this minor difference may tilt the balance (as seen in Tables 6.6 and 6.9). When Shakuntala R's son fell ill, his parents took him to the untrained practitioner in the slum, and then later to a private practitioner in Munirka who had treated him earlier. However, when the daughter fell ill, she was taken only to the former, because the parents felt 'she is less delicate'. Being the biologically stronger sex, many girls manage to survive despite these odds, but this survival takes its toll on their health.

Fertility decline and son preference

In addition there is a simultaneous universalisation of the small family norm. In a situation of poverty where economic security in old age in the absence of welfare schemes is through sons, amongst the two hundred households[9] in the slum talked to at length, all couples wanted at least one son if not two (Table 6.11). Only 13 per cent of the 183 women talked to wanted more than one, i.e. two daughters and 1per cent did not want any girl at all. While one daughter was considered socially necessary for '*kanyadan*', or for the carrying out of certain traditions like the tying of a '*rakhi*', more than 65 per cent wanted two sons. Their logic was, 'if you have two trees, at least one will give you shade' or 'what is the use of one eye'. About 53 per cent of the women wanted one daughter and two sons.

We all understand the significance of these statements. As there is no economic security for the poor in their old age, they still continue to want at least two boys. However, while women may have

Table 6.11
Couples by Number and Gender of Children Wanted

Number of females wanted	Number of males wanted		
	One	Two	Total
Nil	0	1 %(2)	1 %(2)
One	32.5 % (65)	53.5 %(107)	86 %(172)
Two	2 %(4)	11 %(22)	13 %(26)
Total	34.5 % (69)	65.5 %(131)	100 %(200)

Table 6.12
Couples by Achieved Composition of Sons and Daughters

Number of daughters borne	Number of sons borne				
	Nil	1	2	>2	Total
Nil	25.5% (51)	13% (26)	5.5% (11)	4% (8)	48% (96)
1	11% (22)	6% (12)	8.5% (17)	2% (4)	27.5% (55)
2	7% (14)	4% (8)	3.5% (7)	2.5% (5)	17% (34)
>2	3% (6)	3.5% (7)	0.5% (1)	0.5% (1)	7.5% (15)
Total	46.5% (93)	26.5% (53)	18% (36)	9% (18)	100% (200)

had preferences about both family size and sex composition, since there is no control over the sex of the child, they have had to make a trade-off between the desired and achieved family size and composition as seen in Table 6.12. This table indicates a strong son preference. There is the uncertainty of child survival as well. In traditional societies it is the husband's desires, or the social rules that finally determine the number of children in a household. In the given social and economic context furthered in milieu of historical, social acceptance of female elimination, when technology offers a chance of selecting the family composition, there is bound to be a continued threat to females.

Thus, many poor families that may decide that they would rather not have girls any more, have reached what to them is a rational decision. However, we must not assume that this is a free choice for them, nor can we believe that this option is one that confers any power on the woman. In fact, female elimination is a statement on the disempowerment of these poor families and especially the females.

Pressures leading to Sex-selective Abortion

The above helps us to understand why many people are driven to female elimination. I now use qualitative data to detail the experiences of the women from some of these families from the slum to reiterate pressures leading many women to sex-selective abortion. This deals with the question 'what, if any, is the cost of this elimination of the female to the mother? And is there possibly a cost of non-elimination to the mother or child?'

Suman, in Gautam Nagar slum had three daughters. She was a sweeper in a private school and her husband was a helper in a small shop. When she was pregnant for the fourth time she came to me in my capacity as a medical doctor, wanting to know if there was any clinic in her vicinity where she could find out the sex of the foetus. She pointed out that she and her husband could not take good care of more than four children and both their families wanted her to have at least one son. Where should such a woman go? Do any of us have the moral right to decide for her what her course of action should be unless we are going to be there for her once she has another daughter, if that is what the baby is? The problem with an argument like this is that the family planning programmers use this too, as do mercenary doctors who carry out female foeticide. But that does not detract from the validity of the problem—for this will remain as long as boys are considered more necessary than girls.

Krishna on the other hand had the perfect family—one boy and one girl. However the boy fell ill and died in hospital and she was left with only one daughter. Due to family pressure Krishna had to conceive another child. This was another girl. She went into a depression and did not talk for more than a week. Later she confided that her husband was threatening to leave her unless she managed to have a boy! Luckily she had a boy the next time around!

Another woman, Pushpa, stated, 'It is better to die than to be born a girl'. Pushpa had no daughters. She was married to a man who did not earn much and they were poor, with her parents stepping in almost on a monthly basis with financial assistance. She always pointed out that she would not be able to marry her daughters into good families, as her husband would not be able to provide a good dowry! She also wanted to go out and work but was not allowed to. So she stayed at home and brooded on the injustices of her life. Nor would her family allow her to leave him–so she stayed on and made unhappy, bitter comments like the one above.

Similarly, when the author was visiting the Christian Medical College, Vellore in July 2003, a case presentation was made. It was about a literate woman (educated till grade 10 and English-speaking to boot!) in a village who had given birth to third daughter. When her husband threatened to leave her she allegedly jumped into a well with her newborn infant. The child died, she survived. The question was—who was guilty for the child's death–she herself, her husband, her in-laws or the community—and whether the case should be reported, in which situation she would be found to be guilty of homicide. These are difficult questions to answer. We all know that the position of a woman with no son is intolerable. In fact, the *Artha Shastra* allows remarriage of a man if his wife fails to provide a male heir, and even states that women are only for getting sons.

The issue that we need to understand is—what is the situation of some of the women who go in for female foeticide? And what happens to girls who are not eliminated? This understanding is important because while foeticide is an unpleasant reality, we can only deal with it effectively once we realise the multiple pressures on, and the compulsions of many of the people who practise it. This realisation is required for us to carry on the war against foeticide at its different fronts. These stories therefore are not in support of female foeticide or infanticide but to unveil the multiple levels at which one needs to intervene to bring about changes in such a deep-rooted social phenomenon. They also illustrate the need to be non-judgmental and sensitive to the feelings and the dilemmas among people that lead to female foeticide and infanticide. It is these larger issues that need to be dealt with before we can make a dent in the problem. In such a situation, a technology that offers people the option to know the sex of their child, is bound to be misused. Today, access to ultrasound and abortion amongst the poor, and financial ability to pay for procedures for sex determination during pregnancy for the better-off, may also be promoting the purging of females. It is stated that abortions following amniocentesis accounted for 1 per cent of female foetuses conceived between 1981 and 1991–though no study has carried out a class differential on this procedure. Das Gupta and Bhat (1998) have concluded that 4.2 million female deaths, 0–4 years of age occurred in excess of those warranted by official figures, and that there was sex-selective abortion of 1.2 million female foetuses (cited in Banerjee and Jain 2001).

While the PNDT Act has been amended, it is important for us to also know just how many states have amended the statement in their state population policies that those families with more than two children should have negative incentives. Within an overall pressure for a two-child family in the present social environment, if women who have at least one daughter say they need to find out the sex of the foetus because they cannot afford to have more girls while trying to have a boy, what does one do? How can we regulate the private sector where most of the amniocentesis is being carried out? (Jesani 1998). How does one address a situation where despite their lack of logic, the utilitarian and social arguments still continue to thrive? The challenge lies in demolishing the subtle mechanisms of these victimising discourses (Arora 1996).

III

Examining Solutions Offered for Arresting Further Decline in Sex Ratios

Empowerment through Employment

Much has been written on the empowerment of women through employment. Ester Boserup has discussed how the status and standing of women are enhanced by economic independence and others have tried to link the neglect of girls to the higher economic returns for the family from boys. But a question that has been raised is whether it is female work force participation that enhances women's status, or is it areas where women have higher status that have higher numbers of employed women? (Banerjee and Jain 2001)

Policy measures suggested to empower women invariably consist of schemes of more work for them. There is much debate on this link between empowerment and work—for example the patterns of employment available to women and the status of this employment in society, duration and conditions of work, wages, etc. Trends and patterns in employment will thus indicate if any improvement in work conditions of women is occurring, that may in the long run, empower them and add value to their lives. On the other hand, some jobs may increase women's drudgery and exploitation and help maintain the *status quo*. Data from the 1991 Census and the 1996 NSSO reveals certain facts. While the Census did note an increase in female workers as compared to male workers this increase was in rural areas and in sub-contracted work (Kundu 1999). This indicates a pushing of women into the informal and marginal sector with worse conditions of work and decreasing work security. The increasing percentage of women in such labour could mean a situation where employers are not prepared to provide full-time employment. Thus the increase in irregular work for women could indicate their helplessness, and could be in the nature of a distress reaction (Mukhopadhahya 1999) and not a sign of their empowerment. Jhabwala and Sinha (2002) also show through studies that women's employment is adversely affected due to introduction of mechanisation, informalisation and casualisation and sub-contracting which brings their wages to barely Rs 500 per month whereas minimum wages are Rs 1,500. Kundu (1999), points out that even among women in regular work, it is noted that they earn 20 per cent less than male workers or only as much as male casual workers. Hence even an increase in regular women workers does not necessarily indicate higher wages or better working conditions for women.

The 1999–2000 NSSO data also show a decline in the worker population ratio especially for women. It also reveals that in the rural areas women have moved from transport-storage-communication to construction (Chadha and Sahu 2002). Chadha and Sahu also stated that the withdrawal of children and adolescents from the urban labour market is in favour of education. However, by means of a time use survey done in 1998–1999, Hirway (2002) has refuted this assumption. She states that this fall in worker population is actually a result of the increasing share of unpaid component of work. According to her, many workers, especially women, have withdrawn from the labour market and are taking up activities such as producing goods for home consumption, etc., which are all part of coping strategies. This, she states, seems to indicate deterioration in the quality of employment, i.e. an increased employment with low productivity and low wages and an increased burden on women who are carrying out unpaid, domestic work.

Bringing in New Legislations for PNDT

Additionally, we need to question our use of technology. There are two issues to be discussed here. Firstly, the ultra-sonogram can only tell the sex of the foetus around the age of five months after which abortion is illegal. It is thus through amniocentesis and chorionic villus biopsy that sex can be determined earlier and the cost of this is such that it is easier for the well-off rather than the poor to use it. We need to take cognisance of this fact as this agrees with the indications of decreasing 0–4/6 ratios amongst the better-off. This seems to point a finger at the private practitioners catering to this group. In addition we need to keep in mind the issue that if it is not a question of killing girls because of inability to feed them, our social and cultural norms need deeper examination if we want to stop this trend. After all the world average for FMR is 1045 and even higher in the more developed countries. But in India obviously economic development is not commensurate with social development and we need to study and understand this phenomenon.

Secondly, foeticide has been possible only because of the development of a certain kind of technology. This was a technology that was developed basically for eugenic reasons. Amniocentesis was introduced in India in 1975 by the All India Institute of Medical Sciences, and was designed and promoted for detecting abnormalities in the foetus. Interestingly, of the 11,000 couples who initially volunteered for the test, most were more interested in the sex of the child than the possibility of genetic abnormalities. Most women who had two or more daughters and learnt that the foetus was a female went on to have an abortion (Chhachhi and Sathyamala 1993 cited in Sudha and Rajan 1999). The Indian Council of Medical Research therefore ordered that the use of amniocentesis be restricted to suspected cases of genetic disease. The use of pre-natal sex diagnosis for the purpose of abortion was made a penal offence between 1977–1985. This ban on government clinics merely led to a commercialisation of technology, and private clinics with this facility, multiplied rapidly.

However, the conceptualisation behind a pre-natal determination test is eugenic and is an area for much ethical and philosophical debate. We also need to question the hypocrisy of a society that on one hand insists on using terms like 'differentially abled' to prevent discrimination against certain groups and on the other hand produces technology to destroy them. Is that very different from the custom of deifying the girl child on one hand and having a long history of female exploitation and elimination on the other? This is cultural iatrogenesis—an unwanted by-product of diagnostic and therapeutic progress where attempts at solutions become part of the problem—a self-reinforcing loop of negative institutional feedback, that Ivan

Illich (1976) called medical nemesis, that has occurred in response to medical hubris.

IV

Tackling the Problem _____

Our data has revealed that female elimination is not merely due to economic compulsions but that the problem is pervasive across class and region. It is rooted in our very culture and social, economic and political processes. Should we then not enlarge our debate to include these larger social, cultural and political issues that continue to affect the girl's life even if she survives? Interestingly this is the very period when some women are ostensibly being elected to posts in *panchayats*, and newspapers write eulogies on our women entrepreneurs. Simultaneously, Parliament continues to stall the reservation bill for women and we increasingly read about rape and other forms of violence towards women. These contradictory situations are extremely significant for they seem to indicate that actions of individual women, no matter how radical, cannot alter social values that are creating an entrenchment of a bias against women.

While groups are working at attempts to raise awareness on gender, the PNDT Act has also been amended. However, the contention of this paper is that while it is necessary, ultimately legislation is not sufficient to prevent female elimination. Nor can it be a substitute for cultural changes and consciousness raising at a countrywide level. Efforts to tackle this problem cannot be fragmented but need to be comprehensive. Not only do we have to tackle and control our technology, we need to improve the social position of women. There can, therefore, never be a simple approach to tackling this problem. The issue of female elimination cannot be witnessed in isolation from the social, cultural and economic context of people's lives. It is important to realise that one of the issues history has revealed is that this practice was embedded in many of the larger processes that increased the value of the male and devalued the female. While we need to question and tackle the poverty that can often push families into getting rid of daughters, we need to study in depth, the frightening new phenomenon that is rearing its head—the increasing elimination of the girl child in richer households. We need to question our very paradigm of development.

Notes

1. This primary data is from a study carried out by the author over a five-year period in the Gautam Nagar slum of Delhi on a sample of 50 per cent of the 3,000 households in the slum. Two hundred pregnant women from these selected households were followed up once a month from the fifth month of pregnancy onwards till six weeks after delivery. Data collected included information on women's daily lives, their employment patterns, their control over their bodies, as well as their perceptions and experience of pregnancy.

2. It is interesting that even Kerala that is so often held as a model of development and where there is said to be empowerment of women and gender equity, as indicated by lower fertility rates and high levels of female literacy, seems to have a 0–6 FMR lower than some other states!

3. Interestingly, when we talk of female deaths subsequent to the foetal or infancy stage, it is maternal mortality that moves centre stage. Data however reveals that amongst medically certified deaths in 1998, only 1.4 per cent of total female deaths were due to complications of pregnancy. About 17.4 per cent females died due to infectious and parasitic causes and 4.9 per cent died of anemia. Also 11.3 per cent died of suicides and 6.5 per cent died of burns, which would be mainly dowry related deaths, while 10.3 per cent died of causes originating in the perinatal period that can include female infanticide. (However, perinatal deaths increased from 8.2 per cent in 1996 to 10.3 per cent in 1998, which indicates increasing discrimination against the girl child.) GOI 2002.

4. The term elimination/female elimination has been used instead of female foeticide, female infanticide or even higher female mortality in later life to indicate female deaths that are due to women's secondary status in the family with its attendant disadvantages for survival.

5. I would like to clarify at this point that many upper class families share many of the compulsions of the poor women. The overall social pressures are in many ways similar for all women to a large degree. This is important as the reader must not assume from the stories related that it is only the poor who practise female foeticide.

6. However, we need to keep in mind that while the British may have mentioned this bias extensively, it has over time, existed in almost

all societies-including theirs. Interestingly, not only have women been always considered inferior to men and their contributions to work or otherwise trivialised, they have also been simultaneously worshipped and reviled.

7. In a situation of poverty, where survival is at stake, these women who believe that their only value is in sustaining their families, willingly forego their own needs. It is an irony of life, that the very social structures, culture and kinship patterns that form an integral part of the survival mechanism of the community in the slum, can be detrimental to the women, to the extent of affecting their existence. Patriarchy and the fight for survival leech the very life from these women's bodies.

8. The remaining 58 per cent are housewives. I have opted not to use the term unemployed for these women though they are not employed in financially remunerative work.

9. Seventeen households were interviewed twice, since the women in these households became pregnant twice. The advantage of this was that the statements of these seventeen households served as a method of checking if people's perceptions about the number of desired children changed with time. It was seen that responses were not dependent on the number of children they had. The answers the families therefore seemed to be giving when asked about the ideal family size and composition was a social response.

References

Agnihotri, S. B. 2000. *Sex Ratio Patterns in the Indian Population: A Fresh Exploration*. New Delhi: Sage.

Agnihotri, S. B. 2003. 'Survival of the Girl Child: Tunnelling out of the Chakravyuha', *Economic and Political Weekly*, 33 (41): 4351–60.

Arora, D. 1996. 'The Victimizing Discourse: Sex Determination Technologies and Policy', *Economic and Political Weekly*, 31 (7): 420–24.

Athreya, V. and Chukatha, R. S. 2000. 'Tackling Female Infanticide: Social Mobilization in Dahrmapuri 1997–1999', *Economic and Political Weekly*, 35 (49): 4345–48.

Banerjee, N. and D. Jain. 2001. 'Indian Sex Ratio Through Time and Space: Development from Women's Perspective', in Mazumdar, V. and N. Krishnaji (eds.), *Enduring Conundrum: India's Sex Ratio*, pp. 73–119. Delhi: Rainbow Publishers.

Chachhi, A. and C. Sathyamala. 1983. 'Sex Determination Tests: A Technology Which Will Eliminate Women', *Medico Friends Circle Bulletin*, 95: 3–5.

Chadha, G. K. and P. P. Sahu. 2002. 'Post Reform Setbacks in Rural Employment: Issues That Need Further Scrutiny', *Economic and Political Weekly*, 37 (21):1008–2026.

George, S. A. Rajaratnam. and B. D. Miller. 1992. 'Female Infanticide in Rural South India', *Economic and Political Weekly*, 27 (22): 1153–56.

Government of India. 1973. *Survey of Causes of Death (Rural): India Annual Report 1970*. New Delhi: Office of the Registrar General of India.
———. 1982. *Survey of Causes of Death (Rural): India Annual Report 1980*. New Delhi: Office of the Registrar General of India.
———. 1988. *National Plan Perspective for Women: 1988–2000*. pp. 97–111. Delhi: Department of Women and Child Development, Ministry of Human Resource Development.
———. 1992. *Survey of Causes of Death (Rural); India Annual Report 1990*. New Delhi: Office of the Registrar General of India.
———. 1996. *National Sample Survey Organization, Round 52*: July 1995–June 1996.
———. 1997. *Survey of Causes of Death (Rural); India Annual Report 1995*. New Delhi: Office of the Registrar General of India.
———. 2000. *National Sample Survey Organization, Round 55*: July 1999–June 2000.
———. 2002. *Survey of Causes of Death (Rural); India Annual Report 1998*. New Delhi: Office of the Registrar General of India.
———. 2003. *Provisional Population Totals, Paper I of Census 2001*. pp. 141–70. New Delhi: Registrar General and Census Commissioner of India.
Harriss-White, B. 1999. 'Gender Cleansing', in R. Sunder Rajan (ed.), *Gender Issues in Post Independent India*, pp. 124–53. New Delhi: Kali for Women.
Hirway, I. 2002. 'Employment and Unemployment Situation in the 1990's: How Good are NSS Data', *Economic and Political Weekly*, 37 (21): 2027–35.
Illich, I. 1976. *Limits of Medicine; Medical Nemesis: The Expropriation of Health*. London: Marion Boyars.
Jesani, A. 1998. 'Banning Pre-natal Sex Determination: The Scope and the Limits of the Maharashtra Legislation', in Lingam, L. (ed.), *Understanding Women's Health Issues: A Reader*, pp. 219–28. New Delhi: Kali for Women.
Jhabwala, R. and S. Sinha. 2002. 'Liberalization and the Woman Worker', *Economic and Political Weekly*, Review of Labour 37 (21): 2037–44.
Krishnaji, N. 2000. 'Trends in Sex Ratio: A Review in Tribute to Asok Mitra', *Economic and Political Weekly*, 35 (14): 1161–63.
Krishnaji, N. 2001. 'The Sex Ratio Debate', in V. Mazumdar and N. Krishnaji (eds.), *Enduring Conundrum: India's Sex Ratio*, pp. 33–34. Delhi: Rainbow Publishers.
Kundu, A. 1999. 'Trends and Pattern of Female Employment', in T. S. Papola and A. N. Sharma (eds), *Gender and Employment in India*, pp. 52–70. New Delhi: Vikas Publishing House.
Malobika. 1993. Girlhood in Rural Uttar Pradesh and its Implications for Health—*A Study of Two Villages in Allahabad District*. Unpublished M. Phil. Dissertation. New Delhi: Centre for Social-Medicine and Community Health, Jawaharlal Nehru University.
Mukhopadhyaya, S. 1999. 'Locating Women Within Informal Sector Hierarchies', in T. S. Papola and A. N. Sharma (eds.), *Gender and Employment in India*, pp. 206–22.New Delhi: Vikas Publishing House.
Premi, M. K. 2001. 'The Missing Girl Child', *Economic and Political Weekly*, 36 (21): 1875–80.

Sen, I. 2001. 'The Indian Sex Ratio: Patterns in Time and Space', in V. Mazumdar and N. Krishnaji (eds.), *Enduring Conundrum: India's Sex Ratio*, pp. 120–42. Delhi: Rainbow Publishers.

Siddhanta, S. D. Nandy. and S. B. Agnihotri. 2003. 'Sex Ratios and 'Prosperity Effect' What do the NSSO Data Reveal?', *Economic and Political Weekly*, 33 (41) October 11–17: 4381–4404.

Snehi, Y. 2003. 'Female Infanticide and Gender in Punjab: Imperial Claims and Contemporary Discourse', *Economic and Political Weekly*, 33 (41): 4302–05.

Sudha, S. and I. Rajan. 1999. 'Female Demographic Disadvantage in India 1981–1991: Sex-Selective Abortions and Female Infanticide', *Development and Change*, 30 (3): 585–618.

Swaminathan, M. A. Mangai, and S. Raja Samuel. 1998. 'Confronting Discrimination: Some Approaches to the Issue of Female Infanticide', *Search Bulletin*, 13 (3): 64–74.

The Times of India. 2003. New Delhi: 21 October, p. 1.

Viswanath, L. S. 1973. 'Female Infanticide Among the Lewa Kanbis of Gujarat in the Nineteenth Century', *The Indian Economic and Social History Review*, 10 (4): 386–404.

Health Policy, Plan and Implementation: The Role of Health Workers in Altering the Sex Ratio

7

Reema Bhatia

A sex ratio that is lower for women is an indicator of a socio-economic situation unfavourable to females. It indicates the ratio of women to men in a given population. The definition of sex ratio used here is the number of females per thousand males. A lower sex ratio is said to be indicative of a lower status for women. The reasons for a sex ratio that is unfavourable to females could be due to a greater undercount of females relative to males, greater emigration of females, more adverse mortality conditions for females than for males, and sex ratio at birth becoming more favourable to males than in the past (Premi 2001).

In the initial Census, a lower female count was attributed to an incomplete enumeration, particularly in the northern and north-western regions of the country. Premi (*ibid*) points out that differential male and female undercount has narrowed down from 1951, 1971, 1981, and 1991. He indicates that this reason is not substantial enough to explain the imbalance in the sex ratio. In addition, statistics on international migration for India are scarce and are not sufficient to explain the unfavourable sex ratio (*ibid*). In most populations, the world over, sex ratio is favourable to females. In India, South Asia, West Asia, and Africa, the situation is different. In India the overall sex ratio has been favourable to males, and since 1901 the sex ratio has fallen from 972 to 933 in 2001 (Government of India 2002 a).

The state has sought to overcome these imbalances by seeking to empower the disadvantaged. The policies, plans and legal measures of the government are a statement of this intent. It becomes the social and moral responsibility of the state to try and rectify these imbalances. Since a sex ratio unfavourable to women is attributed to poor health of women (among other things), interventions in the sphere of health are one of the ways through which the government seeks to improve the status of women.

This paper focuses on the manner in which the government intervenes through the health services in the rural areas in the state of Punjab and the impact of this on the number of women. Punjab is one of the most prosperous states of India. In 1996–97 Punjab had a per capita net state domestic product of Rs 18,1213 at current prices; second only to Goa. Only 12 per cent of the total population of Punjab is below the poverty line. The figure for India is 36 per cent. Agriculture is the single largest sector of the economy with 83.5 per cent of the total geographical area under cultivation (International Institute of Population Sciences 2001). In addition, Punjab is a patriarchal and patrilineal society. An agricultural economy is indicative of a society with son preference.

Given the predominantly agriculture based economy, the economic prosperity of Punjab and the nature of kinship relationships, it is critical to examine the extent to which the implementation of the health programmes has imbibed the intent and objective of the health policies and the Primary Health Care approach adopted by the Government of India in 1978. The focus would be on examining the implementation of the programmes in the field, by the health workers in the backdrop of patriarchy and economic prosperity. The paper examines the implementation of the policies and plans only in as much as they are relevant to the issues being discussed. The paper does not comment on the sex ratio as a technical aspect. The paper is based on data collected through intensive fieldwork for about eighteen months in a Primary Health Centre, in Roopnagar district in Punjab.

Health Programmes Relevant to Women's Reproductive Health

The path that India set out for herself for attaining health for all, envisioned a hierarchical referral system imparting health care to the people. The health services sector in India functions in the context of the Primary Health Care approach. Planning for health services started with the planning era in 1951. The broad objectives of the policy of health care delivery system are to provide universal coverage and to enable the whole population to have access to the services. It aims at providing comprehensive, preventive, curative, and rehabilitative health services for those who require them. To ensure that services from primary to specialised level are accessible to all, decentralisation is emphasised. Such a health care is to be provided through a health team composed of health professionals, administrative, technical and paramedical staff.

Interventions in the sphere of health are through health programmes directed specifically towards women, viz: Maternal and Child Health Services, Reproductive and Child Health Project (RCH) and the Family Welfare Programme. The programmes aim at providing complete and adequate care to women in terms of their reproductive health. The Family Welfare programme aims at providing better MCH services to women, encourage institutional deliveries and spacing between children. Since 1996 the Target-Free Approach has been introduced and it has been renamed as the Community Need Assessment Approach (CNAA) from 1997. The aim is to encourage decentralised participatory planning. The Universal Immunisation Programme (UIP) aims at achieving universal immunisation and reducing the mortality and morbidity resulting from vaccine preventable diseases. With effect from 1992, the Child Survival and Safe Motherhood Programme, with the assistance of World Bank and UNICEF, has been introduced to supplement the gains of the UIP. Iron and folic acid tablets are being regularly supplied to mothers and children. The RCH project funded by the World Bank aims at looking after the reproductive health of women and encouraging the participation of women in planning for their own health. The World Bank Project aided India Population Project–VII was started in 1991 to improve the quality of Family Welfare and MCH services in the state by providing trained manpower and buildings for both imparting training and for the working environment and residences within the villages.

These programmes are not merely restricted to the curative aspect but are also directed towards health education. The health education component of these programmes is addressed by the Information, Education & Communication Activities (IEC). Through health education, the government aims to positively intervene in improving the status of women in the sphere of family planning and maternal and reproductive health. There has been an improvement in living conditions and medical facilities throughout the country. This has led to a greater survival of both males and females. However, in spite of programmes directed specifically to women's health, the sex ratio indicates a situation unfavourable to females. The National Health Programmes being implemented by the Directorate of Family Welfare in Punjab are given below:

Family Welfare Programme

It is a 100 per cent centrally sponsored programme. The National Health Policy aims at stabilising the growth of population and for that purpose the goals have been set to curtail both fertility and mortality so as to achieve a Net Reproduction Rate of unity. The Government of India has implemented the target-free approach towards family planning from the year 1996–97. There are no specific targets for various methods of family planning but family planning services have to be provided to the public as per their requirements. An action plan has been prepared to motivate the couples for family planning through spacing and the use of terminal methods in the age group of 20–29 years with low parity.

In order to provide better MCH services all pregnant women are required to be registered for ante-natal care; high-risk mothers are to be referred for better care; institutional deliveries are to be encouraged; high-risk babies are to be referred to institutions for treatment.

In order to take health services beyond the pursuit of targets the Government of India introduced the Target Free Approach (TFA) all over India on 1st April 1996 and under the system of decentralised participatory planning. TFA has been renamed as Community Needs Assessment Approach (CNAA) from 1997. Under this approach, planning of family welfare services will be formulated in consultation with the community at the grassroot level. Decentralised participatory planning implicates close association of the community and its opinion leaders such as *Village Pradhans, Mahila Swasthya Sanghs*, primary school teachers etc., in the formulation of the PHC-based family welfare and health care plan. Each state has to prepare an Annual Action Plan in the beginning of each year and circulate it at various levels (GOI 2002 b).

Universal Immunisation Programme

In 1974 the WHO launched the 'Expanded Programme on Immunisation (EPI)' against six most common preventable childhood diseases viz. Diphtheria, Pertusis, Tetanus, Measles, Tuberculosis and Poliomyelitis. The UNICEF, in 1985, renamed it as 'Universal Child Immunisation' (UCI). There is no difference between the two, the goal was the same i.e. to achieve universal immunisation by 1990. The government of India launched the EPI in 1978 with the aim of reducing the mortality and morbidity resulting from vaccine-preventable diseases and to achieve self-sufficiency in the production of vaccines. UIP was started in India in 1985. It has two components; immunisation of pregnant women against tetanus and immunisation of children against the six EPI target diseases. The aim was to achieve 100 per cent coverage of pregnant women with two doses of tetanus toxoid (or a booster dose) and at least 85 per cent coverage of infants with three doses each of DPT and OPV and one dose each of BCG and the measles vaccine by 1990.

The department of health, Punjab is trying to immunise all newborn infants against the above six preventable diseases. Immunisation days have been fixed and services are provided through the health care delivery system on these days.

The strategies to eradicate poliomyelitis include strengthening routine vaccination coverage and supplementing routine immunisation services with National Immunisation Days, i.e. Pulse Polio Immunisation. In the first phase, pulse polio immunisation days were observed on 9th December, 1995 and 20th January, 1996. Punjab too was a part of the nationwide campaign. The aim is to immunise children up to 5 years of age against Polio. The campaign is held regularly every year on pre- fixed National Immunisation Days.

Maternal & Child Health Services (MCH)

MCH services are provided for the health and care of mothers and children. The government provides these services by organising prenatal and well baby clinics. The small family norm is propagated through home visits and by ascertaining the confidence on the survival of a few but healthy children. With effect from 1992 Child Survival and Safe Motherhood Programme, with the assistance of

World Bank and UNICEF, has been introduced to supplement the gains of the UIP. Regular supply of iron and folic acid tablets for mothers and children is being made. Vitamin A solution is being administered twice a year to children upto three years of age so as to prevent night blindness. Efforts are being made to control diarrhoea and Acute Respiratory Infections (ARI) through the distribution of ORS packets and through efforts to control pneumonia. The programme is introduced as part of the overall strategy to reduce infant mortality to below 60 per 1,000 live births, childbirth to below 10 per 1,000 population, reduction of percentage of low-birth-weight babies to less than 10 per cent and maternal mortality to below two per 1,000 live births by the year 2000.

Reproductive & Child Health Project (RCH Project)

The RCH Project, funded by the World Bank, was launched in the ninth plan period. The Project has three major components:

a) Decentralised Participatory Planning,
b) Institutional Strengthening,
c) Programme Implementation Enhancing.

These components are being implemented in the state on two tiers:

a) District sub-project for Sangrur District,
b) State-wide component.

The main objectives of the project are:

a) Provision of family planning services in terms of access and choice;
b) Prevention and management of unwanted pregnancies;
c) Intervention to reduce infant mortality;
d) Prevention and management of Reproductive Tract Infection (RTI) and Sexually Transmitted Infections (STI);
e) Establishment of effective referral and follow up services.

World Bank Projects

The World Bank Project aided India Population Project–VII, was started in 1991 in Punjab. The project meant to improve the quality of Family Welfare and MCH services in the state by providing trained manpower and buildings, both for imparting training and for the working environment and residences within the villages. Under the project Sub-Centre buildings, Lady Health Visitor residential quarters, PHC training annexes have been built.

Information, Education & Communication (IEC) Activities

The Director, Health Services, Family Welfare is responsible for state wide planning, implementing and monitoring of Family Welfare, UIP (including Pulse Polio immunisation), MCH, World Bank Project and Primary School Health Check-up Campaign. The director is supported with a statewide IEC organisation, which starts from the grassroots with the *Mahila Swasthya Sanghs* (MSS) and is officially managed by IEC professionals from block to state level. The IEC component of the family welfare programme uses newspapers, radio, television, and all other means of communication to support community participation.

20-Point Programme

In addition to the five-year plans and programmes, in 1975 the government of India initiated a special twenty-point programme. The programme was described as an agenda for national action to promote social justice and economic growth. On 20th August, 1986 the existing programme was restructured. The government spelt out its objectives as 'eradication of poverty, raising productivity, reducing inequalities, removing social and economic disparities and improving quality of life.'

At least three of the twenty points are related directly or indirectly to health. These are:

a) Health for all;
b) Two-child norm;
c) Expansion of education.

There are thus at least seven programmes that are directed towards women's health directly or indirectly.

I

The various health care programmes are to be carried out at all levels of the health care delivery system. The articulation of the policies and plans takes place at the level of the union and state government and various other planning and advisory bodies. The allocation of resources, the setting of priorities and goals are all articulated at this level. These decisions are then conveyed to the secondary level of the health care delivery system i.e. the district authorities. A mere articulation of policies and plans and allocation of resources is meaningless unless they reach the people and the community. The community is the ultimate beneficiary of this entire planning and implementation process. It is at the level of the community that the primary level of health care is the most vital. It is at the primary level that the health care services are delivered through a network of Community Health Centres (CHC), Primary Health Centres (PHC), Subsidiary Health Centres (SHC), and Sub-Centres (SC). The intent of the state is conveyed through these programmes at various levels to ensure an equitable all round healthy development of all women.

Staff to provide health care at the paramedical level was introduced as and when the various vertical disease control programmes[1] were introduced. The health workers in their present form were introduced on the recommendations of the Kartar Singh Committee Report in 1977 (GOI 1973). The scheme was adopted in the Sixth Plan period (1978–1983).

At the lowest level in the health services sector is the Multipurpose Health Worker (MPW). Each health worker looks after a population of 5,000 people. The health workers operate from a sub-centre located in a village. Each sub-centre looks after four to five villages. The sub-centres are under the Primary Health Centre (PHC), which looks after a rural population of 30,000. The policy and the plan documents have visualised the workers as implementing the programmes by staying with the people of the sub-centre area and becoming one of them. These workers are meant to be staying in the sub-centres in the villages. Their duty structure is such that they are implementers of all the national health programmes. The health workers posted at the sub-centre go from door to door imparting health care to the people in the rural areas. The MPW health workers scheme was conceptualised in a manner to ensure that they provide health services to the people in an integrated manner. The worker is supposed to identify and treat people suffering from TB, malaria, goitre, sprains, leprosy etc. The identification of the person suffering from any disease, the initial treatment, and then, if need be, the final decision to refer the patient are all the official responsibilities of the MPW. In addition, he is also meant to educate the community about healthy living. In short, he is responsible for the health (mental, physical and emotional), of the 5,000 people living in his sub-centre area.

In the field, it becomes difficult to supervise the workers as they do not sit in one place but are constantly on the move as per their schedule. After training, the workers are posted to a sub- centre and they are then expected to build a rapport with the community, live within the community and discharge their duties. The workers carry out their duties by touring the areas under the sub-centre on a daily basis. This involves visiting thirty to thirty five homes by the ANM (Auxiliary Nursing Mother) and 100–120 homes by the male worker on all working days. This means that the ANM comes back to the same house after two months and the male worker revisits the same house after fifteen days. Nowhere else in the health hierarchy in the urban as well as in the rural areas does anybody come into such a close contact with the people on a daily and prolonged basis. In the policy and plan documents they are envisioned as the foundation of the entire structure of the health services in India. In a sense, they are the torch-bearers of India's vision of Health for All. They thus form a very vital link in the chain for imparting health care to the people.

Given their importance in India's vision, it is important to study the workers. Hence, the paper focuses on these health workers (men and women) and the manner in which they implement the various health programmes in the field. Is their implementation in the spirit of the noble intent of promoting equality of both sexes or do they get implemented in a mutated and modified form? Such an analysis becomes important given the dismal sex ratio of 874 (as per the 2001 Census) females per thousand males in Punjab. This is lower than the sex ratio of 882 in 1981 and is lower than the sex ratio of 933 (GOI 2001) for the country as a whole. Analysis of the sex ratio in the sphere of health may help to pinpoint some of the causes for the lower number of women in all age groups in North India. It is only by identification of the shortcomings that viable solutions can be found.

II

Factors Influencing the Implementation of the Programmes _____

Thrust on Targets

An examination of the manner in which the programmes get implemented in the field revealed that the Family Welfare Programme, to
a large extent, is the major one that is carried out in the field at the
cost of all other programmes. The other programmes that get implemented to some extent are those for which targets have been set. The
health personnel at all levels admit the fact that the entire thrust of
the health care services at the village level is confined to the achievement of targets; targets that have been set for family planning,
immunisation and making of malaria slides by the male workers.
The entire focus of their beat programme too is on pursuing these
targets. The performance of the worker is judged on the basis of his/
her targets met. The entire effort of the worker is directed towards
meeting targets at the cost of the rest of the health services. The
target-based approach meant that health care services have been
reduced to the pursuit of targets.

Since the worker's job involves extensive touring of the rural
areas it becomes difficult to monitor his/her work. It becomes difficult for the superiors to judge the worker's performance on the basis
of his interaction with the people on his beat programme. The difficulty stems from the fact that for the doctors or health superiors to
assess the workers' performance it is necessary for them to tour with
the workers, which is physically a difficult task. They have to also
work out the logistics in a way that the workers are present in the
village at the time of the check. The worker can always claim to have
just left the village to meet a prospective client for sterilisation. The
only way that a worker's performance can be assessed is through the
targets achieved by him/her. A good worker is one who achieves his
targets and a bad worker is one who is unable to achieve his targets.
There are no other reliable criteria to judge the workers as being good
or bad. Since the yearly reports are submitted in April, family planning is popular from September to March. There is generally a rush
to get as many cases as possible during this period.

The workers who do not achieve their targets are liable to be penalised. Penalties included public reprimands at the monthly PHC meetings and extreme measures like withholding or cutting of pay and spoiling of annual reports of the workers with less number of cases.

There was thus a fierce competition among workers for their cases of sterilisation. Workers were very careful to guard their case so that nobody else could encroach and make it their own. There were bitter fights and arguments in case this did happen.

As far as the temporary methods of family planning like copper-T, oral pills and condoms were concerned, there was an unwritten and unspoken acknowledgement of the fact that most of the data was fabricated. Many workers, in fact, felt that temporary methods of family planning should be excluded from their duty list since they constituted nothing more than figures to be cooked up for their reports. The workers neither advocated spacing between children through the use of temporary methods nor was it an option, which was acceptable to the average villager. People in any case did not adopt any temporary methods for family planning till they had the desired family composition, which necessarily included at least two sons. Temporary methods of family planning were never a real option in the minds of the workers. In reality, the workers only promoted sterilisation as the method of family planning.

There was a feeling among the workers that since their work was informally evaluated in terms of the number of cases they had, it should be made formal, and their promotions should be on this basis. One ANM went so far as to say that there was no need to do any work at all as it really boiled down to the number of 'cases' each worker had. It was not too difficult to get cases since they could be had for a price from the General Hospital.

The phrase, 'family planning' was, at an informal level, just another term for sterilisation. In order to achieve targets workers advocate female foeticide because if the desired family size and composition is met then it is easier to persuade women to go in for sterilisation.

Informal Targets

Even though the target-free approach has been adopted, there continues to be an emphasis on targets. A communication from the Civil Surgeons Office at the district headquarters to the PHC in 1996–97, states that in order to bring down the CBR by one unit per thousand population per year, the performance should be of the order of: Sterilisation: thirty-six per year and IUD: sixty per year, in a population of 5,000. It further states,

> Since the authenticity of the data available is not very high, it is worthwhile to give sufficient grace/margin to the performance to account for this factor. Based on this formula and the safety margin given, the expected level of achievement for the district should be twenty-four per year of sterilisation and forty per year of IUD in a population of 5,000. Of course, these methods will be supported by two other spacing methods, which are quite popular, i.e. oral pills and use of conventional contraceptive. It is further supplemented by MTP services where again elimination of one birth per MTP is ensured. During the year 1995–96, a total of 2,006 MTPs were done. (Government of Punjab 1997).

This was categorically conveyed to the workers by the Senior Medical Officer of the PHC and the District Family Planning Officer (DFPO) at a meeting held at the PHC to explain the target free approach to the workers. To achieve the targeted birth rate it was important for them to achieve the sterilisation target of three to four per month or thirty six in a year and sixty copper-Ts in a year, that is five in a month. It was also conveyed to them that some emphasis was also to be given to temporary methods of family planning since they were equally important. The reaction on the part of the workers as far as the target-free approach was concerned was that things continued to be the same as far as their work is concerned. They felt that nothing had changed except that they were now more liable to be pulled up for non-achievement of the 'targets'. The emphasis on targets continued to be verbally conveyed to the workers. The feeling amongst the workers was that their task had become more difficult since the cases now had to belong to their area of operation. This, in effect, meant that the workers could now no longer buy motivation slips registering them as the motivators for sterilisation from the General Hospital; they would now have to meet the targets from within their own sub-centre area.

III

By introducing the target-free approach and by emphasising that the targets have to be from the sub-centre area of the worker the government is trying to ensure two things. Firstly, it is trying to ensure that the worker in the field genuinely tries to control fertility by temporary methods of family planning. Secondly, by limiting the cases to the area of the worker, the government is further trying to put a stop to the corrupt practice of buying false motivation slips to falsely show the worker as the motivator for a particular sterilisation. At an informal and oral level, the SMO at a monthly meeting conveyed to the workers that in reality it was sterilisation, which would help them to achieve the desired rates.

Cultural Framework

As per the official discourse, the rules say that the workers should work towards promoting a family with two children only. The workers on the other hand, by virtue of being a part of the same patriarchal society, have modified and negotiated the rules to fit in with the fertility behaviour and desires of the people. It is within the context of this culturally-determined fertility behaviour framework that the workers try to meet their targets for family planning and sterilisation.

In a patriarchal society like Punjab, where descent and succession is through the males, a son is very important. Sons are considered assets for their parents whereas daughters are a burden (Hershman 1981). Sons are considered as a support in old age, as a means of salvation. According to mythology, cremation at the hands of a son ensures a direct passage to heaven. On the other hand, a daughter is considered a burden. A daughter's marriage entails dowry giving which is an economic burden on the parents. After marriage, she goes to live with her husband and his family and the parents have no rights over her fertility. A son on the other hand continues to stay with his parents. His marriage brings in dowry into the family. His bride, i.e. the daughter-in-law, produces a male heir to carry forward the name of the lineage. Typically, within a year of marriage a woman's childbearing years start. Her childbearing years continue till she bears a minimum of two male children. The number of children she has is not important, what is important is the number of male children she bears. The interval between children too is dependent on the number of male children she has. If the last child borne is a male then the birth interval for the next child is longer. If the last child borne is a girl then the attempt for the next child starts almost immediately. Her child-bearing decisions are not hers. Her husband and in-laws make decisions for her. In addition, the male child, till he reaches a certain age, is considered vulnerable to supernatural dangers, hence he is surrounded by a number of superstitious beliefs. He has to be protected from the evil eye.

A woman is considered to be unestablished in her husband's lineage until and unless she bears male children. It is through a son that a woman is secure in her in-laws' house. A son is the key to a woman's establishment in her husband's descent group. In Punjabi kinship, a son is considered to be very important for the continuation of the lineage. In the event of a woman becoming a widow without any male heirs, she is sent back to her natal home. She is not given any share of her husband's property. His property is in fact divided among his collateral. In the event of the widow having sons of the right age, she may gain control of the estate. In some cases a woman is known to adopt the son of her sister and in extreme cases even an uxorilocal son-in-law. The first-born is surrounded with a lot of taboos, since he is prone to mystical dangers. Special care is taken to ward off the evil eye during the time of the first three to five years of his life.

A look at the profile of a village under the PHC somewhat underlines the importance of a male child. As per the Anganwadi Worker's register the village had a population of 983 with 509 males and 474 females. The sex ratio for the village as a whole is 931. Out of a total of 113 households, there are 24.7 per cent Jat households and the number of Scheduled Caste (Harijans, Jhoors and Valmiks) households is 75.22 per cent. Thus the majority of the population is of Scheduled Castes. The age and sex-wise population of children in the village is given in Table 7.1.

Table 7.1
Children in the Village by Age and Sex

Age Groups	Boys	Girls	Total
0–6 Months	10 (52.63)	9 (47.36)	19 (13.47)
6 Months–1 Year	10 (62.5)	6 (37.5)	16 (11.34)
1–3 Years	38 (67.8)	18 (32.14)	56 (39.7)
3–6 Years	31 (62)	19 (38)	50 (35.46)
Total	89 (63.12)	52 (36.87)	141 (100)

Note: Figures in brackets indicate percentages.

From Table 7.1 what emerges is that the maximum number of children are in the age group of 1–3 years followed by the age group of 3–6 years. The number of boys in all the age groups is higher than the number of girls. The sex ratio (i.e. the number of women per 1,000 males) for the above age groups is 584 in the village. In all the age group categories of children, the caste-wise break up is presented in Table 7.2.

A comparison of Table 7.2 with Table 7.1 indicates that for 85 Scheduled Caste households (Harijans, Valmiks and Jhoors) there are 119 pre-school children. This means that there are 1.4 pre-school

Table 7.2
Caste-wise Distribution of Children by Age

Age Groups	Scheduled Castes	Others	Total
0–6 Months	16 (84.2)	3 (15.78)	19 (13.47)
6 Months–1 Year	16 (100)	0 (0)	16 (11.34)
1–3 Years	45 (80.35)	11 (19.64)	56 (39.7)
3–6 Years	42 (84)	8 (16)	50 (35.46)
Total	119 (84.39)	22 (15.6)	141 (100)

Note: Figures in brackets indicate percentages.

children per household. For the 28 Jat households there are 22 pre-school children, which means that there are 0.7 children per household. This indicates that the number of pre-school children per Jat household is half of the number of pre-schoolers in scheduled caste households. This is significant in the light of the lower number of girls as compared to the number of boys amongst the pre-school children.

IV

Given the importance of the son in a family it is but natural that the health workers are not looked at in a positive light. This is truer since the primary task carried out by the workers is that of family planning. The workers are therefore not viewed positively; they are known as the 'bacha band karanwale' or child stoppers. The MPWs tend to target the eligible couples i.e. the men and women in the age group of 16 years to 45 years. Sons and son-bearing is surrounded by a lot of superstitions and taboos. Any suggestions to stop child bearing particularly in the absence of a son are therefore considered to be inauspicious. A woman's position is jeopardised without a son. Any number of daughters, even after many years of marriage' does not secure her position in the house. In such a scenario, even the thought of trying to stop the birth of a son is fraught with dangers and supernatural sanctions. The senior kinswomen exercise complete control over her fertility. They frown upon any attempts to control her fertility. They resort to all means to dissuade the MPWs. They range from name calling to shooing away the workers. Some young women in the village do adopt temporary methods of family planning but this is very rare, generally without the consent of the senior kinswomen and on the sly. But given the low status of the daughter-in-law in the family, particularly if she is a new entrant to the family, there is a tendency to avoid doing things that would jeopardise their already vulnerable status.

The health of women is not of any concern to anyone, including the women themselves. There is only one aspect of a woman's health that is important and that is her son-bearing. Other aspects of a woman's health are invisible. The only time her health is important is after son-bearing. In case a daughter is born, she starts her chores the very next day. Her guilt-ridden conscience does not let her rest beyond a day or so. It is only after bearing a son that she can legitimately rest. Psychologically too, she is at rest that the guilt of having borne a daughter does not rest heavy on her conscience.

There are generally no voluntary cases of sterilisation. The cases are motivated through repeated visits. It generally takes three to four years to motivate a case. In the process another child or two may be born. Some women adopted temporary methods of family planning, generally on the advice of the workers or on the advice of a satisfied, known female user. Temporary methods are adopted only if they have the requisite number of sons (while they made up their minds to go in for sterilisation) or while they wait for their sons to grow up to a safe age.

Given the kind of supernatural sanctions and beliefs that surround the male child and the preferred family composition, the workers have to be cautious in their approach. The health workers first gauge whether the desired family size and composition has been achieved or not. It is only then that they approach the prospective client. They have to be careful not to be considered as casting an evil eye on the male child.

The workers too do not approach couples for sterilisation, till they have a minimum of two sons. The workers feel that sons are very important and it would not be right for them to approach a couple till their family is 'complete' with sons. The workers sympathised with this need and in fact did not advocate fertility control to those who did not have the requisite number of boys. In reality, they only target those people who already have two sons above five years old. The workers too felt that the need for two sons was very valid. The poorer families compromised at one son if they had three to four daughters. The few Muslim families in the area did not accept family planning at all, as it went against their religious beliefs. As one worker put it, 'The government should think of the futility of family planning. Without a male child, there is no point in asking them to undergo sterilisation. "Operations" should only be carried out after two to three male children. The slogan for family planning should be for three children.'

V

The health workers' family composition also reflected the same belief. Their own family composition is the same as that of the people they serve (Table 7.1). They practise what they preach. They preach limiting family size by MTPs and sex selection. The health workers themselves and their family members too follow the same practices.

Table 7.3
Number of Children of the MPWs

Number of children	Male MPWs	Female MPWs	Total
Zero daughters	1 (6.25)	5 (22.7)	6 (14.6)
1 Daughter	5 (31.25)	4 (18.18)	9 (21.9)
2 Daughters	5 (31.25)	4 (18.18)	9 (21.9)
More than 2 daughters	4 (25)	5 (22.7)	9 (21.9)
0 Sons	2 (12.5)	1 (4.5)	3 (7.3)
1 Son	4 (25)	7 (31.8)	11 (26.8)
2 Sons	5 (31.2)	6 (27.27)	11 (26.8)
More than 2 sons	1 (6.25)	1 (4.5)	2 (4.8)

Note: The percentages have been calculated out of a total of 41 married workers (19 male and 22 female workers).

An analysis of Table 7.3 shows that out of 41 married workers, 26.8 per cent have one or two sons. An equal number of workers have one or two daughters. All the workers have sons and those who do not have sons have not yet adopted methods of family planning. None of the male workers follow the two-child family norm that they are supposed to propagate to the public as part of their duties. Seven workers have two or more than two sons. All these workers also have a minimum of one daughter. Two male workers have more than two daughters and four of them have two daughters. As far as the female workers are concerned, eight of the female workers have two children. Of these eight, two have daughters only. Out of these two, one has not yet adopted any method of family planning since she intends to have another child as she put it '*Rab di mehar rahi taan agli baar munda hoyega. Ik munda taan hona chahida hai*' (If God is kind, next time I will have a son. There should be at least one son).

As far, as the other six are concerned, two have one son and one daughter, the other four have two sons only and no daughters. As far as the other ANMs are concerned, eleven of them have more than two daughters and one son. Three ANMs have been married for the past two years and have only one child, two have one daughter, and one has one son. These ANMs have not yet completed their families. The above data shows that the majority of the workers do not practise the two-child family norm that they are supposed to propagate to the public. None of the male workers has only two children. All of them by their own admission felt the need for having sons, irrespective of the number of daughters they have in the process. Some of them felt the need to have a minimum of two sons; 31.2 per cent had two sons and 6.2 per cent have more than two sons. At least some of the female workers who have two sons admitted to having used the ultrasound technique to determine the sex of the foetus. They also admitted to having undergone MTPs when the foetus was a female one. They have also taken some 'medicines' for having a male child.

As far as the number of children is concerned, none of the male MPWs have only two children and eight of the ANMs have only two children. The majority of them have a minimum of two sons.

One of the ANMs, who has daughters, had recently returned from maternity leave after the second daughter. Almost all the male and female health workers, including the Block Extension Educator (BEE), sympathised with her for having borne a second daughter.

They also remonstrated with her for being foolish enough not to use the latest technology (i.e. the ultrasound technique), when she herself was in the same field. As one of the male workers put it:

Asi koi lokaan to judaan taan nahin. Asi samajh sakde hain mundey kinne jaroori han. Sarkar sanu kahandi hai ki kaho do bachhe hone chaida han. Vaise taan aey gal galat taan nahin. Agar vakhiya jaye taan ajkal de jamane vich do bache apni pasand de hone koi mushkal taan nahin. Ajkal taan ultrasound karana badi hi sokhi gal hai. (We are not different from the people we serve. We can understand how important it is to have sons. The government asks us to say, have two children. This is not an incorrect thing to propagate. On the other hand, come to think of it, it is not difficult to have two children of your choice in today's world. These days it is very easy to get ultrasounds done.)

Another ANM had stopped family planning motivation altogether since one of her 'case' had lost both sons in an accident. She felt morally responsible for it since the lady could not have any more sons, since she had undergone tubectomy (she had two daughters). To quote the ANM,

Lokaan de bache koi sade ghar khaan taan nahin aande. Asi onahan nun bache rokan layi kyon kahiya. Rab ton dar ke rahna chaihda hai. Mundey tan sade honde han, budhapey de sahara han. Kudiyaan taan parayi hundiaan han, byah kar chali jaaniyaan hain. Main taan bahut galt kita, oda operation vi karaat ta, hun o' chah kar vi mundey nu janam nahi de sakdi. Casean di ki hai, apne case pure karan de hor vi tarikey han. Asi tan sollanh sector de aspatal to case kharid lende han. Koi mushkal nahin, sab kar de han. (Peoples' children don't come to our house to eat. Why should we tell them to stop children? One should be God-fearing. Sons are your own; they are the support for your old age. Girls are not yours, after marriage they leave. I made a big mistake in getting her operated, now even though she wants sons she cannot bear them. Cases are not a problem; there are other ways to complete my 'cases'. I go to the hospital and buy 'cases' from the government hospital. It is not difficult, everyone does it.)

This means that the ANM felt that the health workers were not responsible for bringing up other people's children. The workers should not propagate family planning as it was against God's will. He (God) who gives will also provide. For those clients of her sub-centre area, who had a minimum of two children (inclusive of one daughter), she recommended sex-determination and sex-selection of the foetus through ultrasounds and abortion of the female foetus.

These quotes illustrate that the workers do not feel it is correct to propagate the two-child norm. On the other hand, they do feel that planning a two-child family, with only male children was possible. It was possible through sex determination tests. In case the foetus was a female, then one could go in for abortions. Some workers felt that because of family planning their respect had gone down. She felt that asking people to limit the size of the family was an amoral practice. They could not ask people to stop having children if they do not have sons. The worker felt that sons are an important part of the family, daughters after marriage, in any case, go to their husbands' homes. Daughters cannot compensate for the loss of a son. The family composition of the female workers shows that their independent economic status has not translated into social independence. The women workers continue to attach importance to a son. Their attitude and their fertility decisions and behaviour are very significant since they themselves are meant to educate the population about the importance of family planning and the equality of the male and the female child. For the female worker, economic independence and an occupational status (in the health sector) have not made a difference in their own family composition and planning.

VI

Middle Path

The workers have negotiated the bureaucratic rules by finding a middle path. They have adapted their operational styles in a way that has modified the governmental definition of family planning from limiting fertility to limiting the number of girl children.

In the field the only programme that actually gets carried out is the family planning programme (and not the family welfare programme). The phrase 'family planning' means two things. For the government it means controlling fertility by limiting the number of children to two, irrespective of the sex of the children. For the people and the workers too it means planning families, but in a different way. It means having a minimum of two sons. For the latter category, it does not mean controlling fertility by limiting the number of children to two. The majority of the workers feel that a family size of three children is a comfortable one. Having one daughter in the quest for two sons is acceptable or one son and two daughters are also tolerable. The workers do not feel that there is anything wrong with foeticide. They empathise with the people and identify themselves with their thinking. As one of the workers said, 'we are not different from the people whom we serve'. All the workers try to help those couples that have daughters and have been unable to bear sons. They guide them about the 'effective methods' of getting sons. The workers empathise with the need for having sons. Some quotes from the villagers further emphasise the widespread practice of female foeticide.

> A Saini Mother-in-law: When my daughter-in-law was pregnant for the second time then the ANM came to us and said that she knew a doctor in a town near the PHC who could tell us if the child was a male child or not. She then took my daughter-in-law and me to Mohali for a test. The child was a boy. She now comes to us and tells us to get the operation done.

> Pregnant Jat lady: When I was pregnant for the third time the ANM told me to get a test done. I went to a town near the PHC for the test. Since it was a girl I got it removed. I already have two daughters.

As we have seen, above approximately 39 per cent of the workers have two or more male children. All the male workers have more than two children and only eight out of the 25 ever-married female workers have only two children. Only two male workers and four female workers had no sons. Their families were not yet complete and none of them by their own admission was using any method of family planning, i.e. they were still trying for sons. All the other workers had a minimum of one son (27 per cent had only one son). The workers, on the other hand, are also aware of the two-child norm, which they are supposed to propagate as a part of their official duties. The workers have found a middle path between the need to have sons and the need to limit the family size.

Participation in MTP and Sex Selection (Corrupt Practices)

At an unofficial and informal level, sex determination of the unborn foetus through ultrasounds and subsequent MTP of the female foetuses had emerged as a popular method of family planning. Depending on the economic standing of the family, the workers on their own initiative, recommended various techniques to have sons. These vary from 'safe scientific' techniques like ultrasounds to determine the sex of the foetus to religious techniques like visiting holy men such as the 'Sant in Niholka' and going to quacks for abortions.

To quote one ANM 'All intelligent people get ultrasounds done'. However, this was an option that was available only to the higher income groups. It was fast becoming popular among the land-owning Jat families. The workers reported that there were normally two to three ultrasounds and MTPs per month, per sub-centre. Subsequent to MTP, people get their names deleted from the list of pregnant ladies. The ideal family composition according to the workers is further dependent on the economic status of the family. They feel that poor families in which there is limited income and that too, in most cases, is dependent on daily wages; it was not possible to plan families through sex-selection tests. At times in the quest for sons, the family size in extreme cases may even go up to seven daughters, as was the case in one family. The desired family composition was that of a minimum of two sons in the family. This was irrespective of the number of girls born in the endeavour. If the family is a landed family of Jats, then at times the family size is limited to only two children. The Jats, by virtue of their better economic status, are able to afford sex selection procedures. Thus, the family size is automatically limited to two sons.

Unsafe Methods

The poorer people who were unable to afford MTPs went to quacks, often with fatal results. One such quack was a lady known as the 'Chanalon wali Dai' (the dai of the village Chanalon). Prior to setting up a private practice, she used to sweep and mop in a doctor's clinic. She now has a very successful practice. She is very popular among the people in the PHC area. It was reported that she used very crude methods for MTP. These methods consisted of methods like insertion of sticks dipped in kerosene oil into the uterus. This often led to ruptured uteruses. People however feel that it is not safe to go to quacks like the 'Chanolon wali Dai' for MTPs since they could prove to be fatal.

They are well aware of the fact that repeated MTPs are not good for a woman's health and that sex-selection tests are illegal. However, given the desire for sons and the planning of families to have a minimum of two sons, the workers have rationalised in their own minds that MTPs are a safer option. They feel that even though MTPs are not good for a woman's health, there is no harm in undergoing multiple MTPs for lack of a better option. The thinking is that choosing the desired sex composition of the children is the right way to plan families. It is only after this that a woman should go in for sterilisation.

The workers were aware of these practices since many such serious cases come to them or go to the government hospital in the neighbouring town for help. The workers dissuaded people from visiting such quacks, since it could prove to be fatal. They felt that if some people could not afford ultrasounds and MTPs at a doctor's clinic, they should carry the pregnancy to full-term. These people had no options but to try for a son till they had the number of sons that they wanted.

The desire for a son was so intense that some people even took loans to undergo ultrasounds and MTPs. The workers felt that the next time that they wanted a son they should follow the 'correct' methods to have a son. The 'correct' methods included sex-selection techniques and having special medicines. One male worker ran a very successful private clinic in a town neighbouring the PHC. His speciality was a medicine for bearing sons. He made a certain preparation at home with herbs, gold and other secret ingredients. He varied the amount of gold (a costly ingredient) in the medicine according to the economic status of the client. Reduction in the gold quantity somewhat reduced the effectiveness of the medicine. Substitutes for gold were also available but they were not as effective as gold. Nevertheless, he claimed to have a 90 per cent success rate.

The workers were aware that sex-selective termination of pregnancies was illegal and had an adverse effect on a woman's health yet they did nothing to stop such practices. As one doctor said,

We know that sex-selective abortions are illegal and are bound to adversely affect the health of the woman. However, if we do not send people to the 'right clinics' then it becomes more fatal for them. It is like choosing between the devil and the deep blue sea.

The workers as well as the doctors help the people by recommending some 'good' ultrasound clinics. In some cases, the workers escorted the people to these clinics on their own scooters or mopeds. A lot of workers act as middlemen and get a commission of 25 per cent (of the ultrasound fee), per case from the doctors who carry out these procedures. Some of the workers charged Rs 100 per case. In some cases, particularly if the woman and her family are poor, the workers either reduced their fees or entirely waived it.

There were instances of doctors at the PHC and at the mini-PHCs[2] conducting ultrasounds and MTPs. The clinics were run by the doctors themselves or their family members. The workers reported the case of a husband-and-wife doctor team posted at the PHC, indulging in this practice. The wife had been suspended for indulging in private practice while still in government service. She subsequently resigned and now has a very successful private practice in Mohali. Her husband continues to be in government service. He now helps his wife's practice by recommending her to those keen on ultrasounds and MTPs. This doctor had built quite a reputation for himself and every Friday he took potential MTP cases to his wife's clinics in his own car. The workers themselves were party to this and helped him to get 'cases'. Those workers owning scooters and mopeds and living in towns and cities near the PHC even took people to the clinic. He reportedly paid the workers Rs 100 per case. The brother and sister-in-law of this doctor were also doctors and were employed in the same PHC. They too contributed to this practice. This entire set of four doctors comprised the sons and daughters-in-law of a recently retired Director, Health Services.

These doctors were erratic in showing up for duty at the rural dispensaries at which they were posted. When they did show up for duty it was observed that it was for a very short while and basically to meet some potential family planning case. Nor did they attend immunisation camps. Closeness to the power structure meant that they could be lax in their routine work. They were able to manipulate the rules to suit their own ends. Closeness to the power structure gave this set of four doctors a kind of immunity. This gave them immunity against punishments. In case the wrong practices of the doctors were reported the doctors were known to have used their 'approach' to waive off the punishment. As a result, the doctors were not very particular in the performance of their duties. Manipulation of the rules meant that they were able to ensure that they were attached to hospitals in a town near the PHC, on special duty for extended periods of time. Such postings ensured that they spent the minimum amount of time in the rural areas.

The workers were well aware of this fact and they knew that nothing could be done about it since the doctors were very highly-connected. This set of four doctors could carry out illegal practices such as MTPs because of their high-powered connections. At times, in the evenings, according to one of the villagers, the doctors even carried out MTPs at the rural dispensaries. The surveillance at the remote dispensaries was very minimal and no one reported such illegal practices since the workers too were a part of this nexus.

By implication, it means that MTPs are inevitable in the desire to have the right kind of family planning. In the quest for the right family composition, coupled with the desire to limit the number of daughters, people were ready to undergo as many MTPs as desired. The guilt of conceiving a daughter is tremendous. The act of giving birth to one doubles the guilt. The woman is made to feel guilty for the crime of conceiving a daughter. One ANM's quote about a woman who underwent an MTP when the ultrasound test showed the foetus to be female was very eloquent. She said,

> *Kaal tak taan aidi jaan suki pai si ki ik hor kudi hoi taan aide gharvalaian ne ainu chadna nahin. Hun vekho, kal hi taan kudi girake aiyee hai, te aaj tapdi phir di hai. Kyonki aide tid vich kudi si dar de maare peed vich vi aaram nahi kar sakdi.* (Till yesterday she was scared out of her wits that if she has another daughter her household members would have made life hell for her. Look at her now, just yesterday she committed foeticide and today she is jumping about. The fear and guilt of carrying a daughter will not let her rest today, even though today she must be in great pain.)

The workers can well identify with these feelings, as they themselves are a part of the same social fabric. Their approach and the reaction of the people to them, because of interaction with them over a period, all reflected the way in which the workers had negotiated the official rules to fit in with the ground reality.

VII

Conclusion

Family planning in the official formal jargon means controlling fertility. At the level of the people, it means controlling the number of daughters that the couple has. The number of daughters that a couple has, as we have seen above, is controlled through the process of ultrasounds and foeticide. The doctors and the entire health hierarchy share an understanding that family planning and/or control of fertility is not possible till a couple has the desired number of sons. The above mentioned communication from the Civil Surgeon's office clearly conveys that they too understand that MTPs are quite common and popular as methods of family planning. The district health headquarter is aware of this reality and conveys it by saying that one birth per MTP is controlled.

It is this kind of an understanding of family planning that the entire health hierarchy in Punjab, including the health workers, identifies with. The doctors and the rest of the health services hierarchy is aware of the fact that in Punjab, temporary methods of family planning are not adopted till the desired family composition is achieved. The desire to have sons is something with which the health hierarchy at all levels identifies with. The traditional social structure is manifested in the primary health care delivery system at the hands of the health functionaries. The Senior Medical Officer too is party to this reality when she conveys to the workers that the only way to bring down the birth rate is through sterilisation. The MPWs too belong to the same Punjabi society. They therefore, share many of the cultural beliefs and values of their clients. Their socialisation has been in the same environment. They are thus a part of the same social structure. They too avoid targeting women who do not have a son. It is only if the woman has had five to six daughters and if she is very weak that the MPWs suggest sterilisation. These days they suggest ultrasounds to women in their third pregnancy, if the earlier children are daughters. In some cases they may target for ultrasounds in the second pregnancy itself.

The people followed the advice of the health department in the case of wrong health education too. This was most striking in the case of sex-selection practices. The health workers are meant to be agents of positive change but they end up propagating wrong practices. Not only the health workers but also the doctors advocate and practice illegal procedures of sex selection. The message that thus gets conveyed to the community is that there is nothing wrong in these practices. In order to meet targets the entire health hierarchy is pushing people towards attaining the desired family composition at the fastest possible rate. Motivating a family for sterilisation takes up to four to five years. Sex-selection practices have emerged as one of the ways of encouraging sterilisation. The desired sex ratio at the macro level and at the micro level in the households is different. The health personnel at all levels help people attain the desired sex ratio, while at the same time trying to keep the number of children per family down. The disastrous consequences are reflected in the low sex ratio at the national level.

Even though MTPs are not illegal, abortion-seeking behaviour has to be viewed in the broader context of the status of women and gender dynamics and the broader implications for the sex ratio of the nation. It is this violence and the ethical issues involved that need to be addressed.

It is a case of son preference versus daughter dis-preference. There is not just a son preference but there is also a daughter dis-preference that leads people to take extreme measures like elimination of unwanted female foetuses. Thus, what emerges is that science and technology are not external to culture but are very much a part of culture. Science and technology have become a part of the culture in the sense that they are abetting a desire for sons and the lack of desire for daughters.

Initiatives and efforts taken to address women's issues have been inadequate, distorted, vertical, and top-down and have rarely emerged out of concern for women's health. The only solution being offered for women's health is for maternal health. This too is extremely limited and is restricted to distribution of iron and folic acid tablets and to tetanus toxoid injections. Here too only those women who have been targeted for sterilisation by the health workers receive iron supplements to pump up their haemoglobin levels prior to a sterilisation operation. Poverty, illiteracy, and a rural background, further compound the marginalisation of women. The household factors like its type, gender, and generational control also contribute to her marginalisation.

There has to be a direct attack on son preference as a way out of this maze created by science and technology. There have to be well-developed links between rights of women, as a part of culture, and female autonomy.

There is a total lack of a supportive structure to empower women. That can only be achieved through cooperation of different departments working in the rural areas and through the involvement of people themselves. Female autonomy should be the prime focus.

Economic empowerment of women can lead to female autonomy. Structural reforms like land ownership can also do the trick. It is only then that the shackles of patriarchy can be broken or modified to suit women too.

Notes

1. The Centre at different points of time to control major public health problems faced by the country launched major disease control programmes. These programmes are the National Tuberculosis Control Programme, National Leprosy Control Programme in 1955, National Malaria Control Programme in 1953, National Family Planning Programme in 1952, etc. Each programme was assigned to separate Deputy Directors or Assistant Directors at the district level. The health staff to run these programmes was introduced as and when the programmes were introduced. All these programmes were run independent of one another, in a vertical manner. It was in the sixth plan that the functioning of these independent health workers was integrated and they were renamed multipurpose workers.

2. Theoretically a PHC is supposed to look after a population of 30,000. In reality the population under a PHC is three to four times this figure. In order to better manage the population under a PHC the government has introduced mini-PHCs. A mini-PHC looks after a population of 30,000 and has a medical officer, a pharmacist, a staff nurse, a laboratory technician and two class-IV employees (i.e. a peon and a sweeper, etc.). In addition, it also has two-three beds in order to admit patients.

References

Government of India. 1973. *Report of the Committee on Multipurpose Worker under Health & Family Planning Program: (Chairman, Kartar Singh)*: New Delhi.

———. 1976. Report of the Committee on Medical Education & Support Manpower: (Chairman, Dr. Shrivastava). *New Delhi*.

———. 1981. *Report of the Sub-Group on Health Services Organization to Achieve Health For All by 2000 AD.* Ministry of Health and Family Welfare: New Delhi.

———. 1983. *National Health Policy–1982*. Ministry of Health & Family Welfare: New Delhi.

———. 1986. *Job Responsibilities of Staff of the Primary Health Centre.* Ministry of Health and Family Welfare: New Delhi.

———. 1993. *National Family Health Survey–Punjab*. Population Research Centre: Centre for Research in Rural and Industrial Development: Chandigarh.

Government of India. 2001. *National Population Policy–2000*. Ministry of Health and Family Welfare: New Delhi.

———. 2002a. *National Health Policy of India*. Ministry of Health and Family Welfare: New Delhi.

———. 2002b. *Annual Report 2000–2001*. Ministry of Health and Family Welfare: New Delhi.

Government of Punjab. 1997. *Action Plan for Family Welfare and Health Care and MCH for the Year 1996-97*. Communication from the Civil Surgeon's office to the PHC: Rupnagar.

———. 2001. *Health Program*. Directorate of Health and Family Welfare, Punjab: (Downloaded from the Official Website of the Health and Family Welfare Department).

Hershman, Paul. 1981. *Punjabi Kinship and Marriage*. Delhi: Hindustan Publishing Corporation.

International Institute for Population Sciences, 2001. *National Family Health Survey India (NFHS-2): Punjab*. Mumbai: International Institute for Population Sciences.

Premi, M. K. 2001. 'The Missing Girl Child', *Economic and Political Weekly*, 36(21): 1875–1880.

Adoption:
Born to Live

8

Rashmi Kapoor

One of the most common, if not universal, features of human societies is inequality between individuals and social groups. The inequality between men and women has been wrongly attributed to be inherent in nature.[1] This artificial construct of natural superiority of male over female gets translated into social inequality. As a consequence of inequality between sexes, females have been relegated to an inferior position and are quite often subjected to covert or overt aggression.

In everyday life, women may be subjected to discrimination but, ironically, both men and women worship female deities with great devotion. According to Hindu mythology the mother goddess is identified as *shakti,* which literally means energy. She is the primary source of creation and she is worshipped in this form by women as well as men. Another interesting visual aspect of the Indian religious tradition related to female deities is the celebration of *Durga Navami Puja.* Small girls who have not yet attained puberty are worshipped to propitiate the mother goddess. Thus the situation is a perplexing one as there is a co-existence of two opposing tendencies towards women. In the sacred realm she is *shakti,*[2] the energising principle and in the secular sphere she is just the opposite, weak and inferior (Das 1980). Adding on to the confusion is the fact that despite young girls being worshipped in order to propitiate the mother goddess, many parents show hostility towards girls by killing small, baby girls and female foetuses, neglecting, mistreating or abandoning children, mostly girls, so as to get rid of them. Also, there is no denial of the fact that there are other childless couples who adopt children and take children for foster care, predominantly girls, out of choice and not out of compulsion. Parents, who disown children, give others an opportunity to become parents by making their own an unrelated child.

This article discusses the age-old practice of female infanticide and female foeticide. The article will also elaborate on the contemporary practice of adoption and then it will be compared with the ancient Indian practice of adoption. The article also seeks to find answer to the existence of the paradoxical situation of coexistence of female infanticide and female foeticide and that of adoption, predominantly of girls, in the same socio-cultural milieu.

Every known society of the world acknowledges the importance of children. To bear children after marriage does not require any special decision by the couple. A primary expectation from a married woman is that she will become pregnant soon and bear children. Typically, a woman knows of no acceptable role for herself than that of wife-mother. Childbirth immediately dispels the stigma of barrenness of a couple, especially that of a wife. The first child's sex is secondary, more important is the couple's fertility (Patel 1994). There are also reports of the improvement of status of women after childbirth (Jacobson 1970, Mandelbaum 1976, Patel 1994). Thus a woman is valued for the children that she bears. The religious rites she participates in are also predominantly related to increasing her fertility.

A woman requires to bear children to prove her womanhood, man desires children to attain full manly state and hence dignity. Even grandparents are eager to have grandchildren as their status gets enhanced in society. The whole family is desirous of having children. By bearing children, it is fulfilling both of the social expectations and personal desire (Oakley 1982). In the situation where society attaches so much importance to children, inability to conceive is a traumatic shock. It is perceived as a disruption in the normal course of an expected life cycle.

The paradox of the situation is that when Indian society attaches such great importance to children, at the same time a large number of children are exterminated either before or after birth, and many are abandoned by parents. Not surprisingly, the children who are victimised are mostly female children. The major cause of aggression and neglect of a girl child can be attributed to the preference for a son over a daughter. The reasons for such an attitude are more a result of the socialisation process of traditional social expectations and appropriate social behaviours and not a consequence of individual choice. Preference for a son invariably gets translated into the subordinate status of girls and may lead to discrimination. The near universal desire and preference for a son may be due to socio-cultural, economic or religious reasons, or combination of some of these.[3] The main cause of population problem is not only the desire to have a son but due to poor health conditions child mortality is high. To have at least one surviving male, a woman has to have five to six children.

Socio-cultural Reasons _____

In Indian society, sons are needed for the transmission of family property. Girls can inherit family property but then the rights pass from her natal family to her family of procreation, which may not be acceptable to many people. Therefore, a son is required to keep the property within the family.[4] Besides, in certain communities there is evidence of parents being subjected to humiliation within the society if they have more girl children (Sunanda 1995).

Dowry system is one such social evil which is a major cause of occurrence of many other social evils. Fear of inability to meet dowry demands leads to killing of girls, abandoning of girls, occasionally selling girls, foeticide, and infanticide by parents themselves. The inability of parents is a source of much humiliation by society. Also, a fear of losing one's daughter in a dowry death or having to face physical and mental torture for not bringing adequate dowry also looms large.

Economic Reasons _____

The most important economic reason is poverty and depression. As noted above, fear of large dowries and high cost of nurturing a girl child force parents to resort to certain inhumane acts. Girls are perceived as a liability, the fact which is responsible for the degradation of her status even prior to her birth. On the other hand, expenditure for marriage of a son is not as much as is for the daughter. Rather, it is financially advantageous for the family, as the bride brings in dowry.

Another important reason for a desire for sons is that they provide an economic support and security in the old age of parents. Sons are expected to stay with the family forever and help them in their twilight years.

Religious and Ritual Reasons _____

The need to have sons is reinforced in religion as well. The son enables the father to pay off the debt he owes to his ancestors. The son offers *pindas*[5] to the ancestors and thus helps in giving salvation. The necessity of having a son is strengthened further when a son is required to perform the rite of lighting the funeral pyre of the father and observe the ancestral (*sraddha*) rites for the father after his death. Daughters are not allowed by religious law to perform any Vedic rites. Therefore for begetting a son, any number of girls born before him are sacrificed.

A strong preference for a son automatically assigns lower status to girls, which very often results in the discrimination against them. Discrimination at times leads to mistreatment, aggression and neglect. The discrimination of the girl child takes an extreme, violent and cannibalistic form when a child is killed either before or after birth, merely because of the fact that she is a 'female'.

It is when socio-cultural and religious justifications support such a negative attitude that people indulge willingly in heinous acts like female foeticide and female infanticide. These acts have social approval and persist despite being fatalistic.

An age-old barbaric act of killing newborn female babies is called female infanticide. It is still widely practised among many communities in India.[6] Another similar practice of exterminating unwanted female foetuses in the womb itself is called foeticide. This practice is also becoming very common and has been made possible by the use of modern science and technology in medicine. The fruits of modern science and technology are thought to be a boon to mankind as they provide a cure for many dreaded diseases. But this boon of mankind has been abused and put to use for destruction of human beings by using it for intentional killing of female foetuses and thereby dismantling the myth of neutrality of science. This undesirable use of medical technology is unscrupulously tempering with the womb even before the birth of the baby. Another act of hostility shown towards girls is that of neglect and, in extreme cases, abandonment. Neglect does not apparently look very harsh but can result in delayed mortality. These acts of aggression and discrimination against girls legitimise the social customs sanctioned by the whole society, which is already skewed heavily towards sons.

It is not only in the early years of life that girls face such hostility. When girls grow up, they quite often face the traumatic experience of rape, wife-beating, bride-burning and are occasionally forced to be a *sati*. These acts, against the will of women, are enacted with a purpose. These are not manifestations of prejudices only but demonstrate 'commodification' of women who can be put to use according to requirement. Some of these aforementioned acts of inhuman torture of women are comparatively of recent origin and endemic to modern society. The acts of aggression against women in traditional society and their persistence in contemporary society demolish the view that the status of women has improved in India as a result of modern and secular influences.

Infanticide, or murder or deliberate neglect of the girl child to induce death is considered female infanticide. In general parlance, female infanticide understood today is the intentional killing of the girl child after birth. It has been known to occur in many human cultures (Miller 1997). In India it has been practised for the last few centuries. The first discovery of female infanticide in India was in 1789 among the *Raj Kumar* clan of *Rajputs* in Jaunpur District, eastern Uttar Pradesh (*ibid.*). The East India Company was governing the country at that time. It felt that a legislation must be enacted to ban the gruesome practice.

The Bengal Regulatory Act XXI of 1795 and Regulation Act VI of 1802 declared the practice of female infanticide as murder. Almost one century after the official discovery of the cases of female infanticide in India, an Act abolishing its practice was passed. This Act was known as the Act VIII of 1870 and was popularly known as 'Female Infanticide Act'. This act was formulated when reports reached the British government showing that villages and tribes 'without even one female child', are increasing (Miller 1997). Initially strong measures were not taken. Later on the Act was actively enforced during the period 1876 to 1906. Unfortunately, it was slowly buried due to political pressure from the groups practising it on one side and half-hearted efforts made by the British to implement it on the other side.

From the available evidence it is clear that female infanticide in 19th century India was practised primarily in the higher social groups of the North,[7] though this point is also debatable (Miller 1997). Other areas where it was widely prevalent were pockets of northeastern India, where it was practised by the tribal Nagas, in the southern area by the Todas of the Nilgiri Hills and the tribal khonds in Orissa.

During the British period, before the ban on infanticide, people were not reticent to admit the murdering of their female offspring. They never regretted having murdered an infant, rather they rationalised the act by demonstrating that the birth of a girl child meant that the family will perish or be ruined. The birth of a female child was considered a misfortune for the parents. It was a situation when the whole community needed to sympathise with them and support them in dealing with their misfortune. Female infanticide had complete social approval.

Child sex ratios along with male/female mortality ratio are perhaps good indicators of female infanticide in contemporary India. The 1991 Census shows that 54 districts, located within just seven states, have a child sex ratio of less than 900 (Behlary 1995). This shows that lesser number of females survive as compared to males. Data of several other child sex ratio studies and juvenile mortality rates in different parts of India support this finding.

A review of juvenile mortality statistics of two studies in the Ludhiana District of Punjab (Khanna study of Wyon and Gordon 1971, The Narangwal Study of Kelly 1975, Miller 1997) reflect the existence of female infanticide. The Khanna[8] study shows the death of 168.4 females infants to 164.6 male infants and Narangwal study

Table 8.1
Juvenile Mortality Statistics from North India

Sex	Sex differentials in infants (0–1 years) Mortality rates (deaths per 1000 birth)	
	Khanna study (1957–59)	Narangwal study (1969–70)
Female	168.4	196.0
Male	164.6	125.0

Sex	Sex differentials in childhood mortality rates (deaths per 1000 population per year)	
Female	36.9	58.0
Male	19.4	29.0

Sex ratio at death during childhood
(Sex ratio–males per 100 females, *reproduced as in the study*).

Age	Narangwal
0–1 Months	126
0–5 Months	114
6–11 Months	73
1 year	62
1–4 year	71

Sources: Wyon and Gordon 1971: 186, Kelly 1975: 132.

shows the deaths of 196.0 females infants to 125 males as shown in Table 8.1. In both the studies, the higher death figures of female infants than those of the male are not natural. The childhood mortality rates, i.e., deaths per 1,000 population per year, in both studies, show female mortality rates almost twice as high as male mortality rates. In the Khanna study, the male mortality rate is 19.4 whereas the female is 36.9. The Narangwal study shows male mortality rate to be 29 per cent and female mortality to be 58 per cent (Table 8.1). Sex ratios at death during different periods of childhood also show wide variations. Ratios at different childhood periods also indicate that the number of deaths of male children is more only in early childhood, from 0–5 months (Table 8.1). Thereafter deaths are preponderantly of females. After the first two months of birth, cultural factors begin to operate to the disadvantage of females, resulting in higher female mortality rate and hence adverse sex ratio.

Another statistical data (Table 8.2) regarding sex ratio by age group shows that only during the childbearing years, that is, approximately between the age of 20–40 years, lesser number of female deaths occur as compared to other periods of life.[9] One may speculate that since a woman is valued more for the children she bears, she is more cared for during that period, hence lesser mortality. Other-

Table 8.2
Sex Ratio (FMR) by Age Group, 1901 to 1971

Age group in year	1901	1911	1921	1931	1941	1951	1961	1971
0–4	1078	1030	1035	1023	1004	990	992	979
5–9	955	999	960	912	945	965	955	943
10–14	924	817	822	884	903	936	877	885
15–19	929	930	916	991	928	944	929	882
20–24	1092	1078	1075	1023	986	969	1051	998
25–29	980	968	968	952	984	958	974	1007
30–34	967	961	954	901	943	927	929	975
35–39	882	853	841	973	914	897	872	909
40–44	969	949	945	869	902	882	891	848
45–49	882	849	823	863	898	884	855	836
50–54	997	917	954	889	904	902	974	847
55–59	919	884	860	945	935	936	861	866
60 and above	1149	1092	1040	994	958	1001	1000	936
Unspecified	1174	1267	–	–	–	–	863	1071

Source: Veena, Shatrugna 1984.

wise, during other periods of life, the female mortality rate is much higher than that of males. It is interesting to note that over a period of seventy years, the trend has remained the same (Table 8.2).

Similar are the findings of Premi and Raju (1998) of his study of female infanticide in Madhya Pradesh. Table 8.3 shows that the sex ratio at birth is 837 females to 1,000 males which decreases, if we consider the sex ratio of live births. The sex ratio of live births is 775 females to 1,000 males. This ratio further decreases if one analyses the sex ratio of existing children which is, 500 females to 1,000 males. Thus with increase in age the child sex ratio decreases drastically

Table 8.3
Sex Distribution of Children at Birth and 0–6 Years of Age in MP, 1998

	Total reported birth	Born alive	Now alive	Sex ratio at birth	Sex ratio of live birth	Sex ratio of existing children
Male	166	151	136	1000	1000	1000
Female	139	117	68	837	775	500

Source: Premi and Raju 1998: 94.

All the above studies of sex ratio of various regions of India show that female mortality is higher for all age groups, except during the childbearing years when it is marginally better. Though male mortality is higher in the first few months, after which social factors put a higher premium on male infants to the disadvantage of females. Perhaps the pressure to conform to the social expectations is so strong that people indulge willingly in the unethical practice of female infanticide.

According to Kelly (1975) the large sex differentials in infant and childhood mortality found in the northern states are responsible for their very low sex ratio. The magnitude of female disadvantage in chances of survival seems to be large enough to explain a major part, and sometimes the entire excess of males, in the population of the North-Western areas of the sub-continent. Thus both higher mortality among girls, perhaps due to their mistreatment and maternal mortality of women, are major factors in higher female than male mortality (Visaria 1961).

Alarming is the fact that in India, the sex ratio has steadily been declining over the years as can be seen in Table 8.4 (Ravindra 1991).

Table 8.4
Number of Females per Thousand Males in India

Year	1901	1911	1921	1931	1941	1951	1961	1971	1981	1991	2001
Sex Ratio	972	964	955	950	945	946	941	930	934	927	933

Source: Ravindra 1991: 4.

The high mortality rate for women indicates that more women are dying either due to natural causes beyond the control of humans or are dying an unnatural death by being killed (like bride-burning, female infanticide, mistreatment, etc.).

While variations in the sex ratio at the time of conception can be attributed to biology, sex ratio after that is more under the influence of culture and society. Many cultures define which will be the 'superior' sex in terms of survival. Sex-selective infanticide is such an example where certain societies systematically kill infants because of the sex of the infants. According to Miller (1997), culture provides the motivations for infanticide, whether they are seen by the people involved as ritualistic (Benedict 1972), economic (Granzberg 1973), or ecological (Freeman 1971). 'Culture "invents" the reasons for which some children who are born are not desired' (Miller 1997: 44).

Foeticide

Foeticide is the practice in which the sex of the foetus is determined with the help of ultrasound, scans and in-vitro sex testing and the foetus is killed through abortion. Female foeticide is, when with the help of medical technology, the sex of the foetus is determined and, if found to be female, aborted. It is also called sex-selective abortion.

There are several ways to determine the sex of the child in the womb itself. These are amniocentesis, ultra-sonogram and chorion villa. These are safe, medical technologies which are mainly used to detect any genetic anomalies. In recent years, all these tests have become synonymous with sex determination tests in India.

A commonly held view is that people who are rich and educated do not indulge in practices like female foeticide. The paradox of the situation is that the incidence of female foeticide is confined to the affluent and highly educated sections of our society (Arora 2002). It has gained popularity among the urban, educated middle classes.

The poor, illiterate and rural people of India are still not aware of such dimensions of medical technology which threaten the very right of a girl child to live. The gravity of the situation can be estimated by the news that according to the Campaign Against Female Foeticide (CAFF), 90 per cent of the estimated 3.5 million abortions in India each year are to eliminate girls (Hughes 2003).

Modern science has been accused of introducing the modern practice of female foeticide after the sex determination test. But ancient India appears to have been quite familiar with the practice of abortion (Chhabra & Nuna). The first reference to abortion is seen in the *Atharva Veda* as early as 2000–800 B.C. Chandrashekar notes in the text *Brihadyogalarinigini*, thought to be written around the first century B.C., '...several contraceptive recipes are given including a method for the occlusion of the cervix' (1974: 23). This suggests the existence of the practice of abortion then too. Interestingly the three Sanskrit medical classics, written respectively by Susruta, Charaka and Vaghbata I, which comprise the main body of knowledge of ancient Hindu medicine, deal with abortion and miscarriage amongst other reproductive issues (*ibid.*). He further observes that almost all ancient Hindu writers and law givers, including Manu, dealt with the subject, often at length. This indicates more than a sporadic existence of the practice over 4,000 years. The 17th century work of Acharya Lolinbaraj, a well-known Ayurvedic physician of his times, provides the means of tackling an unwanted pregnancy when used with caution (*ibid.*). The elaborate and extensive treatment of the topic by the ancient writers probes the mind of the reasons for prevalence of such practices then.

While practices of infanticide and foeticide are widely prevalent, its acceptance by people who are committing it is denied. There are several indicators that can substantiate its existence. The most important indicators are primary and secondary sex ratios. Primary sex ratio is sex ratio at the time of conception whereas secondary sex ratio is a sex ratio at the time of birth. 'There is a misconception that the primary sex ratio or sex ratio at the time of conception would be roughly balanced, i.e. fifty-fifty chance of either a boy or a girl' (Miller 1997: 38). On the contrary, most findings indicate a high (preponderance of males) pre-natal sex ratio. This preponderance of males reduces gradually throughout gestation. Miller concludes that scholars assume that female embryos are more hardy than the male, which more often abort spontaneously.

The fact that the male foetuses are destroyed in a larger number, is substantiated by more number of male still-born babies. Perhaps due to larger size, the male suffers greater stress. The above findings are highly speculative as the study of primary sex ratio is at a very crude level of development. The secondary sex ratio, or sex ratio at birth shows that males tend to slightly outnumber females at birth (Miller 1997). The higher rate of still-born males and higher death rate of male infants in the first year of life evens out things. Indeed by age one, the proportion of the sexes is equal in the West (Miller 1997). From the above observations it is apparent that nature has its own way of balancing sexes in a short time from conception to age one. The variation in the sex ratio later on in life is more clearly regulated by the cultural constructs that define which will be the 'superior' sex in terms of survival.

The deviation from the normal will indicate sex-selective abortion. Certain surveys conducted in states like Madhya Pradesh and Punjab indicate that the number of females born in several areas is a great degree less than the number of males, indicating the abortion of female foetuses (Premi 1998, Ravindra 1991). A study conducted in Ludhiana in Punjab tried to find out the secondary sex ratio (SSR) which is defined as the number of males born for hundred females. The following were the results as in Table 8.5.

The data shows that over the period 1981 to 1988, the number of males born to every hundred females is gradually increasing. Similar are the findings of Premi (1998) in his study of M.P. His data shows that in 1998, 151 males were born alive as compared to 117 females born alive (Table 8.3). These evidences prove the prevalence of female foeticide in M.P.

Recent statistics of female-male sex ratio of 793 females to 1,000 males in Punjab are very alarming. The scourge of foetus killing has become so deadly that there are no brides in scores of villages in the region (Table 8.6). Still girls continue to disappear in the notorious 'Kuri Mar' (girl-killer) region of Malwa (Sharma 2006). The omi-

Table 8.5
Secondary Sex Ratio: Males to 100 Females

Year	1981	1982	1983	1984	1985	1986	1987	1988
SSR	105	105	113	113	113	112	114	122

Source: Ravindra 1991.

Table 8.6
Female-Male Sex Ratio in Punjab, 2001

Towns	Fatehgarh Sahib	Bhatinda	Mansa	Sangrur
Females	28,147	63,738	41,395	112,358
Males	37,312	81,773	53,117	143,227
Sex Ratios	754	779	779	784

Source: Sharma, Shradhha 2006.

nously skewed ratio has brought together the gurudwaras, the government and the women to fight this age-old, barbaric practice to save its girls now.

In the light of the earlier discussion that female foetuses have more chances of survival than male, the data from MP and Punjab shows otherwise. The substantial increase in the number of male births is a good indicator of sex-selective abortion of females, particularly in the latter part of the 1980s, when sex determination tests were becoming very popular.

Infanticide and foeticide are the acts which have been institutionalised and have social approval. They are deliberate efforts to exterminate female babies as early as possible in their life. Those who do not have a heart to kill their daughters, neglect them. Neglecting a baby is far from killing one, but it can shorten a child's life and the traumatic experience can leave a permanent scar. Neglect along with child abuse, if carried too far, can be fatal. 'Child abuse is an act done to harm the child whereas in the case of neglect, harm comes to the child because something is not done which should have been'(Miller 1997: 45). Neglect has been rarely discussed as an expression of discrimination or a form of infanticide. But Harris (1975) has included conscious and unconscious neglect as a form of infanticide along with homicide and malign aggression. Unlike other forms of infanticide, aggression or neglect may not always be fatal.

Adoption of Children: The Study of an Adoption Home

Abandoning children is a case of neglect, a neglect of extreme order. Children, both male and female, are being abandoned in increasing numbers because of changing societal norms and values as a result of modernisation, industrialisation and urbanisation. These processes brought about a fundamental change in the traditional family system. The joint family system gave way to the formation of nuclear units. Nuclear families cannot always cope with the stress and unforeseen circumstances and may breakdown in such situations, leaving children helpless. Wars and other forms of institutionalised violence and terrorism lead to unprecedented number of deaths within a family, or physically separates or tears apart its members. Children are either orphaned, or lost or abandoned as they do not have parents to take care of them.

Still another reason for abandoning children is when wives are deserted by husbands. In the absence of their husbands, women are more vulnerable and many times they are not able to take care of their children physically and financially. Besides, decline in traditional values has led to an increase in the crime against women such as rape and infidelity, leading to illegitimate children being born out of wedlock. These unwanted, illegitimate children are deserted. Even natural calamities like earthquakes, floods and droughts render many children homeless.

Abandoned children often reach adoption agencies which are actively involved in the rehabilitation of such children. The role of adoption agencies has become a crucial one as adoption is seen as a possible answer to the problem of child destitution and institutionalisation in India. They try to identify parents who, by choice, adopt abandoned children to provide them with a secure home. They not only promote adoption but take a more holistic approach to the concept of child welfare, with the broader aim of preventing destitution. Therefore, adoption should be seen as a part of a larger network of child welfare services.

There are twelve adoption agencies in Delhi. All these agencies are coordinated by Voluntary Coordinating Agency (VCA). The Delhi VCA is the Coordinating Voluntary Adoption Resource Agency (CVARA). One of the adoption agencies is the Delhi Council of Child Welfare (DCCW). It was established initially to assist in the care of thousands of children who had been displaced during the partition of India in 1947. It was in 1978 that a home for abandoned children called Palna (literally, cradle) was established at the DCCW to help in the adoption of these children. The adoption programme at Palna was started in keeping with the maxim that 'every child needs a family'.

Palna is not funded by any organisation or government agency. It is maintained by the registration fee it charges from the adoptive parents. In addition, there are donations in cash and kind. Outside the gates of DCCW, a cradle is kept for parents to abandon their child in complete anonymity. Most of the infants in this agency are received in the cradle. Sometimes destitute or abandoned babies are located by the police or found by the public and are brought to the police station. Unwed mothers often give up their claims on their babies by signing the document of relinquishment.

The abandoned and destitute child is admitted to the children's home. A medical examination is done and the child is given a name, an identity. If the child is found fit, the process for his adoption begins. In most cases, predominantly because of infertility, couples opt to form a family by having children through the socially accepted method of adoption. It is parenthood by adoption rather than by procreation.

Adoption is a more complex, social institution than the formation of a natural family that involves only the natural parents and the child. Adoption can be seen as a triad-involving the child, the birth-parents and the adoptive parents. The birth-parent's rights and responsibilities are transferred onto the adopted parents. Thereby, adoption establishes a fictitious relationship between a child and the adoptive family socio-legally (Kapoor 1996).

The *Encyclopedia Britannica* (Vol.1) defines adoption as a family experience. It confers the privileges of being parents upon the childless, and advantages of having parents upon the parentless. Adoption is predominantly a legal procedure and indicates complete transfer of the child from natural parents to the new family (Gokhale 1976, Manooja 1993). A family is created by the state rather than through a biological process, but is socially recognised. The social relation so formed does not coincide with a physical bond. The father of the child may not be his biological father (Kapoor 1996).

In the present day scenario, adoption agencies have become a link between children available for adoption and adoptive parents. It is not that all adoptions are taking place through adoption agencies. People often go in for private adoptions and inter-family adoptions similar to the practice prevalent in traditional India. Only related children were adopted as heredity and blood of the child is seen as very important. Now also, the reasons for adopting a known child are still the same. Such adoptions very frequently lead to disharmony within the family over inheritance rights and conflicting emotional ties. The adoptive parents face a situation where they never really feel that the child belongs to them totally. Private adoptions not only are a grave breach of law, but also of responsibility to the child. In some instances, a large sum of money is said to exchange hands. Most important is the fact that no legal follow-up is ensured. In an unfortunate situation, the child can become a victim.

Though adoption takes place within the family domain, it has wider social implications. The status of the child in the adoptive family is created by the state, where it did not exist before. The induction of the child into a new family affects the family socially, psychologically and legally. Therefore, it is imperative to research the issue of adoption from a socio-psychological perspective. A statistical data and analysis of adoption service in India would provide an insight into the contemporary practice of the adoption. It will help in understanding the trends of adoption practice at present and the future prospects of the service in India. Secondary data was collected from the files of Palna at the DCCW and CVARA[10] in order to reflect on the trends in the child adoption services in Delhi from 1993–2003. A profile of the children adopted, and of the adoptive parents, has been prepared.

The statistical data collected from the files of Palna for the period 1978 to December, 2003 shows that there has been a steady increase in the number of adoptions. But remarkable is the increase in the adoption of girls in India. The comparative figures of male/female adoption from 1978–2003 are given in the Table 8.7. Out of a total of 1,148 adoptions during 1978–2003, the number of adoption of girls is 753 (65.60 per cent) and that of boys is 395 (34.4 per cent). Thus a larger percentage of the total adopted children comprises female children. This trend is very significant in a society where the birth of a female child is frowned upon, and female foeticide and female infanticide is practised undeterred. There are parents who willingly adopt girls. The parentage of most of these abandoned children is not known. So there is a double stigma attached, one of unknown parentage and secondly, that the sex of the child is female. The appreciating fact is that the adoptive parents are living in the same endemic zone of society as those who are hostile towards female children. They are also exposed to the same community strictures and social taboos.

On speculating on this major change in attitude, one can say that it may be due to the changing social norms and growing acceptability

Table 8.7
Number of Indian Adoptions, 1978–2003

| Year | Indian Adoption | | | | Total Children |
	Male	Per cent	Female	Per cent	
1978	4	66.6	2	33.33	6
1979	5	62.5	3	37.5	8
1980	8	80.0	2	20.0	10
1981	6	50.0	6	50.0	12
1982	4	44.5	5	55.55	9
1983	10	66.6	5	33.33	15
1984	10	38.5	16	61.53	26
1985	4	22.3	14	77.77	18
1986	8	38.1	13	61.90	21
1987	15	45.5	18	54.54	33
1988	13	46.5	15	53.57	28
1989	10	25.7	29	74.35	39
1990	15	34.9	28	65.11	43
1991	16	30.8	36	69.23	52
1992	8	14.6	47	85.45	55
1993	22	32.4	46	67.64	68
1994	28	37.4	47	62.66	75
1995	17	25.8	49	74.24	66
1996	21	36.9	36	63.15	57
1997	27	34.7	51	65.38	78
1998	23	30.7	52	69.33	75
1999	16	24.7	49	75.38	65
2000	30	40.0	45	60.00	75
2001	20	34.5	38	65.51	58
2002	28	55.6	63	44.44	91
2003	27	29.0	38	71.05	65
Total	395		753		1148

Source: Delhi Council of Child Welfare.

of an abandoned or destitute child and lesser stress on the origin and identity of the child. Besides, one should not undermine the role of fruitful counselling by the staff of the agency in bringing about a small but meaningful change in the attitudes of the prospective parents. Earlier, fewer Indian parents were coming forward to adopt abandoned children due to the stigma attached to illegitimacy and apprehension about heredity and blood. Now with the help of counselling, not only are abandoned children being adopted in more numbers, but the adoption of girls is increasing significantly.

The period from the late 1980s and early 1990s is of great interest as it was the time when the use of amniocentesis and other sex pre-selection tests were at a peak. This was because parents had the facility to determine a child's sex, and if the foetus happened to be female, parents had an option to abort it. This implies that unwanted pregnancies could be terminated and so a fewer number of children should have been abandoned. But the data does not reflect this trend. On the contrary, the number of adoptions after this period increased substantially. The availability of sex pre-selection test shows no appreciable change in the number of abandoned babies. Thus, it implies that most children who are abandoned, are either from outside the groups who can avail the fruits of medical technology, or are those children who are not planned or are the ones born out of wedlock.

The reason may be that the facility of these highly specialised tests being expensive may be only within the reach of only reasonably well-off people and more so in urban areas. Others are neither aware nor have the resources to go for them. Therefore unwanted children born in such families may still be abandoned. In the absence of data, it is difficult to verify it. It may be a conjecture to say that the substantial increase in the number of adoptions in the year 1993 (108) as compared to only 81 in 1992 (Table 8.7), and thereafter a continuously increasing trend in adoption may be due to the enactment of stringent laws against sex-selective abortion. They may have acted as a deterrent in early the 1990s, resulting in fewer abortions and hence more number of unwanted children available after that period. The limited data are only indicative of the trend and not conclusive.

Since most of the infants are received in the cradle, very little background information of the child is available. Quite often agencies are not even aware of the date of birth of the child. An approximate date of birth of the child is established by the growth of the infant by the doctor and that is considered to be his actual date of birth for all legal matters. Background information of only those children are available who are either relinquished by the parents themselves or babies who come from the hospitals. Hospital babies have an information tag attached to the wrists giving the time and date of birth.

Age of the Adopted Child

Data of earlier studies (Bharat 1993, Kapoor 1996) show that most of the children received by the agency are between the age of 0–3 months. But children in a wide range of ages are abandoned. The

Table 8.8
Adopted Child's Age at the Time of Adoption, 2003

Age group	Number of children	Per cent	
0–3 Months	6	9.24	84.6%
3–6 Months	15	23.07	
6–9 Months	22	33.86	
9–12 Months	12	18.46	
1–2 Years	4	6.15	15.30%
2 +	3	4.61	
Not Clear	3	4.61	
Total	136	100.00	

Source: Coordinating Voluntary Adoption Resource Agency, 2003.

percentage of older children is quite low and they are mostly placed with foreign parents.

Age at the time of adoption is very important for the adoptive parents as most Indian parents prefer to adopt very young babies. The data from CVARA for the year 2003 in Table 8.8 shows that about 84.6 per cent of babies were adopted when they had not attained the age of one year and only 15.38 per cent of those adopted were above one year. The reason for preference for a younger baby is that it is believed that it is easier to form a bond with the child when it is young. Some parents, who keep adoption a secret, prefer a new born baby so as to pass him off as their biological child.

Table 8.9 shows that most of the couples who want to adopt are mainly in the age group of 31–40 years (approximately 74.26 per cent of fathers and 67.64 per cent of mothers). The reason being that for most couples involuntary childlessness leads to adoption. Parents in a hope to have a biological child tend to wait longer. When it becomes clear that it is not possible to have a child of their own, couples decide to adopt.

Table 8.9
Distribution of Waitlisted Adoptive Parents by Age, 2003

Age groups	Adoptive father		Adoptive mother	
	Number	Per cent	Number	Per cent
20–30 Years	1	2.9	33	24.26
30–40 Years	101	74.26	92	67.64
40+	30	22.11	10	7.3
Data Not Known	1	0.73	1	0.73
Total	136	100.00	136	100.00

The incorporation of an unaffiliated person into a family affects not only the familial domain but society at large. Filiation is the relationship created by the fact of being the legitimate child of one's parents. The legitimisation is not social or ritual but jural. In order to recognise an unfiliated child as one's own, adoption has to be carried out according to the laws, as it is a legal binding.

Respecting the religious sentiments of people, adoption comes under the purview of personal laws. But it has to be carried out according to the provisions in the law. There is no secular law of adoption despite secularism being propagated in our country. Adoption of children is carried out according to adoption laws pertaining to the religion of the parents. Hindus can adopt a child under the Hindu Adoption and Maintenance Act of 1956 (HAMA). The personal laws of Muslims, Christians, Jews and the Parsis do not recognise a complete adoption. Persons belonging to these communities, who want to adopt a child, can take a child only in guardianship under the provision of the Guardians and Wards Act, 1890 (The GWA). Under this Act, besides non-Hindus, foreigners can also be appointed as a guardian of the child. The Act deals mainly with the appointment of the guardians and their duties, rights and liabilities. It must be stressed that the GWA only provides for foster care but does not create any such permanent rights in favour of the minor.

In the absence of a uniform law of adoption, a need was felt to have a uniform code for adoption which will have secular orientation and will be uniformly applied to all Indians. This Bill was the Adoption of Children's Bill, 1972. This bill was only an enabling legislation which had 'no compulsive' status. However, the Bill was dropped from the Parliament due to opposition by certain sections of the society.

Surprisingly, the present data shows that all the adoptions that were carried out in 2003 were under the Hindu Adoption and Maintenance Act. The absence of adoption by Muslims and Christians in the data show the lack of suitable adoption law and legislation. This deters the decision to adopt. Members of these communities can only assume guardianship of a destitute child under the Guardians and Wards Act and cannot adopt legally.

Income Levels of the Adoptive Parents _____

The category of the prospective adoptive parents is not a homogenous category as far as incomes are concerned. The income level

Table 8.10
Distribution of Adoptive Parents by Monthly Income, 2003

Income levels (Rupees)	Combined income of mother and father	
	Number	Per cent
up to 10,000	35	25.73
10,001–20,000	42	30.88
20,001–30,000	18	13.23
30,001–40,000	12	08.82
40,000 +	28	20.58
Not Known	01	00.75
Total	136	100.00

ranges from Rs 5,000 to Rs 2,00,000 in some cases. On an average most of the parents belong to middle income levels (Table 8.10).

Most parents (30.88 per cent) are concentrated in the income level of Rs 10,000–Rs 20,000/pm. About 25.73 per cent in incomes below Rs 10,000, about 13.23 per cent in income level of Rs 20,000–Rs 30,000; whereas 8.82 per cent are in Rs 30,000–Rs 40,000. Surprisingly, about 20.58 per cent of parents belong to higher income groups, that is income above Rs 40,000. There is no parent whose income is below Rs 5,000 per month. This can be explained by the fact that the rules for adoption make it mandatory for parents to be earning around Rs 5000/pm or more. Majority of the families, about 52.93 per cent, belong to the middle-income group (Rs 10,000–Rs 40,000). Thus, it is mainly the middle income group that adopts more number of children from this particular agency.

Marital Status of Adoptive Parents

Except one single mother, all others who want to adopt a child are married couples. Single parent adoption is legal in India, but there are few such adoptions taking place. In this sample as well there is only one single mother but her status is not clear, whether she is unmarried, divorcee or a widow.

The data in Table 8.11 shows that approximately 60.29 per cent parents decide to adopt children when they have been married for 6–10 years. About 16.17 per cent of couples decide to adopt within the

Table 8.11
Distribution of Adoptive Parents by Length of Marriage, 2003

Length of marriage	Number	Per cent
Up to 5 years	22	16.17
6–10 years	82	60.29
11–15 years	27	19.85
16–20 years	05	3.67
Total	136	100.00

first five years of their marriage and as little as 3.67 per cent decide to adopt after 16–20 years of their married life. Out of 136 parents in the waiting list there are only two parents who have biological children of their own. One family, which already had a son, wanted to adopt a girl child to complete their family. The second family had two girls who wanted to adopt a male child for obvious reasons. For the rest it was their first adoption.

Preferences of Adoptive Parents

Unlike the biological parents, the adoptive parents have an opportunity, if they want, to express their preference regarding the age of the child they want to adopt. Most adoptive parents prefer a young child, generally below one year. Majority (123, about 90.44 per cent) parents prefer the child to be below six months of age, about 7.35 per cent prefer the child to be below one year (Table 8.12). Two parents preferred the child to be between one–two years and only one adoptive parent asked for the child to be above two years. Generally, it is the age of couples that is the main consideration of the adoption agencies while deciding the age of the child to be given for adoption. Older couples are given older children. Most couples,

Table 8.12
Adoptive Parents' Preference for Child's Age, 2003

Age	Number	Per cent
0–6 Months	123	90.44
6 months–1 year	10	7.35
1–2 years	2	1.47
2 years +	1	0.73
Total	136	100.00

who are above 42 years of age, are given children who are above one year of age.

Out of total data of 136 parents, 62 (45.58 per cent) prefer girls and the preference for boys is 54 (39.70 per cent). There is quite a high number of Indian parents, about 20 (14.70 per cent) who did not express any preference (Table 8.13). This does not mean that the male child has fewer chances of adoption. On the contrary, there is a long waiting queue for the adoption of a male child. Since more girl children are abandoned, their availability is more. Hence many adoptive parents choose to adopt a female child first. If later on they want to adopt a boy, they can do so on a priority basis.

Table 8.13
Adoptive Parents' Preference for Child's Sex, 2003

Gender	Number	Per cent
Female	62	45.58
Male	54	39.70
Either	20	14.70
Total	136	100.00

Table 8.14
Waitlist of Adoptive Parents, 1999–2003

Year	1999	2000	2001	2002	2003
Preference for					
Female child	133	100	111	99	75
	(29.16%)	(31.64%)	(45.86%)	(49.01%)	(46.87%)
Male child	323	216	131	103	85
	(70.83%)	(68.35%)	(54.13%)	(50.99%)	(53.12%)
Total	456	316	242	202	160

The trends regarding the preference of the sex of the child for the period 1999–2003 show that the preference for the female child is increasing. Conversely, the preference for the male child is decreasing. Table 8.14 shows that 29.16 per cent couples preferred a female child and substantially a large number of couples, about 70.8 per cent, preferred a male child in 1999. The preference for the female child increased gradually as 46.87 per cent couples preferred a female child and 53.12 per cent preferred a male child in 2003. The reason for the apparent increase in the preference for girls may be a long waiting list for a male child. In a desire to bring home a child

Table 8.15
Number of Children Arrived in Palna, 1998–2003

Year	Females	Males	Total
1998	190	91	281
1999	179	128	307
2000	139	87	226
2001	146	69	215
2002	111	87	198
2003	94	50	144
Total	859	512	1371

as quickly as possible, prospective parents, who preferred a male child initially, happily accepted a female child who was instead available.

Some alarming trends can also be seen from the data of the last six years of Delhi Council of Child Welfare. Surprisingly the number of children reaching this agency is tremendously declining. Table 8.15 shows that only 144 abandoned children reached Palna in 2003 as against 281 and 307 in 1998 and 1999 respectively. Even the waiting list of parents registered for adoption shows a sharp decline in numbers registering with the adoption agencies. This sharp decline is evident from Table 8.14 which shows, that as against 456 parents who were on the waiting list in the year 1999, there are only 160 who applied in the year 2003. This can be a direct consequence of a growing number of irregular adoptions through private practitioners, nursing homes and unlicensed adoption agencies. This situation can be a dangerous one, as in such cases the child will be an ultimate victim of any improper adoption. There can be legal complications as the child will not have a legal status.

The above observations are very significant because in a male-dominated society, where social norms express the need for a male child, at the same time parents, out of choice, adopt a baby girl. The only plausible explanation for this change can be that the adoptive parents' attitudes may not be identical to those of the biological parents as they are willing to take daughters, because procuring a child becomes most important. The sex of the child remains a secondary factor. This shows the extreme importance of children in our society. The other observation was that there was a drop in both the number of children arriving at the adoption agency and the number of childless couples registering with the agency. This indicates that many people might be opting for irregular adoptions. The reason may be the long procedures at the agencies and the restrictive laws.

The positive changes in the attitude, though small, can be attributed in part to the impact of modernisation and more recent, globalisation. The impact of these processes is more visible in the politico-economic spheres of a society and its individuals. But the social and religious lives of individuals do not remain unaffected. The changes in various spheres of life are bound to have an influence on the traditional, social values of the society, at times modifying it and sometimes altering it, in the process of adaptation to the changing social milieu. So is the case with the attitude towards the girl child, which is showing an appreciable change.

In the backdrop of such a situation when a society is in a flux, where tradition and modernity coexist, conflicting attitudes prevail. Parents do prefer to have a male child initially, for all practical and religious reasons, deeply ingrained in the socialisation process. These social expectations are consciously ignored in the case of non-availability or delay in availability of a male child. The intense desire to become a parent quickly prompts them to adopt a baby girl.

The apprehensions regarding the parentage and sex of the child then become immaterial. The initial preference for a male child seems to be an expression of conforming to the expected traditional, social behaviour. It might not be a strongly held view of the individuals themselves. Besides, with the loosening of social cohesion, individual needs and desires become central, that they prioritise their requirements. They try not to ignore their natural instincts of becoming a parent. This is a crucial step as parents consciously decide to adopt, irrespective of age, sex or parentage of the child. The conscious act for subconscious parental instinct, the love for the abandoned and to give joy to the destitute—the interplay of all these emotions culminate into bringing home a child to complete a family.

Several reasons have been given to rationalise their preference for a son and discrimination against a daughter. Surprisingly these very reasons have been quoted in the ancient Indian texts for preferring a son. Many ancient texts which elaborated on sonship in India, stressed that if a person did not have a biological son, then he should procure one by several methods illustrated. One such socially accepted way of having a son was adoption and an adopted son was called a *dattaka*. To enlarge a family, a *dattaka*[11] was one of the eleven or twelve different kinds of secondary sons that were listed by many ancient *smirti* writers. Some of them were legitimate, some illegitimate, and some had no blood-relationship with the father, therefore regarded as not equal. The large number of secondary sons enumerated by most *smirti* writers, show the desperation of parents to procure a son in his absence.

In ancient India, sons were required for both secular and religious purposes. The *sutras* and *smritis* emphasise the importance of a son for the spiritual welfare of a man. The principal purposes served by the birth of the son were that he enabled the father to pay off the debt he owed to his ancestors and secure immortality and the heavenly world. These religious benefits derived from sons are elaborated by many writers (Jolly 1975, Kane 1946, Kapadia 1947, Mukherjee 1976). The most important secular advantages from sons were the economic utility and the perpetuation of the race through them. These reasons were sufficient enough for people to procure a son by whatever method. In the absence of a male child, the deficiency was made-up by adopting a son who performed all the social, economic and religious acts like a natural born son.

This artificial relationship was socially accepted and legally recognised. Under normal circumstances adoption was not encouraged. The *smritis* tend to describe adoption as an institution for *apad* or times of distress, and hence deplored excessive giving and taking in adoption (Derrete 1977). *Apad* means the inability or the need of the original parents to cater to the needs of their child. The distress so discussed is with reference to the natural parents of the child. The adoption which took place was according to the customary laws.

Secular and religious reasons were often quoted in support of the practice of adoption of sons. Though sons were predominantly adopted, adoption of girls was not unheard of. *Mahabharata* mentions Pritha, the daughter of Sura adopted by Kuntibhoja; Santa, the daughter of king Dasratha was adopted by King Lomapada (Kane 1946). The daughter of Maneka and Vishwamitra was given in adoption (Sunanda 1995). The reasons for which girls were adopted were different from those mentioned for adopting sons. The adoption of girls neither strengthened the family economically nor was religiously required, but it helped the family spiritually to attain *punya* when daughters were given as gift in marriage. The other aim was to strengthen friendship, and as a goodwill gesture girls were adopted (Karve 1953).

Since the birth of a son and the gift of a daughter in marriage were considered to be spiritually meritorious acts, children of both the sexes were necessary to free one from the torments of hell. Keeping these facts in mind, children of either sex could be adopted in earlier times (Manooja 1993). With the passage of time, adoption of a daughter fell into disuse amongst all classes of Hindus except in the case of *devdasis* or dancing girls where it was permitted by custom only (*ibid.*). Given such a situation, girls were adopted only in the absence of a natural born daughter and not to substitute sons. She could not offer *pindas* to the ancestors, nor could she support the family economically.

To recognise jurally an unaffiliated child as one's own, adoption was carried out according to the laws of the land in ancient India. The roots of the Hindu Law lie in the ancient *sastras* of Hindus, which was the law of the land in ancient times (Manooja 1993). It elaborated rules to be adopted while selecting a child for adoption. It also elaborated on the process of adoption. The necessary requisite of the ceremony of adoption was bodily transference of the boy from the natural family to the adoptive family and performance of *Datta Homa* (Bharat 1993, Derette 1977, Manooja 1993). *Datta Homa* is oblation of clarified butter to fire. The adoption taken place according to the customary laws was irrevocable. Nowadays, adoption according to the customary laws in not recognised as legal. Laws pertaining to adoption dominate the whole adoptive process. The Hindu Adoption and Maintenance Act of 1956, the Guardian and Wards Act of 1890 and the Juvenile Justice Act of 1986 are the major Acts governing adoption in India.

Adoption is the creation of fictitious blood relationship. The new parent-child relationship so formed is recognised socially and legally. A permanent parent-child relationship is created which did not exist before. Therefore, adoption that takes place within the family has wider implications for the whole society. It changes the status of the child, affecting his relationship with the members of his natural family, adopted family and society. In traditional India, a son given in adoption did not completely sever his bonds of kinship with the natural family. It created a double paternity and a double affiliation and therefore it was not a complete *sastric*[12] adoption (Derette 1977, Kane 1946, Kapadia 1947). The present day practice of adoption, if carried according to the laws is a complete adoption, where the adopted child takes the place of the biological child legally, and has all the rights of a biological child. It is a complete transference of a child to the parents and is irrevocable.

Adoption, which was treated as a private affair is no longer so. It is the state that has assumed a vital role. The process of adoption is seen as seeking suitable parents for a child-in-need rather than seeking of a child for the prospective parents. The ideology behind the changing attitudes towards adoption has changed as well. Earlier adoption was carried out for the benefit of the adoptive family, then in the last century, the idea of 'charity' motivated parents to adopt children. In recent years, the main concern in the process of adoption is to 'ensure the best interest of the child', thus making it a welfare service for the children. Article 20 of the 'UN Convention of the Rights of the Child' views adoption as a means of providing alternative care for a child who is deprived of his or her family environment and obligation. Though over-riding importance is given to the child, one must not ignore the fact that it leads to the formation of a genuine family unit, where the needs of a child and that of the parents are satisfied.

A comparison of the institution of adoption in the ancient and contemporary times shows that there is a continuity of the institution, but in a different shape and form. The various sources of change like education, industrialisation, urbanisation, uniform legal system, etc., have been assumed to bring about profound changes in the traditional social structure. In India, it succeeded in transforming some and modifying, appreciably, many traditional social institutions. One such institution that continues to exist with modification, is adoption.

Modern societies firmly accept the importance of children but the perspective has shifted from a parent-oriented view to a child-oriented view as children are seen to be the wealth of a nation and their rights and welfare must be protected. The welfare of the child being of prime importance, the practice of adoption is now seen as providing a family for the needs of the child, whereas earlier childless couples were provided with a child to satisfy their needs.

The new reproductive technology, which has separated procreation from sex, has brought hope into the lives of many infertile couples. The success of new reproductive technology has contributed in delaying the decision to adopt for many, or even dismissing adoption as an alternative way to create a family. A recent report that childless NRIs are flocking to India to rent a womb shows that in

India, even in small towns, facilities of in-vitro fertilisation (IVF) are readily available. Anand in Gujarat has seen as many as fourteen commercial IVFS (*Times of India*, 24 February 2006).

Many childless couples prefer surrogacy to adopting a child as they feel that in case of surrogacy the baby is genetically theirs, undermining the fact that surrogacy delinks the genetic and gestational motherhood, a situation which can raise several ethical issues. The other form of surrogacy that disconnects conception from gestation is donated gamete conception. In donated gamete surrogacy, one of the gametes, either the egg or the sperm, is their own and the other is donated. Adoption for them makes infertility permanently visible.

The issue of gender becomes a crucial one in donated gamete conception as argued by Haimes (1993) in *The Issues of Gender in Gamete Donation*. She insists that woman-to-woman egg donation is completely asexual in comparison to man-to-woman semen donation. The latter may convey a sense of 'inappropriate sexuality' or may have 'dubious sexual connotations'. She argues that a female third party is not seen as invasive, or as significant a threat to sociopolitical stability of a family as a semen donor, i.e. the boundaries of the family are less threatened by egg donation than by donated semen (Haimes 1993). Hence, donor sperm is lesser acceptable than the donor egg.

In India, the donated gamete conception is acceptable, but conditionally as long as it is kept secret by all concerned. They have to ensure that the purity and honour associated with the 'biosocial bind'[13] is not compromised (Bharadwaj 2003). According to Bharadwaj the 'biosocial bind' or 'the double conceptual bind' unites the biological and social aspects of reproduction. In case of donated gamete surrogacy, the interested parties collude in recrafting the 'biosocial bind' to mark their offspring as biologically related even when it is not. Such a transgression can be tacitly reconfigured into a legitimate kinship unit. Kinship structures are resilient enough to contain such violations only when they are invisible. Children secretly conceived with donated gametes still remain partially connected and so adoption remains even more undesirable. Bharadwaj further argues that adoption emerges as a problematic alternative as situating the child within the marriage/family visibly depart from the biosocial bind and makes the task of misrecognising the origins of the adoptee extremely difficult.

Hence couples would rather secretly resort to accepting donated gamete conception than choose the option of adoption, an option that evokes widespread fears of making infertility permanently 'invisible' and irreparable upsetting the sacred social and biological triad of mother (womb), father (semen) and the child (foetus). (Bharadwaj 2003: 1879)

Bhargava (2005) provides different reasons for the delay in adoption. She argues that adoption can be understood as an expression of individuality and assertion of difference, both of which can be detrimental in the community where staying connected to the family is of prime importance. The decision to adopt also indicates some autonomy from the social control and social values of the community at large. Those who assert their individuality and defy social control, for them to opt for adoption is easier and sooner. Those who adhere to social norms and customs, show reluctance and reduced communication in the area of adoption which may be seen as an attempt to remain within the confines of a social group. Adoption for them maybe the first instance of expressing individuality. Bhargava believes that asserting individuality by way of adopting may invite some kind of social ostracism or social reprisal in a society where genealogy is at the core of kinship. Hence there is a delay in the decision to adopt, and for some adoption may not even remain as an option. It may be stressed here that adoption is a kind of kinship and not outside kinship. By adopting, one is not breaking the confines but is making the confines more resilient.

A common thread in both the arguments is the strength of oft-repeated phrases like 'adoption mirrors biology', its unreal and has missing blood ties. Both have expressed the coercive nature of social norms and values and anything beyond it will amount to deviation. Being abiding members of the society, infertile couples are compelled to conform as 'docile takers' and not an 'active participant' in the process of management of infertility. There is a need to understand the process of adoption as a proactive process where infertile couples, whose fertility is already very much visible, try to create kinship legally, not as non-conforming persons of the society but by staying integral to the society, and at the same time expressing individuality delimited by broad social roles and expectations.

Adoption is a conscious process for many couples who may not want to explore the option of assisted, reproductive techniques. The presumption that all couples always try these technologies first, failing which they go for adoption, is not always true. It is not necessarily a pre-condition to adoption as people do adopt out of choice. They tend to wait longer only in the hope to have a biological child of their own.

Conclusion

A commonly held view is that religious, secular and economic needs drive people to adopt. This may be true for boys. Adoption of girls does not bring in these advantages. Overarching all these needs is the individual desire to become a parent, even if it meant going tangentially off to the expected cultural and social values. In case of people who choose an alternative of adopting children, especially unknown ones, to form a family, are not barred to do so. Therefore, the overriding principle is neither social conformity, nor traditional, nor secular values. Rather individual's needs and desires guide them. The parental instinct which drives childless couples to adopt and not a social expectation, is a prime mover for adoption. So an abandoned child is adopted out of love and is given another chance to survive, to live in an atmosphere, which is warm and secure.

The various dimensions of the practice of adoption in contemporary India depicts the picture of adoption as an institution which is paradoxical in itself. It internalises a dual process. On the one hand, there are parents who, because of several reasons abort foetuses, kill baby girls or abandon children, mostly girls. On the other hand there are childless couples who need children to complete their families. These childless couples adopt the abandoned children and create a family. There are parents who disown their own children, there are couples who make the children of others, their own

Female infanticide, female foeticide and abandonment of children are persisting in the technologically advanced and socially progressive society of today. The acts are carried out, even when aware of the existence of stringent laws banning them. People are willing to defy them, conscious of the fact that the consequences can be harsh if law takes its course. The reasons for their continued existence may be so strong that people are prepared to defy law. Besides ignoring law, they are knowingly tampering with nature. The fear that playing with nature can cause great havoc is not a deterrent. They even overlook the rights of the children, which are advocated sincerely by all those involved with the welfare of the children

The possible reason being fear for the future of the daughter. A fear is of consequences that a girl might face in adulthood, a fear of parents being drained of their resources because of financial expenses being involved in her upbringing and dowry. These fears quite often drive parents either to kill or abandon children. Thus, conformity to social customs and danger of ostracism in case of nonconformity, pressurise the parents to perform inhuman acts. Recently in January (2003), a horrific case of dowry harassment was brought to light. Not only was the woman brutally tortured but also her daughter was inflicted grievous wounds by her husband, ostensibly for not bringing sufficient dowry. Daughter Shreya is only four years old. She had to go in for three elaborate, reconstructive surgeries to set good the damage. She is said to be probably 'the youngest victim ever of dowry' (Ghosh 2004). Along with the mother, the torture of bringing inadequate dowry was extended to the female child.

The acts of aggression against female children and even against adult females, such as rape, bride-burning, domestic violence, and other such practices as a custom of pre-puberty marriage, prohibition of *pratiloma* (marriage where a woman of higher caste marries a man of lower caste), point that the patriarchal values and normative structure established over 2000 years ago still persist but in a different garb (Desai and Krishnaraj 1990). These symbolic acts relegate a woman to a lower position. Then there are other practices which reinforce her subordinate position. The practices that suggest the control of sexuality of woman like that of marriage at an early age, marriage within the caste, prohibition of *pratiloma* and marriage as a sacrament, whereby a woman is bound in wedlock till she dies, are still operational and alive. These practices are subtle expressions of patriarchal values still holding strong, conveying inferiority of women and at the same time strengthening it.

Abandoning children is a milder form of aggression and prejudice against girls as compared to female infanticide and female foeticide, which are fatal. But there can be no denial that abandoning children, especially girls, is an extreme case of neglect and an indifferent attitude of parents towards their welfare which can again be fatal. The fear psychosis that works behind these acts is not because they are female *per se* but because of the continuity of traditional, social practices and ideologies that have become dysfunctional but retain a stronghold in people's thinking in today's changing society. The elements of such an ideology are falsely implicated to be functional, and so imposed and hence continue.

After carefully analysing various aspects of prejudices against women and deep introspection, the only plausible reason that can be given for its continuance is that people consciously or unconsciously want to believe in the artificial construct of 'male superiority' which is not supported by any scientific evidence. They rationalise the acts by appealing to the social and cultural approvals it gets. But by adoption of girls, adoptive parents are consciously, though slowly, demolishing the preconceived idea of male superiority and trying to re-establish the worth of the girl child.

Notes

1. Aristotle assumed that men were by nature unequal and there was a natural rank order amongst them. He was referring to natural inequalities such as physical strength, intelligence, talent, which can be distinguished from social inequalities. Still it can be argued that natural inequalities, no matter insignificant, provide a base upon which social inequality is built.

2. Veena Das analyses the anthropological meaning of prevalence of the worship of goddesses. She says 'the principle of power finds expression in the goddesses who represent 'shakti', who come to the aid of man and the god in periods of cosmic darkness, by killing the demon who threatens the entire cosmic order.'

3. Due to social, economic and religious reasons, people prefer to have sons. The main cause of population problem is not only the desire to have a son but due to poor health conditions child mortality is high. To have at least one surviving male, a woman has to have five to six children.

4. Sunanda (1995) notes that parents feel that more girls mean lowering of status in the society and that they would be called Pottapayan. Pottapayan is the Tamil word used to denote a male who possesses more female children.

5. Pindas are the cake of boiled rice offered to deceased ancestors in Sraddhas.

6. The imbalance of sex ratio in a few pockets in Rajasthan, Bihar, Madhya Pradesh, Uttar Pradesh, Punjab, Haryana and Tamil Nadu suggest the prevalence of infanticide and female foeticide.

7. In the most infanticide-endemic area, all castes practised it to some extent, but it was clear the higher social groups who were most extreme, preserved no daughter at all.

8. Khanna study was a project carried for over a decade in eleven villages of the Punjab by a team of Harvard researchers and Indian collaborators (Wyon and Gordon 1971). N.O. Kelly's study was 'Some Socio-Cultural Correlates of Indian Sex Ratio; Studies from Punjab and Kerala', conducted in 22 villages.

9. Mortality differentials sex-wise are considered a major determinant of sex ratio in India.

10. CVARA, the Co-ordinating Voluntary Adoption Resource Agency of Delhi, is housed at the DCCW at Qudsia Park, Delhi. When one registers oneself in any agency, the person's name automatically gets entered on to a consolidated waiting list kept updated by CVARA.

11. Most ancient writers and commentators divided twelve kinds of sons into two groups, first six were thought to be heirs and kinsmen whereas last six are only kinsmen. Initially *dattaka* (adopted son) was placed in the second category of secondary sons. In the course of time other forms of obtaining sons like through *niyoga* (the practice of appointing a widow to a relative with a view to beget a son for the deceased) were not approved of, so *dattaka* was exalted to a higher position.

12. The *sastras* tend to regard the adopted son as a member simultaneously of both *gotras*. The severance from the natural family brought about by adoption was only partial and not complete.

13. Aditya Bharadwaj explains that a 'double conceptual bind' unites the biological and the social aspects of reproduction by transmuting the symbiosis between the socially visible aspects of reproduction such as kinship relations and invisible biological aspects of sexual reproduction into a 'taken-for-granted fact'. The cultural 'imaginings' of visible social triad of mother/father/child, as underscored by an invisible biological triangle of womb, semen and foetus, are intimately linked to such cultural conceptions.

References

Arora, S. 2002. *Female, Foeticide and Infanticide*. Delhi: Unpublished Report of Indian Institute of Human Rights.

Benedict, Burton. 1972. 'Social Regulation of Fertility', in G. A. Harrison and A.G. Boyce (eds.), *The Structure of Human Populations*. pp. 73–89. Oxford: Clarendon Press.

Bharadwaj, Aditya. 2003. 'Why Adoption is not an Option in India: The Visibility of Infertility, the Secrecy of Donor Insemination, and Other Cultural Complexities', *Social Science and Medicine*, 56 (9): 1867–80.

Bharat, S. 1993. *Child Adoption in India*. Bombay: Tata Institute of Social Sciences.

Bhargava, Vinita. 2005. *Adoption in India.* New Delhi: Sage Publications.

Bhelary, K. 1995. 'Messengers of Death'. *The Week*, 24 September.

Chandrashekar, S. 1974. *Abortion in a Crowded World.* London: George Allen and Union Ltd.

Chhabra, Rami and S.C. Nuna. 1993. *Abortion in India—An Overview.* Delhi: Veerendra Printers.

Das, Veena. 1980. 'The Mythological Film and its Framework of Meaning: An Analysis of Jai Santoshi Maa', *India International Centre Quarterly*, 8 (1): 43–56.

Derette, J.D.M. 1977. *Essays in Classical and Modern Hindu Law.* Leiden: E.J. Bril.

Desai, Neera and Krishnaraj, Maithreyi. 1987. *Women and Society in India.* Delhi: Ajanta Publications.

Encyclopedia Britannica. 1969. 'Adoption', Vol. 1: 65. United States of America: William Benton.

Freeman, Milton R. 1971. 'Social and Ecological Analysis of Systematic Female Infanticide among the Netsilik Eskimos'. *American Anthropologist*, 73 (5): 1011–18.

Ghosh, Abantika. 2004. 'New Lease of Life for Dowry Victim', *The Times of India*, 23 April.

Gokhale, S.D. 1976. 'Inter-Country Adoptions and Consultancy in Guardianship', *The Indian Journal of Social Work*, 37 (2): 109–20.

Granzberg, Gary. 1973. 'Twin Infanticide: A Cross-Cultural Test of a Materialistic Explanation', *Ethos*, 4: 405–12.

Haimes, E. 1993. 'Issues of Gender in Gamete Donation', *Social Science and Medicine*, 36 (1): 85–93.

Harris, Marvin. 1975. *People, Culture and Nature.* New York: Thomas Y. Crowell.

Hughes, Jane. 2003. 'Indian Soap to Combat 'Boys Only' Culture', *The Observer*, New Delhi, September 7.

Jacobson, Doranne. 1970. *Hidden Faces: Hindu and Muslim Purdah in a Central Indian Village.* Unpublished doctoral dissertation, Columbia University.

Jolly, J. 1975. *Hindu Law and Customs.* Delhi: Bharitya Publishing House.

Kane, P.V. 1946. *History of Dharmasastras*, Vol.3, 2nd ed. Pune: Bhandarkar Oriental Research Institute.

Kapadia, K.M. 1947. *Hindu Kinship.* Bombay: The Popular Book Depot.

Kapoor, R. 1996. *Sociological Study of Adoption with Special Reference to India.* Unpublished Ph.D. Dissertation, University of Delhi.

Karve, I. 1953. *Kinship Organisation in India.* Bombay: Asia Publishing House.

Kelly, Narinder O. 1975. *Some Socio-Cultural Correlates of Indian Sex Ratios: Case Studies of Punjab and Kerala.* Unpublished doctoral dissertation, University of Pennsylvania.

Mandlebaum, D.G. 1974. *Human Fertility in India.* Berkeley: University of California Press.

Manooja, D.C. 1993. *Adoption Law and Practice.* Delhi: Deep and Deep Publications.

Miller, Barbara. 1997. *The Endangered Sex.* Delhi: Oxford University Press.

Mukherjee, S. 1976. *Some Aspects of Social Life in Ancient India.* Allahabad: Narayan Publishing House.

Oakley, A. 1982. *Becoming A Mother*. Oxford: Martin Robertson.

Patel, T. 1994. *Fertility Behaviour Population and Society in a Rajasthan Village*. Delhi: Oxford University Press.

Premi, M.K. and S. Raju. 1998. 'Born to Die: Female Infanticide in Madhya Pradesh', *Search Bulletin*, 32 (17): 94–105.

Ravindra, R.P. 1991. 'Fighting Female Foeticide—A long way to go'. *The Lawyers Collection*, Vol. 2 (3): 1–6.

Sharma, Shradhha. 2006. 'Girl, Uninterrupted', *Sunday Times of India*, New Delhi: 26 February.

Shatrugana, Veena. 1984. 'Women and Health' Research Centre for Women's Studies. Bombay: SNDT Women's University. Reproduced in N. Desai and M. Krishnaraj. 1987.

Sunanda, K.S. 1995. *Girl Child Born to Die in Killing Fields?* Madras: Alternative for India Development.

The Times of India. 2006. 'Maternity for Hire', Editorial. New Delhi: 24 February.

Visaria, P. 1961. *The Sex Ratio of the Population of India*. Census of India, Vol. 1, Monograph 10. New Delhi: Office of the Registrar General.

Wyon, John B. & John E., Gordon. 1971. *The Khanna Study: Population Problems in the Punjab*. Cambridge: Harvard University Press.

PART 3

Representation, Articulation and the State

Female Infanticide, Property and the Colonial State[*]

9

L. S. Vishwanath

The archival records on female infanticide during colonial rule tell us about the castes which practised female infanticide, the societal, and specifically, the institutional ramifications of the practice. They also show how female infanticide was related to caste dominance, status maintenance and dowry avoidance, the complications of British revenue policies for the castes which practised female infanticide and finally, the strategies adopted by the colonial rulers to get rid of the practice.

The paper argues that the efforts of the colonial state to suppress female infanticide is a reminder of the complex relations between state and society. For the land-owning castes, which practised female infanticide, and for the ambitious upwardly mobile castes, the problem of maintenance of socio-economic status was crucial. At the risk of simplifying a complex, social reality, one may say that female infants were sacrificed to avoid heavy dowries and wedding expenses, and to somehow prevent the sale or mortgage of their most precious asset, land. The colonial state was, on the one hand, trying to stop female infanticide and on the other, it complicated matters, so far as status maintenance was concerned, through its revenue policies. It is impossible to say if the female sex ratios worsened during colonial rule compared to the pre-colonial period because we do not have a detailed census on sex ratios for pre-colonial times.

*This is a revised version of the paper presented at a workshop on 'Missing Girls in India: Science, Gender Relations and the Political Economy of Emotions' organised by the Department of Sociology, Delhi University on 30th and 31st October, 2003. I thank Tulsi Patel for inviting me to the workshop.

Since the colonial rulers depended on those they perceived as having local influence to collect taxes and maintain law and order, the earlier generation of British administrators like Monstuart Elphinstone in Bombay Presidency were for caution and against too much intrusion into the most private and domestic proceedings of the superior castes, to stop female infanticide. The cautious approach was given up in the 1830s but re-introduced after the uprising of 1857.

Female Infanticide and Caste

In December 1789, Jonathan Duncan, the British Resident at Benares, first found female infanticide among Rajkumar Rajputs in Jaunpur district of Benaras Division. The discovery was made when he was touring the district to settle its revenues (Kaye 1966: 555). Right from the time of Duncan's discovery, the Rajputs in north, west and central India which means undivided Punjab, Rajasthan, U.P. Malwa and Saurashtra, figure very prominently in the records as a caste which resorted to extensive female infanticide. British officials reported in 1817 that female infanticide was so extensive among the Jadejas, a Rajput clan in peninsular Gujarat, that whole taluks inhabited by the clan were without any Jadeja female children (SRBG 1856: 389). In 1856, an official appointed to investigate female infanticide in Benares Division found, after taking a census in 418 villages, that Rajput female children were deficient in 308 villages; of these, 62 villages, nearly one-fifth, had no Rajput female children below 6 years (Moore 1868: 54–84). The other castes, which the records say, killed their female children, were: the Lewa Kanbis and Patidars of central Gujarat and Jats, Ahirs, Gujars, Khutris and Moyal Brahmins in north India

When the census enumerations were launched in the last quarter of the 19th century, we find that the same castes, which the archival records say practised female infanticide, also figure in the census reports as having low female sex ratios. Perhaps taking the cue from the records, the author of more than one census report refers to the Rajputs and Lewa Patidars as having a 'stigma' or 'a tradition' of female infanticide since 'olden times' (Census 1901, 1921). The 1921 census report classifies castes into two categories, namely castes having 'a tradition' of female infanticide and castes without such 'a tradition' (see Table 9.1). This census provides figures from 1901 to 1921 to show that in Punjab, United Provinces and Rajputana castes such as Hindu Rajputs, Hindu Jats, and Gujars with 'a tradition' of female infanticide, had a much lower number of females per 1,000 males compared to castes without such 'a tradition' which included: Muslim Rajputs, Muslim Jats, Chamar, Kanet, Arain, Kumhar, Kurmi, Brahmin, Dhobi, Teli and Lodha. What is interesting about this census classification is that in Punjab, the Hindu Rajputs are shown as having 822 (1901), 756 (1911) and 796 (1921) females per 1,000 males, while Muslim Rajputs had 883 (1901), 841 (1911) and 864 (1921) females per 1,000 males. The Hindu Jats had fewer females: 795 (1901), 774 (1911), and 789 (1921) compared to

Table 9.1
Sex Ratios of Castes in North India

Caste	Category	Number of females per 1,000 males		
		1901	1911	1921
Punjab				
Jat (Hindu)	A	795	774	789
Khutri	A	808	802	811
Rajput (Hindu)	A	822	756	796
Gujar	A	799	763	778
Jat (Muslim)	B	859	807	820
Rajput (Muslim)	B	883	841	864
Chamar	B	871	836	845
Kanet	B	924	947	936
Arain	B	877	807	830
United Provinces				
Jat (Hindu)	A	852	769	763
Rajput (Hindu)	A	887	873	877
Gujar	A	802	755	785
Brahmin	B	923	899	895
Chamar	B	986	958	960
Kumhar	B	931	941	931
Kurmi	B	970	929	909
Rajputana				
Rajput (Hindu)	A	794	778	722
Jat (Hindu)	A	830	851	840
Gujar	A	834	846	837
Brahmin	B	925	937	920
Dhobi	B	916	962	922
Teli	B	908	930	941
Lodha	B	911	916	895

Source: Census of India (Report), 1921, Vol. 1, Appendix VI.
Notes: A= Castes with 'a tradition' of female infanticide
         B= Castes without 'a tradition' of female infanticide

859 (1901), 807 (1911) and 820 (1921) females per thousand males among the Muslim Jats.[1]

The classification in the 1921 census also seems to suggest that the lower castes which did not own much landed property such as Chamars, Kumhars, Dhobis, Telis, Lodhas and Kurmis had a much higher proportion of females; at that point in time, they did not have 'a tradition' of female infanticide perhaps because the problem of status maintenance through dowry avoidance and female infanticide which clearly existed among the hypergamous and propertied upper castes did not exist among them. However, it is difficult to conclude from this that the lower castes will not or will never practise female infanticide because sanskritisation, acquisition of assets, modern education and dowry adoption can push the lower castes towards female neglect and infanticide. Indeed recent data for the Chamars and scheduled castes in U.P. suggest that the dalit castes are moving in the direction of deficiency of females and possibly female infanticide or foeticide. Thus in 1901, the Chamars in U.P. had a female to male ratio of 986; but by 1981 the female to male ratio among Chamars in the same state had dropped to only 880. Again in 1901, the female to male ratio among SCs in U.P. was 970; by 1981, it was down to 892. Drawing attention to these figures Dreze and Sen (1995: 156) note that 'so far as gender relations are concerned, the scheduled castes in Uttar Pradesh are now more like the higher castes than they used to be'. The records provide information on the lower castes being influenced by the higher, so far as female infanticide is concerned. For example, E. G. Jenkinson, the Officiating Magistrate of Saharanpur district found on investigation in mid-1830s, that the Pureer clan of Rajputs in the district, practised female infanticide. He also found that two other castes, the Tuggas and Kolis who had a 'fair proportion of girls all over the district, practised female infanticide only in one Tehsil. 'They have probably' says Jenkinson 'adopted the practice of female infanticide from the Rajputs in the midst of whom they have been living for so many years' (SRG 1879: V, I&II).

Sex Ratios and Institutional Ramifications

When one examines the female infanticide records, what strikes one is the overwhelming evidence of the dominant castes like the Patidars,

Rajputs, Jats and Ahirs—all of them were hypergamous—trying to maintain their socio-economic status through dowry avoidance and female infanticide. British officials often speak in their reports of Rajputs of high status seeking 'lofty marriage alliances' for their daughters and resorting to female infanticide to avoid substantial dowry payment, which could lead to alienation of their hereditary agricultural lands. Thomason, the Magistrate of Azamgarh district (then part of the North Western Provinces) found in 1836 that 'among a body of Rajputs, numbering 10,000, not a single daughter was forthcoming'. Thomason goes on to state that the Bais Rajputs prefer 'high alliances' which are 'difficult to be obtained, and attended with great expense which they can ill-bear and are almost certain to cause the alienation of the whole or a great part of their hereditary lands. Hence the birth of a daughter is considered a most serious calamity, and the unfortunate infant is very seldom spared' (Brown 1857: 53).

Since the high status, Rajputs had a martial ethos as noted by anthropological studies (Steed 1955: 102–144, Hitchcock 1959: 10-15) they generally did not take advantage of the avenues for social mobility, which opened up during colonial rule. By freezing the political boundaries, the British certainly complicated matters for the dominant Rajput lineages in north India and peninsular Gujarat. Since territorial expansion was ruled out, the Rajputs' only economic resource was agricultural land. A further complication introduced by colonial rule was the stricter mode of collecting land revenue, sale of land for revenue arrears of those who failed or were unable to pay revenue and doing away with the lucrative revenue contract system of pre-colonial times.

B. S. Cohn, after a detailed study of the archival records for the Benares region, found that in the mid-19th century, the Rajputs in the region engaged in a running battle with the auction purchaser to somehow prevent sale of their hereditary lands. Cohn further notes that faced with the prospect of sale of their hereditary lands, the revenue demands of the British and heavy dowry demands from the groom's side, the Rajputs had to make a choice between expensive marriages(s) of daughters and maintenance of their socio-economic status. They chose the latter, avoided heavy dowries and practised female infanticide (Cohn 1987: 183).

As regards the British doing away with the lucrative revenue contract system of pre-colonial times in certain regions (Shah 2002: 44–45) and the complications of this policy for the marriage of daughters, we find the Lewa Patidars of Nadiad, Borsad, Napad and Mahuda parganas telling the Collector of Kaira district, J. Webb in 1849 that:

> Respectable persons give their daughters in marriage incurring the expenses according to their abilities, but amongst our people the expenses are daily increasing; whilst during the former administration (Maratha rule), we used to obtain the management of the villages from the state on our own responsibility and therefore made the collections on our own authority, consequently our means were kept up; at present we have no such means. (MSS 1849: 212)

The interviews of Patidars and Rajputs with British officials point to the new difficulties they faced. The Patidars telling the officials (the members of this caste told the same thing to the Ahmedabad Collector in 1847) of their inability to pay land revenue and large dowries demanded by the groom's side since the revenue contracts were done away with, does provide a clue. However, it is not possible to say what impact this problem had on female sex ratios and if female infanticide was accentuated due to British revenue policies. Figures on female to male ratios for the pre-colonial period, which would enable a comparison with sex ratios during colonial rule, are not available.

We find qualitative and quantitative data in the historical records, which relate sex ratio to the social status of clans, and lineages, which controlled territory during the 19th century. The data reveal that among Rajputs, the clan, which controlled the largest territory and occupied the topmost position in the Rajput hypergamous hierarchy, resorted to very extensive female infanticide. Thus in the mid-19th century, among Rajputs of Benares division, the top position in the Rajput hierarchy was held by the Suryavamshis of Amroha Pargana in Gorakhpur district. They controlled 78 villages and were acknowledged to be the highest by all the Rajputs in the region. A census of 1856 revealed that the Suryavamshis had in the 78 villages, 721 boys to only 129 girls below six years of age. That is, only 15 per cent were girls. The same census also revealed that 10 of the Suryavamshi villages had no Rajput girls and marriage of Rajput girls was a 'rare occurrence' in many Suryavamshi villages. Though placed in a tight spot due to British revenue policies and lack of mobility as noted above, Rajput clans, which ranked below the Suryavamshis, had somewhat better female to male child sex ratios. Thus, the

Rajkumars of Ungli pargana in Jaunpur district controlled 42 villages. They gave the daughters they preserved to the Suryavamshis and had a CSR of 283 boys to 80 girls below 6 years, that is 22 per cent were girls (Moore 1868: 54–84).

In peninsular Gujarat, the Jadejas occupied the top position in the Gujarati Rajput hierarchy and controlled the largest chunk of territory (9,931 sq. ml.) A census of 1,834 showed that in 32 *taluks* where they resided, the Jadejas had 102 males and only 20 females in the age group, one year and below. The same census also showed that Jadeja males of 20 years of age and below, were 1,422, and Jadeja females of all ages were only 603 (SRBG 1856: 445). Female infanticide was no less extensive among the Jethwa Rajputs who held the number two position below the Jadejas in the Gujarati Rajput hierarchy. Alexander Walker, the Resident at Baroda reported to Duncan in 1800 that his enquiries showed that in the family of the Rana of Porbandar, the head of the Jethwa clan, not a single female child had been preserved for more than a hundred years (*ibid.*: 322–60).

The data on sex ratios in the records for the Lewa Patidars and Kanbis reveal that the top stratum in this caste, comprising the Lewa Patidars of twelve villages known as *Baragam* in the Charotar area of central Gujarat, had much worse female sex ratios than other Lewa Kanbis. The Kanbis had 73 to 75 females per 100 males for a major part of the 19th century (Clark 1983: 35); from 1847 onwards, British local officials talk of very low numbers of females in what they called the 'aristocratic' Patidar villages in Charotar. A census of 1872 showed that the number of females in the twelve top-ranking Patidar villages in Charotar, ranged from 39 to 53 girls to 100 boys below 12 years of age (Cooke 1875). The census of 1891, 1901 and 1911 also showed that the Patidar villages in Charotar had a very low proportion of females. For example, the census of 1911 showed that five of the twelve Patidar villages under Baroda had less than 700 females per 1,000 males (Census 1911: 136).

For Sikh Khutris of Punjab, the records again suggest that the top rung in the hypergamous ladder consisting of Bedi Khutris, who claimed descent from Guru Nanak, the founder of the Sikh faith, practised female infanticide more extensively than other Khutris. The information on female infanticide for Bedi Khutris range from Major Lake's report of 1851 to the Punjab Board of Administration that 'the Bedees are an influential caste of Sikh Khutris who have destroyed all their female offspring for the last four hundred years'

(Brown 1857: 45) to figures from the Punjab Correspondence for the years 1848–49 to 1850–51 showing that the Bedi Khutris had 28 boys to only 10 girls in 1848–49, 24 boys to only 6 girls in 1849–50 and 20 boys to 12 girls in 1850–51(Brown 1857: 45).

Though the female infanticide records and later the census refer to low female sex ratios among Jats, Ahirs and Gujars in north India, detailed information on whether the top rung in these castes resorted to more extensive female infanticide than those of lower status is not available. There is information that the princely Jat houses of Bharatpur, Nabha, Jind, Kythal, Patiala and Faridkot practised female infanticide 'extensively' (Brown 1857:49).

Since the Lewa Patidars, the Jadejas and Suryavamshi Rajputs were acknowledged to be the highest in the hypergamous hierarchy in the respective region, they wished to maintain that position. Moreover, the top stratum had restricted options in selecting eligible grooms. Consequently, they practised more extensive female infanticide than others in their caste. The point is that for those at the top of the hypergamous hierarchy, the complications of bringing up girls went beyond dowry avoidance. Going by the reports of British officials in the records, this is how the establishment perceived the extensive female infanticide among the high status Patidars and Rajputs. It seems to me to have substance and it may be erroneous to regard it as the coloniser's perception. As noted before, the British certainly complicated matters for the castes, which resorted to female infanticide; however, it would be simplistic to suggest, as some scholars have done, that the complications contributing to female infanticide were mainly due to British revenue policies or the support to the dominant castes by the political rulers.[2] A close reading of the socio-political history of Gujarat region shows that even during pre-colonial Maratha rule and Muslim rule, there were influential Patidars in the Charotar villages, who were tax collectors and rulers of villages. The Maratha and Muslim rulers tried to be friendly to the Charotar Patidars. Even during pre-colonial rule, the Patidari or Narwadari villages, which paid fixed revenues, enjoyed a higher status than Senja villages inhabited mostly by Kanbis who paid variable revenue (Shah 2002: 29). Hence the complications of status hierarchy, hypergamy and the friendship between the political authority and the local dominant caste existed before colonial rule. Among Gujarati Rajputs, the freezing of the political boundaries giving clans like the Jadejas the highest position among Gujarati

Rajputs, happened before colonial rule. It is not possible to date it precisely but it is safe to assume that the Rajput territorial boundaries got frozen after the conquest of Gujarat by the Mughal Emperor, Akbar which gave the Rajputs of peninsular Gujarat the top position in the regional Rajput hierarchy.

Female-male Sex Ratios: Continuity and Change

Since caste census was discontinued after independence, it is difficult now to relate sex ratios to caste and status within caste, which one could do earlier on the basis of the female infanticide records and the census. Nevertheless, it is possible to point to continuity and change, which arguably has been a core feature of Indian society for millennia. When one compares the information in the records on female infanticide to the region specific census data on sex ratios since independence, one is struck by the fact that though caste no longer figures now in the census, the regions which the records speak as having female infanticide are the same. Thus while the records speak of undivided Punjab as having female infanticide among certain castes, now it is Punjab and Haryana which is shown very consistently, as having not only low but also declining female to male sex ratios since independence. The child sex ratio (girls per 1,000 boys aged 0–6) in Punjab declined from 894 in 1961 to 793 in 2001. In Haryana, the child sex ratio plummeted from 910 in 1961 to 820 in 2001(Premi 2001:1877). Gujarat, Rajasthan and Uttar Pradesh, which figured in the records as areas where a number of castes practised female infanticide, continue to figure as areas with low female to male sex ratios (*ibid.*: 1878). Given the low female to male sex ratios in the Jat dominated districts in U. P. and also in Punjab and Haryana, it is not difficult to surmise that this caste which resorted to female infanticide in colonial times is now practising female foeticide. A look at the districtwise sex ratios for Gujarat from 1901 to 1971, shows that compared to other districts, Kheda district (Kaira during colonial days), which was the site of the Patidar dominance since pre-colonial and colonial times, has not only lower but also declining female to male sex ratio. The sex ratio in Kheda district dropped from 897 in 1901 to 894 in 1971. It was only 865 in 1911 and 875 in 1931(Mitra 2001:178).

A suggestive pattern which emerges from the female infanticide records is that a) the hypergamous castes which practised female infanticide were dominant at the local level in parts of north and west India and b) they claimed kshatriya status and tried to cultivate a martial ideology. It is interesting to note here that the records never refer to trading or merchant castes such as the Banias who were mostly urban-based, as practising female infanticide. Nor do the Kayasths, who were scribes or took to service since medieval times, find a mention. Except in Punjab, the Brahmins do not figure in the records in connection with female infanticide in any other part of north, west or south India though they were dominant in some rural areas.

The records speak of the lower level Rajputs and Kanbis seeking wives from the Kolis or tribals due to shortage of marriageable women at the lower levels of the hypergamous hierarchy. Established brokers were approached who procured women for a fee. Invariably, the lower level Rajputs and Kanbis paid bride price and brokerage. The deal was, however, kept a secret and generally came to light when the woman was ill-treated in her husband's household (MSS 1849, Vishwanath 2000: 83) . At the middle and lower levels of the status hierarchy among Kanbis and Rajputs, families faced a double financial burden of dowry payment for marrying their daughters hypergamously and bride price for marrying sons.

The caste-specific information on female infanticide available in the records and the data on sex ratios for regions, are clearly indicative of how long the practice has been around in certain communities. The first reference to female infanticide among Jats in Punjab is in an 1857 publication by John Cave Brown on Indian Infanticide. The census data for the colonial period and the recent 2001 Census suggests that the Jats in Punjab have been practising female infanticide, now foeticide for over 150 years. For Lewa Patidars and Kanbis of Central Gujarat, the first mention of low female sex ratios goes back to 1847 (MSS 1848: 192–95). The long history of female infanticide in these castes shows how well entrenched the practice is. There is no getting away from the fact that the practice is embedded in the social structure of certain dominant castes. Unfortunately, for reasons of status mobility and possibly other reasons we can guess, the other non-dominant castes are following their bad example. Once we accept the fact that female infanticide is rooted in the social structure of certain castes for a century and a half, the reality that it is not easy to eradicate it also needs to be faced. The colonial rulers' efforts to stop female infanticide may be instructive but perhaps inoperative in democratic India.

Efforts at Suppression and Tenacity of Female Infanticide

The official records on female infanticide do not tell us everything we want to know, particularly how the castes, which practised female infanticide, viewed it. In addition, there is always the problem of an official bias. Despite these limitations, the records show the very different perceptions of the coloniser and the other. While the colonial officials who were called upon to deal with female infanticide in the course of their official career, called it 'inhuman', 'obnoxious' 'barbaric' and 'a crime', the castes which practised female infanticide, in their interviews with the officials, justified it by saying that they killed their female infants because they could not afford huge dowries. This prompted officials like Walker to call the Jadejas an 'avaricious' lot who wished to keep their wealth intact by destroying their female children (SRBG 1856: 322–60). The differing viewpoints[3] bring out the fact that on one side there was a modern, reformist colonial state which viewed female infanticide as an 'obnoxious custom' or a 'crime', which should be eradicated. On the other side, the castes which practised female infanticide had well-entrenched social norms such as dowry, hypergamy, caste endogamy, clan exogamy and so on, which made the marriage of daughters a very complicated affair. These castes did not regard female infanticide as a crime. That there was no meeting ground between these perceptions is evident from the fact that British efforts to stop female infanticide and change the social norms, which contributed to the practice, were a failure. Coercion yielded temporary results. Starting from Duncan's efforts among the Rajkumar Rajputs of Jaunpur district in 1789, to the passing of the Female Infanticide Act in March, 1870, British efforts to stop female infanticide covered a period of nearly hundred years. The continuing low female to male sex ratios among castes known to practise female infanticide, as revealed by the census from 1891 onwards, is proof enough that the British efforts at eradicating female infanticide did not make a dent in the problem.

Jonathan Duncan was an orientalist by conviction. As the Resident at Benares and as Governor of Bombay (1795–1812), he obtained written agreements signed by Rajkumar Rajputs in 1789 and Jadeja Rajputs in 1808. The agreements stated that the signatories would thenceforth desist from killing their female children since such an act was a sin according to the Hindu Shastras and a Puran (PP 1824). How successful Duncan was is clear from Major Ballantine's report of 20th June, 1817, which showed that many taluks in Kathiawad, inhabited by Jadeja Rajputs, had only one female child and some not even one. Ballantine cited the case of Drappa taluka, which contained more than four hundred Jadeja families but 'not a single female child in any of them' (SRBG 1856: 389). As for the Rajkumars, I have earlier referred to the low female to male sex ratios in this Rajput clan as revealed by a census of 1856.

To stop female infanticide, the British tried persuading the castes, which practised it to reduce dowry, and wedding expenses. In the 1840s and 1850s meetings were organised in the North Western Provinces and Punjab to obtain agreements from the castes that they will resort to 'self-regulation' by cutting down on wedding expenditure (Raikes 1852: 39). The agreements did not lead to any concrete result. Later, British officials admitted that the agreements were a non-starter because the 'problem' of hypergamy, which mainly contributed to expensive weddings of girls, had not been addressed (SRG 1879: 50). Perhaps taking a cue from this experience, the British tried to curb hypergamy and encouraged reciprocal marriages to stop female infanticide.

Since the Lewa Kanbis, who sought marriage alliances for their daughters in aristocratic Lewa Patidar families of Charotar, were excluded by the latter unless they offered a huge dowry, the Kanbis formed endogamous circles known as *ekadas* or *gols*. These endogamous circles had rules, which were sometimes written on stamp paper; the rules prohibited the members of the *gol* from marrying their daughter in a higher status family or circle (MSS 1849: 93–102). To counter hypergamy and female infanticide, the British encouraged the formation of *gols* and tried to strengthen the existing ones. British efforts bore fruit in terms of the number of gols formed; by 1872 there were 49 *gols* in Kaira district alone (MSS 1872). However, the *gols* failed to check hypergamy. Ambitious members of the *gols* flouted its rules and married their daughters hypergamously, with large dowries. British efforts to promote the *gols* started in 1847. A census of 1849 showed that there were in British Kaira, 72.84 Kanbi females per 100 males (MSS 1849: 93–95). This moved by 1872 to a sex ratio of 73 Kanbi females per 100 males (MSS 1872). In 23 years, the sex ratio 'improved' by less than one percentage point. It shows the degree of success attained by the British in checking hypergamy and female infanticide by promoting the endogamous circles. The efforts of Wilkinson in 1836 to curb hypergamy to stop female infanticide among the Rajput chiefs in central India and similar efforts of Mcloyd in 1853 among the Bedi Khutris of Punjab, did not yield the desired results (SRG 1879: 50).

That the Female Infanticide Act of 1870 also did not produce any significant result so far as suppression of the practice is concerned, is evident from the census figures and comments of census officials. The author of the 1911 (India) report says: 'The figures for certain communities show that there is still in their case, a great dearth of females but there is very little direct evidence that it is due to actual infanticide and it may equally well be the result of more or less deliberate neglect of girls.' There is evidence that deliberate neglect of girls was there even before the Female Infanticide Act was passed. One is reminded of W. R. Moore's observation in his report of 1856. Designated as the Infanticide Commissioner, Moore was asked to investigate female infanticide in the Benares Division of the North Western Provinces and submit a detailed report. When he asked the Rajputs why they had no female children, they told him: '*Sookh jatain hain*' (they dry up).

The Post-Independence Scenario

When one looks at the knowledge gained about female infanticide and the socio-economic institutions related to it, from the colonial period to the present, it is clearly diminishing knowledge which confronts the researcher and all those deeply concerned with the problem. Based on the interviews of British officials with the castes, which practised female infanticide, the records throw considerable light. The census till 1931, continues to relate caste to female infanticide as the records do, but they are bereft of the kinds of information which the records provide. What we find after 1931, and in the post independence period, is a whole lot of region-wise statistics, which shows that female infanticide, has changed to female foeticide wherever sex determination facilities are available. It is certainly alarming to find that the practice is spreading like wild fire. However, none of the detailed information, which the records throw up on the socio-economic matrix in which female infanticide was located, is now available. This is an important point, which needs stressing in the present day context. It is sometimes assumed that since female infanticide and female foeticide is related to dowry, the problem will be solved once dowry is eradicated through efficient law enforcement or some other method like generating public opinion against it. However, what leads to dowry in the first place, is often not asked. The colonial experience is instructive. From the use of the *Shastra* to coercion, to social engineering, the colonial state tried almost everything to stop the practice. Its failure shows the resilience of the institutionalised norms to which the female infanticide was related and about which we now know so little. It is not surprising therefore, that facile suggestions are being made that this most blatant form of discrimination against females, can be tackled by somehow removing son preference and dowry. Matters don't seem that simple. How does one tackle firmly-entrenched, institutionalised norms of which dowry and son preference are a part? Faced with a daunting task such as removing gender discrimination, the governmental and non-governmental agencies, who are doing their bit to solve the problem, certainly deserve praise and admiration. But we must know what we are up against and here the colonial records and experience are a pointer.

Conclusion

Putting together the information in the records, anthropological studies and other sources, the perception of the analyst of female infanticide during colonial rule is in terms of its caste specificity, hypergamy, hierarchy, status maintenance, dowry avoidance and so on. However, I often ask if that is all there is to analysing the records. Is female infanticide just a matter of a sex ratios and statistics? Were the perpetrators of female infanticide all heartless souls who steeled themselves from human emotions and sacrificed their female infants at the altar of pride and social status to protect their ancestral lands through dowry avoidance? Does not the element of compulsion leading to female infanticide reported by more than one British official give some indication that those who practised female infanticide felt caught up in the social structure of which they were a part? Raising such questions is not to say that the practice is any way justified because of social compulsions. Following Durkheim one may say that there is no wishing away the social compulsions and these need to be addressed to get rid of female infanticide and female foeticide.

Finally, it is necessary to ask if female infanticide, now foeticide in urban centres, is the only one to persist since colonial times. A number of pernicious, social practices concerning women, which the social reformers of the colonial era tried to eradicate, are still with us. *Sati* in U.P. and Rajasthan has been reported; child marriage persists in rural India. The prohibition on widow re-marriage among upper caste Hindus and the sanskritising lower castes, is still to be reckoned with. Given the persistence of these customs, female infanticide and female foeticide, it can be argued that modernity, with its ideology of equality of the sexes, intruded into Indian society without significant changes in the position of women.

Notes

1. The figures in 1921 census do not imply that castes, which convert to Islam, will not practise female infanticide. The records refer to the Pathan Khanzadas of Jaunpur district in N.W.P who practised female infanticide in mid-19th century. The records also mention that the Pathan Khanzadas were Rajkumar Rajputs before conversion and converted to Islam during the medieval period to 'secure to themselves the proprietary possession of a village'.

2. Alice Clark in her paper 'Limitations on Female Life Chances in Rural Central Gujarat', argues that 'partly unwittingly and partly by feigning blindness, British administrators ultimately supported the continuation of female infanticide and female child neglect'. Clarks argument has merit if we take a restricted view only of the colonial period. However, if we go back to pre-colonial rule, it is clear from the studies of scholars (Shah 1964, 2002) that in central Gujarat, the Maratha rulers allowed the Patidars to maintain their high status by permitting them to pay fixed revenues. The British continued the same policy. As I have argued, the complications of status hierarchy and hypergamy existed before colonial rule. Moreover, regardless of the practice of female infanticide by a

dominant caste, the ruling political authority generally took into account the local power of the dominant caste to collect taxes and maintain law and order.

3. Perceptions of female infanticide and ways of eradicating it, varied within the British establishment. Some perceived it as an 'abomination', which should be firmly eradicated since it was their duty as rulers to stop such customs. This view gained ground around the 1830s. The earlier generation of administrators like Jonathan Duncan and Monstuart Elphinstone, were more cautious. They too regarded it as an 'abomination' but favoured a persuasive approach to suppress it. The missionaries, of course, viewed female infanticide, Sati, child marriage and also superstition as a sure sign of the 'decadence' of Hindu society.

References

Manuscript Sources (cited as MSS)
At the Bombay Secretariat Record Office

(i)   Political Department 1848, Vol. 4, 2014 and 2181.
(ii) Judicial Department 1849, Vol. 15, (No. 237 of 1849), Vol. 21
(iii) Political Department 1855, Vol. 61, 1856, Vol. 86, 1857, Vol. 119, 1859, Vol. 110, 1863, Vol. 35, 1867, Vol. 19.
(iv) Judicial Department 1868, Vol. 29.
(v)   Home Department (Judicial) 1872, No. 1604.

Printed Sources
A. Selections from Records of Government

(i)   Govt. Records. 1856 (cited as SRG). *North Western Provinces, Mr. Thomason's Despatches*. 2 Vols. Calcutta : Baptist Mission Press.
(ii) Bombay Govt. Records. 1856 (cited as SRBG). *Measures Adopted for the Suppression of Female Infanticide in the Province of Kattywar*. Bombay: Education Society's Press.
(iii) Bombay Govt. Records. 1869 (cited as SRBG). *Introduction of the Revehue Survey Assessment in the Kaira Collectorate*. No. XIV (New Series). Bombay: Govt. Central Press.
(iv) Bombay Govt. Records. 1875 (cited as SRBG). *Repression of Female Infanticide in the Bombay Presidency* by H. R. Cooke. No. XLVII (New Series). Bombay: Govt. Central Press.
(v)   Govt. Records. 1879 (cited as SRG). North West Provinces. *Female Infanticide*. Vol. V. Allahabad: North West Province and Oudh Govt. Press.

B. Reports

(i)   Moore, W. R. 1868. *Papers on the Subject of W.R. Moore's Investigation and Report Regarding Female Infanticide in the Benares Division*. Calcutta: A Dozey, Home Secretariat Press

(ii) Census of India. Reports 1901,1911,1921 (Appendix VI), 1931. Punjab and United Provinces Census Reports 1911, 1921.

C. Great Britain, Parliamentary Papers (cited as PP), House of Commons Infanticide Correspondence 1789–1820. Paper 426 of 1824.

D. Other Sources

Brown, John Cave. 1857. *Indian Infanticide, its Origin, Progress and Suppression*. London: W. H. Allen.

Clark, Alice. 1989. 'Limitations on female life chances in rural Central Gujarat', in J. Krishnamurthy (ed.), *Women in Colonial India*. pp. 27–51. Delhi: Oxford University Press.

Cohn, B.S. 1987. 'Is There a New Indian History ? Society and Social Change Under the Raj' in B. S. Cohn. (ed.) *An Anthropologist among the Historians: And Other Essays*. pp. 172–99. Delhi: Oxford University Press.

Cooke, H.R. 1875. *Repression of Female Infanticide in the Bombay Presidency*. Bombay: Govt. Central Press.

Durkheim, Emile. 1970. *Suicide*. London: Routledge and Kegan Paul Ltd. (Reprint).

Dreze, Jean and Amartya, Sen. 1995. *India: Economic Development and Social Opportunity*. Delhi: Oxford University Press.

Hitchcock, John T. 1959. 'The Idea of the Martial Rajput', in Milton Singer (ed.), *Traditional India: Structure and Change*. pp. 10–15. Philadelphia: The American Folklore Society.

Kaye, John. 1966. *The Administration of the East India Company*. Allahabad: Kitab Mahal Pvt. Ltd. (Reprint).

Mitra, Asok. 2001. 'Implications of Declining Sex Ratio in India's Population', in Vina Mazumdar & N. Krishnaji (eds.), *Enduring Conundrum: India's Sex Ratio*. pp. 149–98. Delhi: Rainbow Publishers.

Pocock, D. F. 1971. *Kanbi and Patidar: A Study of the Patidar Community of Gujarat*. London: Oxford University Press.

Premi, Mahendra K. 2001. 'Missing Girl Child', *Economic and Political Weekly*, XXXVI (21): 1875–80.

Raikes,Charles. 1852. *Notes on the North-Western Provinces of India*. Originally published in the *Benares Magazine*. VII (XXXIII). London: G. Barclley.

Shah, A. M. 2002. *Exploring India's Rural Past*. Delhi: Oxford University Press.

Steed, Gitel P. 1955. 'Notes on an Approach to a Study of Personality in a Hindu Village in Gujarat', in Mckim Marriott (ed.), *Village India*, pp. 102–44. Chicago: University of Chicago Press.

Vishwanath, L. S. 2000. *Female Infanticide and Social Structure*. Delhi: Hindustan Publishing Corporation.

The Political Economy of Missing Girls in India

10

Vibhuti Patel

I

Selective elimination of female foetuses and selection of male at a preconception stage contributes to more and more 'missing girls'. The legacy of continuing declining sex ratio in India in the history of the Census of India has taken a new turn with the widespread use of new reproductive technologies (NRTs) in India. NRTs are based on the principle of selection of the desirable and rejection of the unwanted. In India, the desirable is the baby boy and the unwanted is the baby girl. The result is obvious. The Census results of 2001 have revealed that with a sex ratio of 927 girls for 1,000 boys, India had a deficit of 60 lakh girls in the age-group of 0–6 years, when it entered the new millennium. Hundred million women have been missing due to femicide (female infanticide, ill-treatment and discrimination) leading to higher mortality rate among women/girls in the first three quarters of the 19th century and in the last quarter of the 19th century, due to misuse of NRTs for sex determination, SD and preconception sex-selection, SP from 1901 to 2001.

Female infanticide was practised among selected communities, while the abuse of NRTs has become a generalised phenomenon rapidly encompassing all communities irrespective of caste, class, religious, educational and ethnic backgrounds. Demographers, the population control lobby, anthropologists, economists, legal experts, medical fraternity and feminists are divided in their opinions about gender implications of NRTs. NRTs, in the context of patriarchal control over women's fertility and commercial interests, are posing a major threat to women's dignity and bodily integrity. The supporters of sex-selective abortions put forward the argument of 'Women's Choice' as if women's choices are made in a social vacuum. In this context, the crucial question is—Can we allow Asian girls to become an endangered species? Asian countries are undergoing a demographic transition of low death and birth rates in their populations. The nation-states in South Asia are vigorously promoting small family norms. India has adopted the two-child norm and China has ruthlessly imposed a 'one child per family' rule. Sex ratios in Europe, North America, Caribbean, Central Asia, the poorest region—sub-Saharan Africa are favourable to women as these countries neither kill/neglect girls nor do they use New Reproductive Technologies for the production of sons. Only in South Asia, the sex ratios are adverse for women as Table 10.1 reveals. The lowest sex ratio is found in India.

There is an official admission to the fact, 'It is increasingly becoming a common practice across the country to determine the sex of the unborn child or foetus and eliminate it if the foetus is found to be a female. This practice is referred to as pre-birth elimination of females (PBEF). PBEF involves two stages: determination of the sex of the foetus and induced termination if the foetus if not of the desired sex. It is believed that one of the significant contributors to the adverse child sex ratio in India is the practice of elimination of female foetuses.' (UNDP 2003: 1)

Table 10.1
Women per 100 Men in the World

Europe & North America	105
Latin America	100
Caribbean	103
Sub-Saharan Africa	102
South East Asia	100
Central Asia	104
South Asia	95
China	94
India	93

Source: The World's Women—Trends and Statistics, UNFPA, United Nations. N.Y. 1995.

II

Historical Legacy of Declining Sex Ratio

Historically, most Asian countries have had a strong son-preference. The South Asian countries have declining sex ratios. In the beginning of the 20th century, the sex ratio in colonial India was 972 women per 1,000 men, it declined by –8, –11, –5 and –5 points in 1911, 1921, 1931 and 1941 respectively. During the 1951 Census it improved by +1 point. During 1961, 1971, 1981 and 1991 it declined by –5, –11, –4, –7 points respectively. Even though the overall sex ratio improved by +6 points, the decline in the juvenile sex ratio (0–6 age group) is of –18 points, which is alarmingly high (See Table 10.2).

India has had a tradition of killing female babies (custom of *dudhapiti*) by putting opium on the mother's nipple and feeding the baby, by suffocating her in a rug, by placing the afterbirth over the

Table 10.2
Sex Ratio in India, 1901 to 2001

Year	Number of women per 1,000 men	Decadal variation
1901	972	
1911	964	–8
1921	955	–11
1931	950	–5
1941	945	–5
1951	946	+1
1961	941	–5
1971	930	–11
1981	934	–4
1991	927	–7
2001	933	+6

Source: Census of India. 2001. Provisional Population totals, Series 1, Paper 1.

Table 10.3
Sex Profile of India's Population

Population of India	102.7 crores
Males	53.1 crores
Females	49.6 crores
Deficit of women in 2001	3.5 crores
Sex ratio (women per 1000 men)	933

Source: Census of India. 2001. Provisional Population totals, Series 1, Paper 1.

infant's face, or simply by ill-treating daughters (Clark 1983). A survey by *India Today* (15.6.1986) revealed that among the Kallar community in Tamil Nadu, mothers who gave birth to baby girls may be forced to kill their infants by feeding them milk from poisonous oleander berries. This author is convinced that the researcher could also find contemporary cases of female infanticide in parts of western Gujarat, Rajasthan, Uttar Pradesh, Bihar, Punjab and Madhya Pradesh. In addition, female members of the family usually receive inferior treatment regarding food, medication and education (Kynch and Sen 1983). When they grow up, they are further harassed with respect to dowry. Earlier, only among the higher castes, the bride's parents had to give dowry to the groom's family at the time of engagement and marriage. As higher caste women were not allowed to work outside the family, their work had no social recognition. The women of the higher castes were seen as a burden. To compensate the husband for shouldering the burden of his wife, dowry was given by the girl's side to the boy's side. Lower-class women always worked in the fields, mines, plantations, and factories and as artisans. Basic survival needs of the family such as collection of firewood and water, horticulture and assistance in agricultural and associated activities were provided by the women of lower castes and lower classes. Hence women were treated as productive members among them and there was no custom of dowry among the toiling masses. Historically, the practice of female infanticide in India was limited among the upper caste groups due to the custom of hypergamy (marriage of woman with a man from a social group above hers) because of the worry as to how to get a suitable match for the upper caste woman (Sudha and Rajan 1999). Prof. Amartya Kumar Sen (2003), in his world famous article 'Missing Women', has statistically proved that during the last century, 100 million women have been missing in South Asia due to 'discrimination leading to death' experienced by them from womb to tomb in their life cycles.

III

Dynamics of Missing Women in Contemporary India

The declining juvenile sex ratio is the most distressing factor reflecting low premium accorded to a girl child in India. As per the Census of India, juvenile sex ratios were 971, 945 and 927 for 1981, 1991 and 2001 respectively. In 2001, India had 158 million infants and children, of which 82 million were males and 76 million were females. There was a deficit of 6 million female infants and girls. This is a result of the widespread use of sex determination and sex pre-selection tests throughout the country (including in Kerala), along with high rates of female infanticide in the BIMARU states, rural Tamil Nadu and Gujarat. Millions of girls have been missing in the post independence period. According to UNFPA and RGI (2003), 70 districts in 16 states and Union Territories recorded more than a 50 point decline in the child sex ratio in the last decade. To stop the abuse of advanced scientific techniques for selective elimination of female foetuses through sex determination, the government of India passed the PNDT Act in 1994. But the techno-docs based in the metropolis, urban and semi-urban centres and the parents desirous of begetting only sons, have subverted the act.

Sex determination and sex pre-selection, scientific techniques, useful when genetic anomalies are anticipated, are used in India and among Indians settled abroad to eliminate female babies. People of all class, religious, and caste backgrounds use sex determination and sex pre-selection facilities. The media, scientists, the medical profession, government officials, women's groups and academics have campaigned either for or against their use for selective elimination of female foetuses/embryos. Male supremacy, population control and money-making are the concerns of those who support the tests and the survival of women is the concern of those who oppose the tests. The Forum Against Sex Determination and Sex Pre-selection had made concerned efforts to fight against the abuse of these scientific techniques during the 1980s.

Amniocentesis became popular in the last 25 years though earlier it was conducted in government hospitals on an experimental basis. Now, this test is conducted mainly for sex determination (SD) and thereafter for extermination of the female foetus through induced abortion carried out in private clinics, private hospitals, or government hospitals. This perverse use of modern technology is encouraged and boosted by money-minded private practitioners who are out to make Indian women 'male-child-producing machines'. As per the most conservative estimate made by a research team in Bombay, sponsored by the Women's Centre, based on their survey of six hospitals and clinics; in Bombay alone, 10 women per day underwent the test in 1982 (Abraham 1982).

This survey also revealed the hypocrisy of the 'non-violent', 'vegetarian', 'anti-abortion' management of the city's reputable Harkisandas Hospital, which conducted antenatal sex determination tests till the official ban on the test was clamped in 1988 by the Government of Maharashtra. The hospital's handout declared the test to be 'humane and beneficial'. The hospital had outpatient facilities, which were so overcrowded during 1978–1994 that couples desirous of the SD test had to book for the test one month in advance. As its Jain management did not support abortion, the hospital recommended women to various other hospitals and clinics for abortion, and asked them to bring back the aborted female foetuses for further 'research'.

Scenario During the 1980s

During the 1980s, while in other countries the SD tests were very expensive and under strict government control, in India the SD test could be done for Rs 70 to Rs 500 (about US $6 to $40). Hence, not only upper class but even working class people could avail of this facility. A survey of several slums in Bombay showed that many women had undergone the test and after learning that the foetus was female, had an abortion in the 18th or 19th week of pregnancy. Their argument was that it was better to spend Rs 200 or even Rs 800 then than to give birth to a female baby and spend thousands of rupees for her marriage when she grew up.

The popularity of this test attracted young employees of Larsen and Toubro, a multinational engineering industry. As a result, medical bills showing the amount spent on the test were submitted by the employees for reimbursement by the company. The welfare department was astonished to find that these employees were treating sex determination tests so casually. They organised a two-day seminar in which doctors, social workers, and representatives of women's organisations as well as the Family Planning Association were invited. One doctor who carried on a flourishing business in SD stated in a seminar that from Cape Comorin to Kashmir, people phoned him at all hours of the day to find out about the test. Even his six-year-old son had learnt how to ask relevant questions on the phone such as, 'Is the pregnancy 16 weeks old?' etc. (Abraham 1985).

Three sociologists conducted micro-research in Bijnor district of Uttar Pradesh. Intensive fieldwork in two villages over a period of a year, and an interview survey of 301 women who had recently delivered, drawn from randomly selected villages in two community development blocks adjacent to Bijnor town, convinced them of the fact that 'Clinical services offering amniocentesis to inform women of the sex of their foetuses have appeared in North India in the past 10 years. They fit into cultural patterns in which girls are devalued' (Jeffery, Jeffery and Lyon 1984). According to the 1981 Census, the sex ratio of Uttar Pradesh and Bijnor district respectively, were 886 and 863 girls per 1,000 boys. The researchers also discovered that female infanticide practised in Bijnor district until 1900, had been limited to Rajputs and Jats who considered the birth of a daughter as loss of prestige. By contrast, the abuse of amniocentesis for the purpose of female foeticide is now prevalent in all communities.

In Delhi, the All India Institute of Medical Sciences began conducting a sample survey of amniocentesis in 1974 to find out about foetal genetic conditions and easily managed to enrol 11,000 pregnant women as volunteers for its research (Mazumdar 1994). The main interest of these volunteers was to know the sex of the foetus. Once the results were out, those women, who were told that they were carrying female foetuses, demanded abortion (Chhachhi and Sathyamala 1983). This experience motivated the health minister to ban SD tests for sex selection in all government run hospitals in 1978. Since then, the private sector started expanding its tentacles in this field so rapidly that by the early eighties amniocentesis and other sex-selection tests became bread and butter for many gynaecologists.

A sociological research project in Punjab in 1982 selected, in its sample, 50 per cent men and 50 per cent women as respondents for their questionnaire on the opinions of men and women regarding SD tests. Among male respondents were businessmen and white-collared employees of the income group of Rs 1,000 to Rs 3,500 per month, while female respondents were mainly housewives. All of them knew about the test and found it useful. (Singh and Jain 1983). Why not? Punjab was the first to start the commercial use of this test as early as 1979. It was the advertisement in the newspaper regarding the New Bhandari Ante-Natal SD Clinics in Amritsar that first activated the press and women's groups to denounce the practice.

A committee to examine the issues of sex determination tests and female foeticide, formed at the initiative of the government of

Maharashtra in 1986, appointed a gynaecologist, Dr. Sanjeev Kulkarni (1986) of the Foundation of Research in Community Health, to investigate the prevalence of this test in Bombay. Forty-two gynaecologists were interviewed by him. His findings disclosed that about 84 per cent of the gynaecologists interviewed were performing amniocentesis for SD tests. These 42 doctors were found to perform on an average 270 amniocentesis tests per month. Some of them had been performing the tests for 10–12 years. But the majority of them started doing so only in the last five years. Women from all classes, but predominantly middle class and lower class women, opted for the test. About 29 per cent of the doctors said that up to 10 per cent of the women, who came for the test, already had one or more sons. A majority of doctors feel that by providing this service they were doing humanitarian work. Some doctors felt that the test was an effective measure of population control. With the draft of the Eighth Five Year Plan, the Government of India aimed to achieve a Net Reproduction Rate of one (i.e. the replacement of the mother by only one daughter). For this objective SD and SP were seen as handy; the logic being a lesser number of women means less reproduction (Kulkarni 1986).

Recent studies have revealed that, in South Asia, we have inherited the cultural legacy of a strong son-preference among all communities, religious groups and citizens of varied socio-economic backgrounds. Patrilocality, patrilineage and patriarchal attitudes manifest in women and girls having subordinate position in the family, discrimination in property rights and low-paid or unpaid jobs. Women's work of cooking, cleaning and caring is treated as non-work. Hence, women are perceived as a burden (V. Patel 2003a). At the time of marriage, dowry is given by the bride's side to the groom's side for shouldering 'the burden of bride'. In many communities female babies are killed immediately after birth, either by mothers or by elderly women of the household, to relieve themselves from the life of humiliation, rejection and suffering. In the most prosperous state of Punjab, the conventional patriarchal preference of male children leads to thousands of cases of sex-selective abortions.(V. Patel 2003b) Recently a man drowned and killed his 8-year-old daughter and also tried to kill his wife for having borne him the girl child. According to the Chandigarh (Punjab) based Institute for Development and Communication, during 2002–03, every ninth household in the state, acknowledged sex-selective abortion with the help of ante-natal sex determination tests (*The Asian Age*, Mumbai, 25 April 2003).

Recently, the Voluntary Health Association of India published its research report based on fieldwork in Kurukshetra in Haryana,

Table 10.4
Sex Ratio and Literacy Rate in States & UTs of India

State	Overall sex ratio	Child sex ratio (0–6 yrs)	Total literacy rate	Male literacy rate	Female literacy rate
India	933	927	65	76	54
Andaman & Nicobar Islands	846	965	81	86	75
Andhra Pradesh	978	964	61	71	51
Arunachal Pradesh	901	961	55	64	44
Assam	932	964	64	72	56
Bihar	921	938	48	60	34
Chandigarh	773	845	82	86	77
Chhattisgarh	990	975	65	78	52
Dadra & Nagar Haveli	811	973	60	73	43
Daman & Diu	709	925	81	88	70
Delhi	821	865	82	87	75
Goa	960	933	82	89	76
Gujarat	921	878	70	81	59
Haryana	861	820	69	79	56
Himachal Pradesh	970	897	77	86	68
Jammu & Kashmir	900	927	54	66	42
Jharkhand	941	966	54	68	39
Karnataka	964	949	67	76	57
Kerala	1,058	963	91	94	88
Lakshadweep	947	974	88	93	82
Madhya Pradesh	920	929	64	76	51
Maharashtra	922	917	77	86	68
Manipur	978	961	69	78	60
Meghalaya	975	975	63	66	60
Mizoram	938	971	89	91	86
Nagaland	909	975	67	72	62
Orissa	972	950	64	76	51
Pondicherry	1,001	958	81	89	74
Punjab	857	793	70	76	64
Rajasthan	922	909	61	76	44
Sikkim	875	986	70	77	61
Tamil Nadu	986	939	73	82	65
Tripura	950	975	74	81	65
Uttar Pradesh	898	916	57	70	43
Uttaranchal	964	906	72	84	60
West Bengal	934	963	69	78	60

Source: Census of India. 2001. Provisional Population totals, Series 1, Paper 1.

Fatehgarh Sahib in Punjab and Kangra in Himachal Pradesh. These have the worst child sex ratio as per the 2001 Census. The study surveyed 1,401 households in villages, interviewed 999 married women, 72 doctors and 64 Panchayat members. It revealed that 'The immediate cause for the practice of female foeticide is that daughters are perceived as an economic and social burden to the family due to several factors such as dowry, the danger to her chastity and worry about getting her married' (VHAI 2003).

In this context, commercial minded techno-docs and laboratory owners have been using new reproductive technologies for femicide for over two and half decades. Among educated families, adoption of the small family norm means minimum one or two sons in the family. They can do without a daughter. The propertied class do not desire daughter/daughters because after the marriage of the daughter, the son-in-law may demand a share in the property. The property-less classes dispose off daughters to avoid dowry harassment. But they don't mind accepting dowry for their sons. The birth of a son is perceived as an opportunity for upward mobility while the birth of a daughter is believed to result in downward economic mobility. Though the stronghold of this ideology was North India, it is now increasingly gaining ground all over India (V. Patel 2003d).

Overall literacy rates in all states and Union territories have gone up as compared with the 1991 Census. Even states and Union Territories with high female literacy, namely Goa, Delhi, Mizoram, Pondicherry, Lakshadweep, Kerala, Andaman & Nicobar, Daman & Diu, and Chandigarh have experienced a decline in the child sex ratio. In a micro-study of Kolkata, the Census Report observes, 'Out of 141 municipal wards, the percentage of child population has declined in 134 wards since 1991. More importantly, the child sex ratio has declined sharply, from a high of 1,011 females per 1,000 male children in 1951 to an abysmal 923 in 2001. This is the lowest child sex ratio for Kolkata in the last 50 years. A major cause for the

Table 10.5
States with Lowest Child Sex Ratio

States	1991	2001
Punjab	875	793
Haryana	879	820
Gujarat	928	878
Maharashtra	946	917

Source: Census of India. 2001. Provisional Population totals, Series 1, Paper 1.

decline is sex-selective foeticide' (Sen 2002). Rates of female foeticide have increased along with the increase in female literacy rates
(Chattopadhyay 2003).

The neo-classical logic of the Law of Demand and Supply does
not apply to the complex social forces where patriarchy controls
sexuality, fertility and labour of women without any respect to her
bodily integrity. Hence, the real life experiences point towards the
contrary. In fact, a shortage of women in Haryana, Punjab and the
BIMARU states has escalated forced abduction and kidnapping of
girls, forced polyandry, gang rape and child prostitution.

It has been noted that the fertility rates in Kerala have declined
over the past few decades and currently the Crude Birth Rate (CBR)
for the state is as low as 17.9 per 1,000 population in 1997. The Infant
Mortality Rates (IMR) is also one of the lowest experienced among
Indian states, about 12 per 1,000 live births in 1997 (RGI 1998). The
indicators of human wellbeing in Kerala are among the best in relation to the different states of India. With modernisation and changing
lifestyles, wrought by both external migration and incomes from
remittances, there has been a qualitative change in the lives of the
people. There has been a proliferation of private health care in the
state and this, in addition to demand-driven factors, has contributed
to the better access to health care in the state. One of the factors
associated with the proliferation of health care facilities, especially
in the private sector, has been the improvement in the availability of
medical diagnostics. Medical personnel have sought the use of such
facilities not only to improve diagnostics, but also to avoid complications of expensive litigation in the light of the inclusion of private
medical practice within the purview of the Consumer Protection Act,
1986. All this has resulted in the increasing trend of the use of medical
diagnostic facilities and an increase in the cost of healthcare for the
consumer. A micro-study in Trivandrum city found that the known
number of ultra-sonographs in the city alone was about 37, of which
only 6 were in the public sector (Sunita and Elamon 2000).

IV

NRTs and Women _____

NRTs perform four types of functions. In Vitro Fertilisation (IVF)
and subsequent embryo transfer, GIFT (Gamete Intra Fallopian

Transfer), ZIFT and cloning assisted reproduction (Nandedkar and Rajadhyaksha 1995). In Mumbai girls are selling their eggs for Rs 20,000. Infertility clinics in Mumbai receive 4–5 calls per day from young women who want to donate their eggs (*The Asian Age*, 11 June 2004).

Contraceptive Technologies prevent conception and birth. Amniocentesis, chorion villi biopsy (CVB), needling, ultrasound and imaging are used for pre-natal diagnosis (V. Patel 2000). Foetal cells are collected by the technique of amniocentesis and CVB. Gene technologies play a crucial role through genetic manipulation of animal and plant kingdoms (Agnihotri-Gupta 2000). Genomics is 'the science of improving the human population through controlled breeding; it encompasses the elimination of disease, disorder, or undesirable traits, on the one hand, and genetic enhancement on the other. It is pursued by nations through state policies and programmes (Heng Leng 2002).

New Reproductive Technologies in the neo-colonial context of the third world economies and the unequal division of labour between the first and the third world economies, have created a bizarre scenario and cut-throat competition among body chasers, clone chasers, intellect chasers and supporters of femicide. There are mainly three aspects to NRT—assisted reproduction, genetic or pre-natal diagnosis and prevention of conception and birth. It is important to understand the interaction among NRT developers, providers, users, non-users, potential users, policymakers, and representatives of international organisations (FINRRAGE 2004).

Assisted Reproduction

The focus of assisted reproduction experts is on healthy women, who are forced to menstruate at any age, backed by hazardous hormones and steroids. The processual dimensions involve: the use of counsellors, techno-docs and researchers to know the details of the personal life of women to delegitimise the victim's experience. There is an utter disregard for the woman's pain, carcinogenic and mutogenic implications and vaginal warts, extreme back pain, arthritis, sclerosis, heavy bleeding, growth of hair on the face, nose, chin and cheeks, joint pain associated with uterine contractions for production of egg-cells, are dismissed as 'mood-swings'. The network between stake groups has only one goal—impregnating women for embryo production, which in the techno-docs' language, is *assisted reproduction*. Embryos and foetuses are used for the cure of Parkinson's disease among influential and wealthy ageing patriarchs. The side effects on women's health are totally ignored. The growth of moustache, deformation of teeth and dietary requirements are totally ignored.

By using phallocentric and misogynist psychologists and psychiatrists, the state and politicians, (ever ready for a plastic smile and neat presentation) have found a ruthless weapon to cretinise, dehumanise, degrade, humiliate, terrorise and intimidate women. Through advertisements in newspapers, poor/needy women are asked to lend their womb for IVF on payment of money. Through websites rich clients are sought.

Elimination of Female Foetuses and Selection of Male at Preconception Stage

Rapid advances in the field of new reproductive technologies has 'created a situation where there has been a breakdown of the moral consensus' with respect to medical ethics and gender justice (Malik 2003). Techno-docs refuse to see the larger contexts, future and gender implications. The sharp remark of the Member Secretary of the Maharashtra State Commission for Women on male pre-selection, represents the concerns of women's rights organisations in these words,

> The attempt at legitimising the vetoing of female life even before it appears, is worse than the earlier abortion-related violence in the womb, precisely because it is so sanitised and relies on seemingly sane arguments against the policing of 'human rights' in a democracy in the intensely personal matter of procreation. This needs to be resisted at all cost. (Thekkekara 2001)

Diametrically opposite views come from Dr Anniruddha Malpani, the most articulate proponent of sex-pre-selection tests. When asked, 'Is it ethical to selectively discard female embryos?' he said, 'Where does the question of ethics come in here? Who are we hurting? Unborn girls?' (Banerjee 2001). My questions are: Can we allow Indian women to become an endangered species? Shall we be bothered only about endangered wildlife, tigers, lions, so on and so forth? Massive resources are invested in OPERATION TIGER. When shall we start OPERATION GIRL CHILD?

Population Control Policies _____

There is a serious need to examine population policies and global funding from the perspective of statisation of the medical market and marketisation of the nation states in the context of the newly emerging culture of the daily changes of sponsors. Financial economists have reigned supreme to generate a moment-to-moment existence among population so that they can get an unending supply of cannon fodder for the NRT experimentation. Budgetary provision on health has a hidden agenda of NRT. The victims are not given scientific details and by labelling them as parasites and beneficiaries, their consent is not sought. It has burdened women with back-breaking miseries. The nation states have been coached to implement the use of NRT in secrecy, in line with the programmes executed by G8 in Thailand, Indonesia, Philippines and Bangladesh. To achieve population stabilisation, 2.1 per cent growth rate of population and NRR, net reproduction rate of 1(i.e. a mother should be replaced by 1 daughter only) are envisaged. These have an inherent sexist bias because it desires the birth of 1 daughter and 1.1 sons. Those who support sex determination (SD) and sex pre-selection (SP) view these tests as helpful to achieve NRR of 1. A recent study in Haryana revealed that out of 160 mothers and grandmothers interviewed by the AIIMS study team, 40 per cent supported SD on the ground that it contributed to population control and prevented families from having a series of females in an attempt that a male was born (Bardia *et al.* 2004). This will further widen the gap between the number of girls and boys in the country.

Science in Service of Femicide _____

Advances in medical science have resulted in sex determination and sex pre-selection techniques such as sonography, foetoscopy, needling, chorion villi biopsy (CVB) and the most popular, amniocentesis and ultrasound have become household names, not only in urban India but also in rural India. Indian metropolises are the major centres for sex determination (SD) and sex pre-selection (SP) tests with sophisticated laboratories; the techniques of amniocentesis and ultrasound are used even in the clinics of small towns and cities of Gujarat, Maharashtra, Karnataka, Uttar Pradesh, Bihar, Madhya Pradesh, Punjab, West Bengal, Tamil Nadu and Rajasthan. A justification for this has been aptly put by a team of doctors of Harkisandas Narottamdas Hospital (a pioneer in this trade) in these words, '...in developing countries like India, as the parents are encouraged to limit their family to two offspring, they will have a right to quality in these two as far as can be assured. Amniocentesis provides help in this direction'. Here the word 'quality' raises a number of issues that we shall examine in this paper (Patanki *et al.* 1979).

At present, ultrasound machines are most widely used for sex determination purposes. Doctors motivated in part by multinational marketing muscle and considerable financial gains are increasingly investing in ultrasound scanners, report George and Dahiya (1998). But for the past quarter century, amniocentesis, a scientific technique that involves taking 15–20 ml of amniotic fluid from the womb by pricking the foetal membrane with the help of a special needle was practised. After separating a foetal cell from the amniotic fluid, a chromosomal analysis is conducted on it. This test helps in detecting several genetic disorders, such as Down's Syndrome, neurotube conditions in the foetus, retarded muscular growth, 'Rh' incompatibility, haemophilia, and other physical and mental conditions. The test is appropriate for women over 40 years because there are higher chances of children with these conditions being produced by them. A sex determination test is required to identify sex-specific conditions such as haemophilia and retarded muscular growth, which mainly affect male babies. Other tests, in particular CVB, and pre-planning of the unborn baby's sex have also been used for SD and SP tests. Diet control method, centrifugation of sperm, drugs (tablets known as Select), vaginal jelly, 'sacred' beads called Rudraksh and recently advertised Gender Select kit are also used for begetting boys (Kulkarni 1986). Compared to CVB and pre-selection through centrifugation of sperm, amniocentesis is more hazardous to women's health. In addition, while this test can give 95–97 per cent accurate results, in 1 per cent of the cases the test may lead to spontaneous abortions or premature delivery, dislocation of hips, respiratory complications or needle puncture marks on the baby (Ravindra 1986).

Debate on the Consequences for Women

In such circumstances, 'Is it not desirable that a woman dies rather than be ill-treated?' asked many social scientists. In Dharma Kumar's (1983) words: 'Is it really better to be born and be left to die than be killed as a foetus? Does the birth of lakhs or even millions of unwanted girls improve the status of women?' Before answering this question let us first see the demographic profile of Indian women. There was a continuous decline in the ratio of females to males between 1901 and 1971. Between 1971 and 1981 there was a slight increase, but the ratio continued to be adverse for women in 1991 and 2001 Census. The situation is even worse because SD is practised by all—rich and poor, upper and the lower castes, the highly educated and illiterate—whereas female infanticide was and is limited to certain warrior castes (Jeffery, Jeffery and Lyon 1984).

Many economists and doctors have supported SD and SP by citing the law of supply and demand. If the supply of women is reduced, it is argued, their demand as well as status will be enhanced (Sheth 1984). Scarcity of women will increase their value (Bardhan 1982). According to this logic, women will cease to be an easily replaceable commodity. But here the economists forget the socio-cultural milieu in which women have to live. The society that treats women as mere sex and reproduction objects will not treat women in a more humane way if they are merely scarce in supply. On the contrary, there will be increased incidences of rapes, abduction and forced polyandry. In Madhya Pradesh, Haryana, Rajasthan and Punjab, among certain communities, the sex ratio is extremely adverse for women. There, a wife is shared by a group of brothers or sometimes even by patrilateral, parallel cousins (Dube 1983). Recently, in Gujarat, many disturbing reports of re-introduction of polyandry (*Panchali* system—one woman being married to five men) have come to the light. In the villages in Mehsana district, the problem of declining number of girls has created a major social crisis as almost all villages have hundreds of boys who are left with no choice but to buy brides from outside (*The Times of India*, 8 July 2004).

To believe that it is better to kill a female foetus than to give birth to an unwanted female child, is not only short-sighted but also fatalistic. By this logic it is better to kill poor people or Third World masses rather than let them suffer in poverty and deprivation. This logic also presumes that social evils like dowry are god-given and we cannot do anything about them. Hence, victimise the victims.

Another argument is that in cases where women have one or more daughters they should be allowed to undergo amniocentesis so that they can plan a 'balanced family' by having sons. Instead of continuing to produce female children in the hope of giving birth to a male child, it is better for the welfare of both the family and the country, that they abort the female foetus and produce a small and balanced family with daughters and sons. This concept of the 'balanced family' however, also has a sexist bias. Would the couples with one or more sons request amniocentesis to get rid of male foetuses and have a daughter in order to balance their family? Never! The author would like to clarify the position of feminist groups in India. They are against SD and SP leading to male or female foeticide. What price should women pay for a 'balanced family?' How many abortions can a woman bear without jeopardising her health?

V

Do Women Have a Choice? Gendered Power Relations and NRTs _____

The search for a 'perfect' baby through genetic screening, ante-natal sex determination tests, pre-implantation diagnosis, commercialisation of sperm and/or egg donation, commercialisation of motherhood and hormonal contraceptives, all these raise many socio-legal and ethical questions. Division of labour among women to control women's sexuality, fertility and labour by utilising homophobia and pitting women of different race, religions, age and looks to suit the interest of NRTs, will serve the interest of patriarchy, medical mafia, pharmaceutical industries, scientists, techno-docs at the cost of vulnerable human beings. If the NGOs don't want to get criminalised, they must dissociate from NRTs and divert the funding for public health, library, education, skill-building, employment generation as a long-term investment and channelise their energies towards formation of self-help groups.

It is important to understand that reproduction has an individual and a social dimension. While examining birth control practices, an individual is a unit of analysis. While examining the population control policies we have to analyse the pros and cons of NRTs, national governments, population control organisations, multinational pharmaceutical industries, public and private funded bodies, medical researchers and health workers who shape women's choice and women's autonomy or control at micro and macro levels. Thus choices are not made in a vacuum. NRT as a choice for some women (educated, career women), can become coercion for others (powerless and less articulate women). Hence it is important to be vigilant about power relations determined by race, age, class and gender while examining implications of NRTs on different stake groups. Power relations in the medical market favour the techno-docs and the clients are not given full details of the line of treatment and its consequences. Respect for diversity, adoption of child/children is a far simpler and more humane solution than subjecting women to undergo infertility treatment. Obsession with the creation of designer baby boys has made the development agenda subsidiary.

It has been repeatedly stated that women themselves welcome the test of their own free will. 'It is a question of women's own choice.' But are these choices made in a social vacuum? These women are socially conditioned to accept that unless they produce one or more male children they have no social worth (Rapp 1984). They can be harassed, taunted, even deserted by their husbands if they fail to do so. Thus, their 'choices' depend on fear of society. It is true that feminists throughout the world have always demanded the right of women to control their own fertility, to choose whether or not to have children and to enjoy facilities for free, legal and safe abortions. But to understand this issue in the Third World context, we must see it against the background of imperialism and racism, which aims at control of the 'coloured population.' Thus, 'it is all too easy for a population control advocate to heartily endorse women's rights, at the same time diverting the attention from the real causes of the population problem. Lack of food, economic security, clean drinking water and safe clinical facilities have led to a situation where a woman has to have 6.2 children to have at least one surviving male child. These are the roots of the population problem, not merely a desire to have a male child' (Chhachhi and Sathyamla 1983).

There are some who ask, 'If family planning is desirable, why not sex-planning?' The issue is not so simple. We must situate this problem in the context of commercialism in medicine and health care systems, racist bias of the population control policy and the manifestation of patriarchal power (Wichterrich 1988). Sex choice can be another way of oppressing women. Under the guise of choice we may indeed exacerbate women's oppression. The feminists assert: survival of women is at stake.

Outreach and popularity of sex pre-selection tests may be even greater than those of sex determination tests, since the former does not involve ethical issues related to abortion. Even anti-abortionists would use this method. Dr Ronald Erricsson, who has a chain of clinics conducting sex-preselection tests in 46 countries in Europe, America, Asia and Latin America, announced in his handout that out of 263 couples who approached him for begetting offspring, 248 selected boys and 15 selected girls (V. Patel 2003a). This shows that the preference for males is not limited to the Third World countries like India but is virtually universal. In Erricsson's method, no abortion or apparent violence is involved. Even so, it could lead to violent social disaster over a long term. Although scientists and medical professionals deny all responsibilities for the social consequences of the tests, the reality shatters the myth of the value neutrality of science and technology. Hence we need to link science and technology with socio-economic and cultural reality (Holmes and Hoskins 1984). The class, racist and sexist biases of the ruling elite have crossed all boundaries of human dignity and decency by making savage use of science. Even in China, after 55 years of 'revolution', 'socialist reconstruction' and the latest, rapid capitalist development, SD and SP tests for femicide have gained ground after the Chinese government's adoption of the 'one-child family' policy (Junhong 2001). Many Chinese couples in rural areas do not agree to the one child policy but due to state repression they, while sulking, accept it provided the child is male. This shows how adaptive the system of patriarchy and male supremacy is. It can establish and strengthen its roots in all kinds of social structures—pre-capitalist, capitalist and even post-capitalist—if not challenged consistently (V. Patel 1984). As per the UN report of 2003, 80 countries had adverse sex ratio leading to deficit of women.

VI

Protests against SD and SP _____

How can we stop deficit of Indian women? This question was asked by feminists, sensitive lawyers, scientists, researchers, doctors and women's organisations such as Women's Centre (Mumbai), Saheli (Delhi), Samata (Mysore), Sahiar (Baroda) and Forum Against SD and SP (FASDSP)—an umbrella organisation of women's groups, doctors, democratic rights groups, and the People's Science Movement. Protest actions by women's groups in the late 70s got converted into a consistent campaign at the initiative of FASDSP in the 1980s. Even research organisations such as Research Centre on Women's Studies (Mumbai)), Centre for Women's Development Studies (Delhi) and Voluntary Health Organisation, Foundation for Research in Community Health also took a stand against the tests. They questioned the 'highly educated', 'enlightened' scientists, technocrats, doctors and of course, the state who help in propagating the tests (V. Patel, 1987). Concerned groups in Bangalore, Chandigarh, Delhi, Chennai, Kolkata, Baroda and Mumbai have demanded that these tests should be used for the limited purpose of identification of serious genetic conditions, in selected government hospitals under strict supervision. After a lot of pressure, media coverage and negotiation, poster campaigns, exhibitions, picketing in front of the Harkisandas Hospital in 1986, signature campaigns and public meetings and panel discussions, television programmes and petitioning; at last the Government of Maharashtra and the Central Government became activised. In March 1987, the government of Maharashtra appointed an expert committee to propose comprehensive legal provisions to restrict sex determination tests for identifying genetic conditions. The committee was appointed in response to a private bill introduced in the Assembly by a Member of the Legislative Assembly (MLA), who was persuaded by the Forum. In fact the Forum approached several MLAs and Members of Parliament to put forward such a bill. In April 1988, the government of Maharashtra introduced a bill to provide for the regulation of the use of medical or scientific techniques of pre-natal diagnosis solely for the purpose of detecting genetic or metabolic disorders or chromosomal abnormalities or certain congenital anomalies or sex-linked conditions and for the prevention of the misuse of pre-natal sex determination leading to female foeticide and for matters connected therewith or incidental thereto (L. C. Bill No. VIII of 1988). In June 1988, the Bill was unanimously passed in the Maharashtra Legislative Assembly and became an Act. The Act's purview was limited only to SD tests, it did not say anything about the SP techniques. It admitted that medical technology could be misused by doctors and banning of SD tests had taken away the respectability of the Act of SD tests. Not only this, but now in the eyes of law, both the clients and the practitioners of the SD tests are culprits. Any advertisement regarding the facilities of the SD tests is declared illegal by this Act. But the Act had many loopholes.

Two major demands of the Forum, that no private practice in SD tests be allowed and in no case should a woman undergoing the SD test be punished, were not included in the Act. On the contrary the Act intended to regulate them with the help of an 'Appropriate Authority' constituted by two government bureaucrats, one bureaucrat from the medical education department, one bureaucrat from the Indian Council of Medical Research, one gynaecologist and one geneticist and two representatives of Voluntary Organisations, which made a mockery of 'peoples participation'. Experiences of all such bodies set by the government, have shown that they merely remain paper bodies and even if they function they are highly inefficient, corrupt and elitist.

Jesani (1988) argues that the medical mafia seemed to be the most favoured group in the act. It has scored the most in the chapter on Offences and Penalties—the last clause of this chapter empowers the court, if it so desires and after giving reasons, to award less punishment than the minimum stipulated under the Act. That is, a rich doctor who has misused the techniques for female foeticide, can, with the help of powerful lawyers, persuade the court to award minor punishment. The court shall always assume, unless proved otherwise, that a woman who seeks such aid of pre-natal diagnostic procedures on herself, has been compelled to do so by her husband or members of her family. In our kind of social milieu, it is not at all difficult to prove that a woman who has a undergone SD test, went for it of her 'free will'. The Act made the victim a culprit who could be imprisoned up to three years. For the woman, her husband and her in-laws, using SD tests became a 'cognisable, non-bailable and non-compoundable' offence! But the doctors, centres and laboratories were excluded from the above provision. The Act also believed in victimising the victim. With this act, the medical lobby's fear that the law would drive SD tests underground, vanished. They could continue their business above ground. A high powered committee of experts had been appointed by the Central Government to introduce a bill applicable through out India to ban SD tests leading to female foeticide.

The Forum accepted that with the help of the law alone, we can't get rid of female foeticide. Public education and the women's right's movement are playing a much more effective role in this regard. Some of the most imaginative programmes of the Forum and women's groups have been a rally led by daughters on 22 November 1986, a children's fair challenging a sex stereotyping and degradation of daughters, picketing in front of the clinics conducting the SD tests and promoting a positive image of daughters through stickers, posters and buttons. For example, 'daughters can also be a source of support to parents in their old age,' 'eliminate inequality, not women', 'Demolish dowry, not daughters', 'make your daughter self-sufficient, educate her, let her take a job, she will no longer be a burden on her parents.' The Forum also prepared 'Women's Struggle to Survive,' a mobile fair that was organised in different suburbs of Bombay. It conveyed this message through its songs, skits, slide shows, video films, exhibitions, booklets, debates and discussions.

VII

Initiatives by the State and NGOs

Twenty years ago a controversy around SD and SP started as a result of several investigative reports published in popular newspapers and magazines such as *India Today, Eve's Weekly, Sunday* and other national and regional English language journals. The article by Achin Vanaik (1986) in *Times of India* revealed that almost 100 per cent of 15,914 abortions during 1984–85, by a well known abortion centre in Bombay, were undertaken after SD tests. All private practitioners in the SD tests, who used to boast that they were 'doing social work' by helping miserable women, exposed their hypocrisy when they failed to provide facilities of amniocentesis to pregnant women during the Bhopal gas tragedy (1984) in spite of repeated requests by women's groups, and many reported cases of the birth of deformed babies as a result of the gas carnage. Thus it is clear that this scientific technique is in fact not used for humanitarian purposes, not because of 'empathy towards poor Indian women' as has been claimed.

Forced sterilisation of males during the emergency rule brought about politically disastrous consequences for the Congress Party. As a result, in the post-emergency period, there has been a shift in policy and women have become the main target of population control. The after-effects of SD and SPs, harmful effects of hormone-based contraceptive pills and anti-pregnancy injections and camps for mass IUD insertion and mass sterilisation of women under unhygienic conditions, are always overlooked by enthusiasts of the Family Planning Policy. Most population control research is conducted on women without consideration for the harm caused by such research to the women concerned (Mies 1986).

In a patrilocal, patrilineal society son preference is highly pronounced. In the power relations between the bride's and groom's family, the bride's side always has to give in and put up with all taunts, humiliation, indignities, insults and injuries perpetrated by the groom's family. This factor also results in further devaluation of daughters. The uncontrollable lust of consumerism and commercialisation of human relations, combined with patriarchal power over women, have reduced Indian women to easily dispensable commodities. Dowry is easy money, 'get rich quick' formula spreading in the society as fast as cancer. By the late eighties, dowry had not been limited to certain upper castes only but had spread among all communities in India irrespective of their class, caste and religious backgrounds. Its extreme manifestation was seen in the increasing state of dowry-related murders.

Pre-natal Diagnostic Techniques (Regulation and Prevention of Misuse) Act was enacted in 1994 by the Centre followed by similar Acts by several state governments and union territories of India after the Maharahstra legislation to regulate pre-natal sex determination tests. This was as a result of pressure created by the Forum Against Sex determination and sex pre-selection. But there was a gross violation of this central legislation.

In response to the public interest petition filed by Dr Sabu George, Centre for Inquiry into Health and Allied Themes, Mumbai) and MASUM (*Mahila Sarvagin Utkarsh Mandal*) fought on their behalf by the Lawyers Collective (Basu 2003), the Supreme Court of India gave a directive on 4 May 2001 to all state governments to make an effective and prompt implementation of the Pre-natal Diagnostics Techniques (Regulation and Prevention of Misuse) Act (enacted in 1994 and brought into operation from 1 January 1996). Now, it stands renamed as 'The Pre-conception and Pre-natal Diagnostic Techniques (Prohibition of Sex Selection) Act 2003'.

Having received the assent of the President of India on 17th January 2003, the Act tightens the screws on sex selection at the pre-conception stage and puts in place, a string of checks and balances to ensure that the act is effective (Kamdar 2003). The Act provides for the prohibition of sex-selection, before or after conception, and for regulation of pre-natal diagnostic techniques for the purposes of detecting genetic abnormalities or metabolic disorders or sex-linked disorders. It also provides for the prevention of their misuse for sex determination leading to female foeticide and for matters connected therewith or incidental thereto. Under the Act, the person who seeks help for sex-selection can face, at first conviction, imprisonment for a three-year period and be required to pay a fine of Rs 50,000. The state Medical Council can suspend the registration of the doctor involved in such malpractices and, at the stage of conviction, can remove his/her name from the register of the council. The Amendment Rules, 2003 have activated the implementation machinery to curb nefarious practices contributing towards 'missing girls'. According to the rules, all bodies under the PNDT Act, namely Genetic Counselling Centre, Genetic Laboratories or Genetic Clinic cannot function unless registered (GOI 2002). The Bombay Municipal Corporation has initiated a drive against the unauthorised determination of gender of the foetus as per the directive of the Ministry of Law and Justice. All sonography centres are required to register themselves with the appropriate authority—the medical officer of the particular ward. The registration certificate and the message that under no circumstances should the sex of the foetus be disclosed, are mandatory to be displayed (V. Patel 2003c).

The shortcomings of the PNDT Act (2003) lie in the criteria set for establishing a genetic counselling centre, genetic laboratory and genetic clinic/ultrasound clinic/imaging centre and person qualified to perform the tests.

- The terms genetic clinic/ultrasound clinic/imaging centre cannot be used interchangeably. But the Act does so.
- Moreover, the amended Act should have categorically defined persons, laboratories, hospitals, institutions involved in pre-conception sex-selective techniques such as artificial reproductive techniques and pre-implantation genetic diagnosis.
- Who is a qualified medical geneticist? As per the Act, 'a person who possesses a degree or diploma or certificate in medical genetics in the field of PNDT or has a minimum of two years experience after obtaining any medical qualification under the MCI Act 1956 or a P.G. in biological sciences.' Many medical experts feel that a degree or diploma or two years experience in medical genetics cannot be made synonymous.
- As per the Act, an ultrasound machine falls under the requirement of genetic clinic, while it is widely used also by the hospitals and nursing homes not conducting Pre-implantation Genetic Diagnosis (PGD) and PNDT.

Ban on the Advertisements of SD and SP Techniques

Another important initiative that has been taken is against any institution or agency whose advertisement or displayed promotional poster or television serial is suggestive of any inviting gestures involving/supporting sex determination. MASUM, Pune made a complaint to the Maharashtra State Women's Commission against Balaji Telefilms because its top-rated television serial's episode telecast during February 2002, showed a young couple checking the sex of their unborn baby. The Commission approached Bombay Municipal Corporation (BMC) and a First Investigation Report (FIR) was lodged at the police station. After an uproar created by the Commission, Balaji Telefilms came forward to salvage the damage by preparing an ad based on the Commission's script that conveyed that sex determination tests for selective abortion of female foetus is a criminal offence. Now there is another battle brewing. The women's groups insist that the ad should be telecast for three months before each episode, while Balaji Telefilms found it too much (*The Indian Express*, Mumbai, 19 May 2003).

Conclusion

We need to counter those who believe that it is better to kill a female foetus than to give birth to an unwanted female child. Their logic eliminates the victim of male chauvinism, does not empower her. The techno-docs do not challenge anti-women practices such as dowry. The logic, 'better spend Rs 5000 for female foeticide than Rs 5 lakhs as dowry for a grown-up daughter,' seeks to kill poor people or third world masses rather than let them suffer in poverty and deprivation. This logic also presumes that social evils like dowry are God-given and that we cannot do anything about them. Hence victimise the victim. Investing in a daughter's education, health and dignified life to make her self-dependent, are far more humane and realistic ways than brutalising the pregnant mother and her would-be daughter. Recently, a series of incidents in which educated women have got their grooms arrested at the time of the wedding ceremony for harassment for dowry, are an encouraging step in the direction of empowerment of girls. Massive and supportive media publicity has empowered young women from different parts of the country to cancel marriages involving dowry harassment. They have provided new role models.

Hence, our slogans are: 'Daughters are not for slaughter',
'Eliminate Inequality, not Women', 'Destroy Dowry, not Daughters',
'Say "No" to Sex Determination', 'Say "Yes" to Empowerment of Women',
'Say "No" to Sex Discrimination', 'Say "Yes" to Gender Justice'.

Philosophical and medical details of NRT need a public debate without an iron wall of secrecy, in all Indian languages as NRT is penetrating even in those areas where you do not get even safe drinking water or food. Technologies for population control are primarily concerned about efficiency of techniques to avert births rather than safety of women. Women have to put up with the side-effects of NRTs. New reproductive technologies are provider/doctor controlled, not women controlled. Hence women's groups repeatedly state that NRTs have an inherently anti-women bias. The petitions filed have not only been accepted but rules have also been formulated for the implementation of Acts. The state governments are also organising state level seminars for doctors from the government and private sectors to focus on raising awareness that sex-selective foeticide is a discriminatory practice (V. Patel 2003e). They are also trying to deal with the issue from the point of view of responsibility of science towards gender justice, medical ethics and human rights (See CEHAT 2003 for more writings). There is a need to clarify the gender-justice position from the anti-abortionist position. Women should have a right to their bodies and unconditional access to abortion is not in conflict with the claim that sex selection and sex-selective abortions are unethical. It is not the abortion which makes the act unethical, but the idea of sex selection (Madhivala 2001).

We have a great task in front of us, the task of changing the mindset of doctors and clients, creating a socio-cultural milieu that is conducive for the girl child's survival and monitoring the activities of commercial minded techno-docs thriving on sexist prejudices. Then only will we be able to halt the process of the declining sex ratio resulting in the phenomenon of missing girls. To correct a gender-imbalanced society we will have to convince doctors and clients, state and civil society that 'Daughters are not for slaughter'.

References

Abraham, Ammu. 1982. 'Sex Determination Tests in Mumbai', Mumbai: *Women's Centre.* (Mimeograph).

Abraham, A. 1985. 'Larsen and Toubro Seminar on Amniocentesis', Mumbai: *Women's Centre Newsletter,* 1 (4): 5–8.

Abraham, A. and S. Shukla. 1983. 'Sex Determination Tests', Mumbai: *Women's Centre Newsletter.*

Agnihotri-Gupta, J. 2000. *New Reproductive Technologies—Women's Health and Autonomy, Freedom or Dependency?* Indo-Dutch Studies in Development Alternatives–25. New Delhi: Sage Publications.

Banerjee, P. 2001. The Battle Against Chromosome X', *The Times of India,* Mumbai: 25 November.

Bardhan, P. 1982. 'Little Girls and Death in India', *Economic and Political Weekly,* XVII (36): 1448–50.

Bardia, A., E. Paul, S.K. Kapoor and K. Anand. 2004. 'Declining Sex Ratio: Role of Society, Technology and Government Regulation in Haryana: A Comprehensive Study'. *Comprehensive Rural Health Services Project.* New Delhi: All India Institute of Medical Sciences.

Basu, A. 2003. 'Sex Selective Abortions', Mumbai: *The Lawyers Collective,* 18 (11) November: 20–23.

CEHAT, 2003. *Sex-Selection, Issues and Concern.* 2003: 59–63.

Chhachhi, Amrita and C. Sathyamala. 1983. 'Sex Determination Tests: A Technology Which Will Eliminate Women', Delhi: *Medico Friend Circle Bulletin,* No. 95: 3–5.

Chattopadhyay, D. 2003. 'Child Sex Ratio on the Decline in Bengal: Report', *The Times of India*, Mumbai: 10 March.

Clark, A. 1983. 'Limitation of Female Life Chances in Rural Central Gujarat', Delhi: *The Indian Economic and Social History Review*, 20 (1): 1–25.

Dube, L. 1983. 'Misadventure in Amniocentesis'. *Economic and Political Weekly*, XVIII (8): 279–80.

FINRRAGE. 2004. 'Women's Declarations on Reproductive Technologies and Genetic Engineering'. Germany: *Feminist International Network of Resistance to Reproductive and Genetic Engineering* and Dhaka: *UBINIG*.

George, S. and R. Dahiya. 1998. 'Female Foeticide in Rural Haryana', *Economic and Political Weekly*, XXXIII (32): 2191–98.

Government of India. 1988. *L C Bill of 1988*. New Delhi: Ministry of Law.

Government of India. 2002. *Handbook on PNDT Act, 1994*, New Delhi: Department of Family Welfare, for use by Appropriate Authorities in States/ Union Territories.

Heng Leng, C. 2002. 'Genomics and Health: Ethical, Legal and Social Implications for Developing Countries', Bombay. *Issues in Medical Ethics*, X (1): 146–49.

Holmes, H. B. and B. B. Hoskins. 1984. 'Pre-natal and Pre-conception Sex Choice Technologies—A path to Femicide', Paper presented at the International Inter-disciplinary Congress on Women, The Netherlands.

IIPS. 2002. *National Family Health Survey, NFHS-2, 1998–99*, Mumbai: International Institute of Population Science.

Jeffery, R., P. Jeffery. and A. Lyon. 1984. 'Female Infanticide and Amniocentesis', *Social Science and Medicine*, 19 (11): 1207–12.

Jesani, A. 1988. 'Banning Pre-natal Sex Determination– Scope and Limits of Maharashtra Legislation', *Radical Journal of Health*, II (4) March: 11–17.

Junhong, C. 2001. 'Pre-natal Sex Determination and Sex-Selection Abortion in Rural Central China', *Population and Development Review*, XXVII (2): 259–81.

Kamdar, S. 2003. 'Sex Selection Law Tightened'. *Times of India*, 6 June.

Kulkarni, S. 1986. 'Pre-natal SD Tests and Female Foeticide in Bombay City— A Study'. Bombay: *Foundation for Research in Community Health*.

Kumar, D. 1983. 'Male Utopias and Night Mares', *Economic and Political Weekly*, XVIII (3): 61–64.

Kynch, J. and A. Sen. 1983. 'Indian Women: Well-being and Survival', Cambridge: *Cambridge Journal of Economics*, 7: 363–80.

Madhiwalla, N. 2001. 'Sex Selection: Ethics in the Context of Development', Mumbai: *Issues in Medical Ethics*, IX (October- December): 12–14.

Malik, R. 2003. ' 'Negative Choice' Sex Determination and Sex-Selective Abortion in India'. *Urdhva Mula*, Mumbai: Sophia Centre for Women's Studies Development, 2 (1) May: 60–84.

Mies, M. 1986. 'Sexiest and Racist Implications of New Reproductive Technologies', Paper presented at XI World Congress of Sociology, 18–22, New Delhi.

Mazumdar, V. 1994. 'Amniocentesis and Sex Selection'. Delhi: *Centre for Women's Development Studies*, Occasional Paper Series No. 21.

Nandedkar, T. D. and M. S. Rajadhyaksha. 1995. *Brave New Generation, Vistas in Biotechnology*. CSIR, Department of Biotechnology. Delhi: Government of India.

Patanki, M. H, D. D., Banker, K. V., Kulkarni and K. P., Patil. 1979. 'Pre-natal Sex-prediction by Amniocentesis—Our Experience of 600 Cases', Paper presented at the First Asian Congress of Induced Abortion and Voluntary Sterilization, Bombay.

Patel, V. 1984. 'Amniocentesis—Misuse of Modern Technology', *Socialist Health Review*, 1 (2): 69–71.

———. 1987. 'Sex Determination and Sex Pre-selection Tests in India- Recent Techniques in Femicide', Bradford: *Reproductive and Genetic Engineering RAGE* II (2) 1989: 111–19.

———. 2000. 'Sex Selection' in Kramarae, C. and D., spender. (eds.) *Routledge International Encyclopedia of Women-Global Women's Issues and Knowledge*, 4: 1818–19.

———. 2002a. 'Adverse Juvenile Sex Ratio in Kerala', *Economic and Political Weekly*, XXXVII (22) June 1: 2124–25.

———. 2002b. *Women's Challenges of the New Millennium*. New Delhi: Gyan Publications.

———. 2003a. 'The Girl Child: Health Status in the Post Independence Period', *The National Medical Journal of India*, 16 (Supplement 2): 42–45.

———. 2003b. 'So Much for Son', Mumbai: *One India, One People*, 6 (11): 45–46.

———. 2003c. 'Sons Are Rising- Daughters Are Setting', Mumbai: *Humanscape*, September 2: 14–16.

———. 2003d. 'Locating the Context of Declining Sex Ratio and New Reproductive Technologies'. *VIKALP- Alternatives*, Mumbai: Vikas Adhyayan Kendra.: 25–40.

———. 2003e. 'Declining Sex Ratio and New Reproductive Technologies'. Delhi: *Health Action*, 16 (7-8): 30–33.

Rapp, R. 1984. 'The Ethics of Choice', *Ms. Magazine*, USA: April.

Ravindra, R.P. 1986. 'The Scarcer Half—A Report on Amniocentesis and Other SD Techniques, SP Techniques and New Reproductive Technologies' Mumbai: *Centre for Education and Documentation*, Health Feature, Counter Fact No. 9.

Registrar General of India. 1998. *Women and Men in India*. Central Statistical Organisation. New Delhi: Government of India.

Sen, V. 2002. '2001 Census of India—Report for Kolkata', *Director of Census Operations*, West Bengal.

Sen, A. 2003. 'Missing Women: Revisited', *British Medical Journal*, 327: 1297–98.

Sheth, S. 1984. 'Place of Pre-natal Sex determination', Larson and Turbo Seminar, also mentioned in *Women's News*, Bombay: Women's Centre.

Singh, G. and Jain, S. 1983. 'Opinion of Men and Women Regarding Amniocentesis', College of Home Science, Ludhiana: *Punjab Agricultural University*.

Sudha, S. and I. Rajan. 1999; 'Female Demographic Disadvantage in India 1981–1991: Sex Selective Abortions and Female Infanticide', *Development and Change*, 30 (3): 585–618.

Sunita, and Elamon, J. 2000. 'Medical Technology: Its Uses and Abuses in Trivandrum City', Thiruvananthapuram: *Achyutha Menon Centre for Health Sciences Studies.*

The Asian Age. 2003. Special Correspondent Report. Mumbai: 25 April.

———. 2004. Mumbai: 11 June.

The Hindu. 2003. 'More Babies Being Abandoned Now', Chennai: 1 April.

The Indian Express. 2003. Mumbai: 19 May.

The Times of India. 2004. Mumbai: 7 April.

Thekkekara, T. F. 2001. 'On the Road to Extinction', Mumbai: *The Indian Express:* 5 December.

United Nations. 2003. *World Population Prospects: Sex and Age Distribution of Population.* The 2002 Revision, Vol. II. New York: UN.

United Nations Population Fund. 2001. *Sex Selective Abortions and Fertility Declining: The Case of Haryana and Punjab.* New Delhi: United Nations Population Fund.

UNFPA and Registrar General of India. 2003. *Missing...Mapping the Adverse Child Sex Ratio in India.* Office of the Registrar General and Census Commissioner of India, Delhi: Ministry of Health and Family Welfare and United Nations Population Fund.

Vanaik, A. 1986. 'Female Foeticide in India'. Mumbai: *The Times of India.*

VHAI. 2003. *Darkness at Noon- Female Foeticide in India.* Delhi: Voluntary Health Association of India.

Wichterrich, C. 1988. 'From the Struggle Against 'Overpopulation' to the Industrialisation of Human Production', USA: *Reproductive and Genetic Engineering–journal of International Feminist Analysis, RAGE,* 1 (1): 21–30.

Female Foeticide, Family Planning and State–Society Intersection in India

11

Tulsi Patel

This essay explores the manner and the processes of the relationship between the technology and the culture of reproduction, mediated by the practice of the Indian state. It focuses on the multi-layered relationship between the state and the society through the ideology, programmes, and their deployment, through the apparatuses of the former, and meanings, practices, strategies and resources around reproduction, including female foeticide, of the latter. It looks into the relationship and the disparity between the lived ideas and governmental structures on the frontiers of human reproduction and its manipulations. It aims to explore the family planning programme's multi-pronged efforts on its own, and in conjunction with other state steered programmes at controlling and curtailing reproduction in the Indian society. The state's visions of itself and of the society, and the state's policies and practices are viewed through its policing mechanisms, after Donzelot's (1979) work on French society. Both state documents and research available on the family planning programme, over this period, is used for the analysis. Also, the society's institutional mechanisms, especially the family and reproductive practices associated with the use of NRTs, especially the use of ultrasound technology to test the sex of the foetus, are viewed through their practices based on data collected in rural Rajasthan and in the Bundelkhand[1] region of Uttar Pradesh and Madhya Pradesh.

Many of these practices are connected with wider material and historical influences mediated through culture. They are often responses to the practices of the state. At the outset I wish to make it clear that I am focusing largely on North India, especially the upper class, middle class and those groups with lower incomes, who cherish middle class aspirations, who are struggling to come out of the shadows of prosperity. The last category of people are those who send their children to schools, universities, invest in finding white collar jobs for them, try to copy middle class consumption patterns and are keen on being seen as sanskritised by emulating upper caste cultural practices, as Shah (2005) discusses for India as a whole. Adopting dowry in place of bride wealth is one of the striking practices adopted by this section of the society. These are, by and large, middle and other backward castes (OBCs). The paper thus speaks for these and the upper castes. The poorest among the OBCs, the lower castes and most tribals, remain outside the purview of this paper, though they are also gradually moving towards the dominant fertility pattern. Similarly, Indians other than those in North India, are not included in this analysis. Especially, South Indian, poorer OBCs and matrilineal communities, might show different pictures on the ground, though the middle class and upper class Indians, as a whole, seem to converge in their views and values regarding family size norms and reproductive outcomes (See Sen 2003 for intra-country variation by region and religion and for other countries in South and South-East Asia). One more arena this paper does not elaborate on is the great deal of impact of the mass media (culture industry) providing easy exposure to urban, middle class values added by increased migration, urbanisation and spread of formal education. While acknowledging their impact on people's perceptions and transformation of values and aspirations, to do justice to their role by attempting to analyse these, would require another paper.

The state is not limited to an actor or a unitary body with interests of its own which do not necessarily reflect those of the society. The state inflects with society in many ways, it directly and indirectly interacts with it. It seems to be close to what Rudolph and Rudolph (1987) describe the Indian state as semi-autonomous or 'constrained', a third actor. The networks that bring the state and society in interaction with each other, are explored. Yet, through its policies and projects, the state does often appear as an entity capable of exercising power over its population. First, the paper provides the contemporary historical context of NRTs and deals with reproduction as a social and political issue. Next, the efforts of the Indian state that views reproduction as a population growth problem, and its ensuing policies and programmes at controlling it are looked at in three separate phases: (a) up to the 'internal political emergency' (1975–77), (b) the post-emergency period, and (c) decentralisation of services for Mother and Child Health since the early 1990s. In the context of FPP, the paper analyses the processes and interaction between the programmes of the state and society's acceptance of contraceptive technologies in independent India. Lastly, it explores why, in spite of all the efforts, there are differences in the state's family size norms prescribed for its citizens and those of the people themselves. However, it does not look into the history of the voluntary efforts of planned parenthood by the socially and the politically influential class in India in the pre-1947 period. Their thought and efforts, mediated also by the impact of the Western birth control movement and the Malthusian ideology, did influence the post-1947 family planning policies.

I

New Reproductive Technology to Diagnose Congenital Abnormalities

Introduced in the 1960s to monitor high-risk pregnancies, foetal-ultrasonography[2] had become by the 1980s, a routine aspect of pre-natal care, not only in most of the industrially advanced countries but also in many others. Advances in medical technology, such as the use of ultrasound and amniocentesis, offer much more reliable antenatal screening and diagnosis than was previously ever possible. These have been critical in transforming the meaning of physiological dimensions of reproduction. This has enabled people to know the previously unknown aspects of a foetus. Technically, amniocentesis is usually combined with an ultra-sonography that is an 'ultrasound guided amniocentesis' (so that the foetus is not touched with the needle). Another diagnostic test, which is seen as having an advantage over amniocentesis, is Chorionic Villus Sampling (CVS). This involves taking a small amount of chorion tissue with the aid of ultrasound, at 9–12 weeks' gestation. It takes about a week for the results to be obtained. But there is a miscarriage risk of two per cent over one per cent in the case of amniocentesis from CVS diagnostic test; in addition, there is an increased risk of limb defects to the foetus. Yet another test is foetal blood sampling. Foetal blood obtained from the umbilical cord, with the aid of ultrasound at an early stage in pregnancy, gives the results in three days. This test too carries a 1.15 per cent risk of foetal loss. Harpwood (1996) informs that foetal blood sampling is seldom used in England for technical reasons.

With an increasing number of women all over the world coming under the fold of antenatal screening since the medicalisation of birth began in the early 20th century, foetal testing has attracted a greater involvement of women in decisions about their treatment and that of their unborn babies. It has given an option to people whether or not to carry through an abnormal foetus. Usually the sex of a child can be determined at 16–20 weeks of pregnancy by sonography and even a couple of weeks earlier by amniocentesis. It is now possible to manage a preconception gender selection (PGS). It involves flow cytometry, pre-implantation sex determination of the embryo, and in-vitro-fertilisation, to ensure the birth of a baby of the desired sex without undergoing abortion. In PGS, X and Y sperms are separated and X sperms are utilised to fertilise the ovum. The method was intended to reduce the risk of diseases related to the X linked genetic disorders, which are far more likely to occur in boys than in girls (who have two X chromosomes).

The most common test in India is ultrasound, colloquially known as 'sonography'and in some rural areas of Bundelkhand as '*untracson*'. By mid-1970s, amniocentesis and CVS were introduced in India for research on the determination of genetic abnormalities. The volunteers in the research were exhilarated to discover their unborn babies' sex and wanted abortions if they carried a female foetus (for details see V. Patel and Sagar in this volume). With the introduction and spread of ultrasound technology by the late 1980s, the sex determination test has gained popularity all over India. After the introduction of these tests, hoardings appeared in different parts of India, encouraging parents to spend Rs 500 now to save 50,000 later. The hoardings were found first in Amritsar in Punjab in the late 1970s, and subsequently in Delhi and large towns and cities of Punjab and Haryana, where the depletion of sex ratios is among the worst in the country. Subsequent scientific advances in biotechnology and genetic research have only added to the depletion in sex ratio, i.e. reduction in the ratio of females to males. Pre-conception gender selection (PGS) is used in India to avoid conceiving girl children. But it is a relatively new, complex and exorbitantly expensive procedure costing between Rs 20,000–50,000 and is not common.

Pregnancy and its Politics

The international recognition of basic human rights after the II WW (European Convention of Human Rights and Fundamental Freedoms, first signed in 1950) laid the foundations for the arguments advanced in support of the rights of pregnant women. Unwanted pregnancies and legalising of abortion were brought under the purview of rights. These matters moved out of the domestic and entered the larger political arena as questions of human rights. The evolution of the shift of emphasis of pregnancy from the micro and the private, to the macro and public political domain, is traceable most directly to the emerging consumer movement of the 1960s and 70s, and even earlier in the early 20th century to the birth control movement. The consumer movement paralleled the second wave of the women's movement that reiterated with force some of the earlier issues it had on its agenda. Operating routinely at the micro political level in the household and the family, the ability or inability to reproduce has cultural meanings. Cultural politics has surrounded the occurrence or non-occurrence of biological events, such as conception, pregnancy, miscarriage, induced abortion and childbirth in all societies. Birth is not merely a biological event, it is also a social event as it creates relationships. The harrowing experiences of childlessness, faced particularly by childless women in rural India (Patel 1994), in Egypt (Inhorn 1996) and in many parts of the world, Inhorn and Balen 2002) are palpable. The ideology of motherhood is pervasive in these societies. The desire for pregnancy and childbirth is a recurrent theme. It is not only that motherhood brings status to a woman but also it is an attribute without which she is useless. She justifies her existence and is privileged only as a mother of son/s (see Patel 1994 on how disconcerting and disheartening births of 'daughters only' can be). North India, particularly certain dominant castes, has been notorious for its violence against women, especially for female infanticide in the past until the early decades of the 20th century

(Panigrahi 1972, Vishwanath 2000). The region is also infamous for female neglect (Miller 1981, Das Gupta 1987, Wadley 1993). The incidence of female infanticide is increasingly surfacing in certain pockets in the Southern states of India as well (Bumiller 1990).

The all-India fall in sex ratio disfavouring the girl child aged 0–6 years of age (927 girls for every 1000 boys), especially when the overall sex ratio has marked a slight improvement between 1991–2001 (933 females for 1000 males) signifies the abuse of NRTs. Ultrasound has become synonymous with the sex determination test in India. To examine the fairly widespread diffusion of pre-natal diagnostic screening, especially ultrasound technology in Indian society, I am drawing on the village ethnographic data collected in three parts between 1980–87 in rural western Rajasthan. Later on, survey data was collected in 14 districts in Uttar Pradesh (U.P.) and Madhya Pradesh (M.P.), i.e. in Bundelkhand region between 2002–05. The data in U.P. and M.P. was collected through focus group discussions (FGDs) and unstructured interviews with NGO directors, workers, other government organisations and people in general. The data in Bundelkhand was collected during brief visits to towns and villages to study domestic violence. Sporadic brief visits have been made to the Rajasthan village several times since. Case studies have also been collected during the 1990s in a few towns and cities in Rajasthan. It adopts the multi-sited ethnographic method as it follows the practice of NRTs in these locales, while dealing with the related state policies and practices with this institution.

II

The Spread of Foetal-ultrasound and the PNDT Legislation _____

Since 1994 the use of pre-natal diagnostic techniques (PNDT) for non-medical purposes is illegal in India, especially to test the sex of the foetus. The Pre-natal Diagnostic Techniques (Regulation and prevention of Misuse) Act 1994, provides for the regulation of the use of PNDTs for the purpose of detecting genetic or metabolic disorders or chromosomal abnormalities or certain congenital malformations or sex-linked disorders. It aims at prevention of the misuse of such techniques for the purpose or with the intention of sex determination leading to female foeticide. PNDTs include all gynaecological or obstetrical or medical procedures and techniques such as ultra-sonography, foetoscopy, taking or removing samples of amniotic fluids, chorionic villi, blood or any tissue of a pregnant woman for being sent to a genetic laboratory or genetic clinic. All genetic laboratories and clinics are to be registered, even advertising of these facilities is an offence. The PNDT Act 1994 was passed owing to large-scale feminist protest in India against reported abuse of the test for sex identification leading to abortion of female foetuses. This has been an achievement for the Indian feminists (see Vibhuti Patel in this volume for more on this). As if the 1994 PNDT Act was not enough, soon the still newer technology of pre-conception sex selection arrived on the Indian scene. The sex of the desired baby could now be chosen even before conception by separating the sperms having x and y chromosomes. In order to prevent the misuse and abuse of the new technology for pre-conception sex selection, an amendment in the PNDT Act 1994 was brought about in 2002 and implemented from 2003. The 1994 Act now stands renamed as 'The Preconception and Pre-natal Diagnostic Techniques (Prohibition of Sex Selection) Act' (see Appendices 2, 3 and 4). The Act prohibits sex selection before and/or after conception. It regulates but does not deny, use of pre-natal diagnostic techniques, such as ultrasound, for the purposes of detecting genetic abnormalities or other sex-linked disorders in the foetus. A person who seeks help for sex selection can face, under the Act, at first conviction, imprisonment for a period of three years and can be required to pay a fine of Rs. 50,000. The State Medical Council can suspend the registration of the medical practitioner involved and, at the stage of conviction, can remove his/her name from the register of the council. The National Population Policy (GOI 2000) includes among its aims, gender-balanced population stabilisation. Hospitals are supposed to refuse to declare the sex of the foetus even if people are curious and often keen to learn. People both in urban and rural areas are aware of the ban. Unlike the openness about foetal tests prior to the ban, they are shrouded in secrecy presently.

Notwithstanding the PNDT Act and its amendment, the 'public secret'-like sense with which the issue is infused, is enough to indicate that something is the matter between the state and the population about these tests. The information about the sex of a foetus is possible to obtain through tests in private clinics/hospitals but at a very high cost perhaps because of its non-permissibility clubbed with its popularity in Indian society. On the ethical front, sex identification tests are culturally understood to mean that they are conducted for having 'desirable sex composition' of children in families or simply put, elimination of female foetuses. There is little open encouragement or acceptance of the practice. Son preference is intensive as it is extensive in India and also in South Asia as a whole. It does mean that the less preferred sex remains less numerous, whether through infanticide, neglect or foeticide. These practices are not openly accepted though these are open secrets given away to a long standing and keen observer and careful listener of local language. Despite its widespread prevalence, there is something about the practice that is encircled with a great deal of hesitation in discussing it. It is an act having a mixed meaning associated with it, it is both good and bad at the same time, bad enough to keep it shrouded and good enough to continue the practice. When people perceive a sense of conspiracy about their action, they do not want others to know about it. Yet, NFHS-II, a survey conducted in 1998–99 found that 13 per cent of the pregnant women (8 per cent from rural and 31 per cent from urban areas) self-reported having gone for pre-natal sex determination during the last pregnancy, amounting to about 3.6 mn. women having access to the technology (reported in Jha et al 2006). 'In the popular perception, pre-natal diagnosis has become associated with sex selection rather than the discovery of genetic abnormality' (Wertz and Fletcher 1993: 1363). Let us see below how half a century of pushing of contraception and abortions along with governmental efforts to transform people's reproductive behaviour, has influenced thought styles and predispositions towards contraception and sonography.

III

India's Family Planning Programme (FPP) and Popularity of Sonography _____

The Indian state's insistence on people's conscious identification with its policies and activities did attempt to reach the private, i.e.

reproductive and the familial domain. Modern contraception has been one of the several paths for people to accept the state's call for controlling their fertility and having a small family. In the initial years of the FPP since the beginning of 1950s, the state tried to bring down the desired number of children couples wanted to have. The efforts continued with little success and over time, but only very gradually, some positive though highly differential response was traceable. There was little demographic indication until the 1980s that the rate of fertility in India was on the decline. Not all population groups and categories were equally stubborn. But the rural, the poor, the illiterate, the Muslims, and slum dwellers were hardy showing their preference for fewer children compared to the educated, urban and salaried sections of the society. The educated and professional class of Indians were among the first to accept the message of the small family norm. This group also preferred non-terminal contraceptives, such as IUDs, oral pills and condoms for spacing births. This however, did not show any visible impact in national population figures in the short run, though over time, class and educational group differences in fertility became apparent. The intrepidity of the high fertility sections of the population was a cause for concern and continues to remain more or less so for the Indian state, which can be seen from the population and health policy documents. As NRTs have found favour with most people across economic and social categories, and as sex ratio is declining all over India, the paper explores the state-society relations in general, rather than for any specific group in particular. The role of the state in surveillance and in attempts at moulding society's ideas about reproductive behaviour, can be seen in the background of FPP.

The Small Family Norm in India's Modernisation and Development

The state's insistent efforts to encourage adoption of modern technology in reducing or even averting births began long before the inroads made by amniocentesis and ultrasound technologies. India is the first country in the world to have started its official Family Planning Programme (FPP), sponsored by the government of India in 1951, soon after it set off on its path of planned economic development after gaining political independence. FPP began with the first Five Year Plan. The worldwide scare of population explosion, and in its wake, an explosion of problems for the whole world, had been seriously heeded to by India (Patel and Purewal 2005). Right from its inception, India's FPP had been a programme for population control. The goal was to stabilise population consistent with the requirements of national development. Primary Health Care services also started with the planning era in 1951 with the broad objective to provide universal coverage and to enable the whole population to have access to health services (Bhatia in this volume). It was recurrently mentioned in official documents that if success was not achieved in containing the ticking time bomb of population growth, all efforts at reduction of poverty and unemployment would go awry. The then prime minister, Nehru had in one of his speeches at the inaugural meeting of the Coordination Board of ministers of river valley projects, New Delhi, on 13th October,1954, stated that as there were 360 million individuals in the country, it had 360 million problems (GOI 1958). In fact, his speech is titled, 'Three hundred and Sixty Million Problems'. Soon after independence, the perception of the Indian state was that rapid economic growth is necessary to compete in the world economy, like the perception of several other states too (Gerschenkron 1962). This required planned and sustained state intervention. The state as an engine for modernisation of the society needed to have control of the development process. State's direct intervention into family life and reproduction thus followed.

Approaches to the Small Family Norm

As officials and leaders of the country saw population as a problem, they wanted the state to chalk out policies to plan people's families to control the country's population growth and thereby to control its problems. The norm of small family (the Indian family then conceived erroneously as consisting only of parents and their unmarried children) as an ideal family, has been propagated from 1951 onwards and several measures adopted by the FPP in India through the means of mass media and the widespread network of the country's health care programme.

Two prominently different phases of the FPP are clear from the experiences of the programme since its inception in 1951. The first phase is until 1977 and the second one begins after 1977. The great divide in the flow of FPP came with the fall of the government soon after the political emergency between 1975–77 owing to the excesses of vasectomy and stringently forced quotas on every government employee, to recruit people for contraception, mostly sterilisation. The excesses of the family planning programme during the political emergency in 1975–77 threatened not only all health workers at each level but also all other government and private sector employees with withheld salaries, promotions, hard transfers, etc. unless they met family planning targets. During the emergency period, hardly any part of India remained untouched by the population control programme. Sterilisation figures shot up manifold during the emergency in 1975–76, majority of them being vasectomies. From trying to force couples, to find volunteers, and to conditional treatment of patients only if they agreed to sterilise or accept IUD insertions, the pressure was enormous on government and private establishment employees. Tarlo (2000) vividly describes the varying means adopted by the displaced people to adhere to the sterilisation dependent plot allotment in resettlement colonies in Delhi during the emergency. Sterilisation (*nas bandi/uperason/baccha band karno*), condom (*Nirodh*) and IUD (copper-T/*loop*) became household names in India. The emergency period sticks out as a sore point in the history of India's FPP as the public (government employees as well as other citizens) backlash brought about a total change in the government's approach to FPP.

Treating the emergency as a watershed, the first phase, i.e. the period up to the emergency was primarily the male-oriented phase, while the post-emergency phase focussed on the female. Haney's (1998) paper explicates the re/distributive outcomes of welfare states to illuminate gendered ways of resource allocation. The gendered stress in the FPP approach brought about a great deal of change in the ways of population stabilisation. Gender became the hinge on which the shift of FPP's emphasis rested after the emergency. We shall see below how the state's notion of the small family through FPP evolved during the two phases. The family, in its household dimension, goes through phases of demographic progression and regression. The associated economic and other human and social resources too either deplete or accumulate during these phases. This process view of the family has not been borne in mind by the state in its model of the small family it set out for people to adhere. The connections and contradictions between the hierarchies of the household and the state in the socio-cultural field of reproduction, are located in concrete material and historical terms.

a) FPP Until the Emergency: Small Family as Three Children Family

Three main means through which health workers were to spread the message of the desirable small family of up to three children (*do ya teen bacche, hote hain ghar mein achhe*) were: 1) Clinical, 2) Extension and motivation, and 3) Target and incentive. During the first and second five year plans (1951–61) the programme adopted the clinical and cafeteria approach. Health workers, through the primary healthcare network, were to provide advice and information to couples on the rhythm method, jellies, diaphragms, foam tablets, etc. as and when people approached the health staff in the state run clinics. A few committed citizens ran private clinics in a couple of big cities like Bombay (now Mumbai) and Madras. But the response of people to fertility control, was less than enthusiastic. Therefore there was a shift in the programme's implementation strategy. Rather than waiting for people to come to the clinics, it was considered proper to go to people and take both the information and the contraceptives (pills, condoms, IUDs and sterilisation) to people's door steps. A greater responsibility of awareness generation was assigned to health staff during the third five year plan through the extension approach. The workers now had to carry the information and persuade couples to adopt family planning methods. The focus was to alter the preferences of people regarding the number of children they wanted to have. But for this to happen, health workers themselves had to be convinced before hand. Nevertheless, the Total Fertility Rate (TFR) had to be brought down from over five children per woman to three children per woman.

This was also the period when numerous KAP (knowledge, attitude and practice) surveys were conducted and the question of the number of children one desired or did not want, became widespread throughout India. The demand for children, the notion of unwanted children etc. also came up during the KAP and later surveys. Talking about sexual life and control of the number of children, was no longer a taboo subject for restricted and private discussion in decent society as far as KAP surveys were concerned.

Reproduction, especially reduction of the number of children was part of the mass media and social studies and co-curricular activities in educational institutions. Parents with several children were shown to be deprived of food, clothing and children's schooling, in contrast to parents who had fewer children, through posters, hoardings and radio broadcasts. Not only would their family budget go awry but their irresponsible behaviour as parents with a string of children made the nation's budget and planning for development difficult. Thus for the development of the nation, a small family (therefore a happy family) was ideal towards which parents were exhorted to strive. Such clippings were shown in movie theatres, before and during the intermission, prior to and even for years after the spread of television in India. Radio was similarly deployed to convey the message that a small family with not more than three children was a desirable family. Food scarcity during the 1960s in India, prior to the Green Revolution, aggravated the desirability of the small family all the more. It was a hot topic for debate and elocution competitions in schools and colleges. The Malthusian gloom was feared both by the state and the educated class to be fast approaching during the 1960s.

The popularity of the population control programme among the health workers began through the target-cum-incentive approach. By the mid 1960s, the impatience of the government, to control population growth within a stipulated period, led to target oriented sterilisation and IUD camps. The health workers employed by the government were given targets to achieve. They were also provided incentives for motivating and bringing cases for contraceptive adoption. Target cum incentive approach made the workers look for possible cases who could be persuaded to accept contraception. Sterilisation thus became the most important means of population control. There was a clear shift to population control through reduction in birth rate within a stipulated period. The method changed to target-oriented camps and one-time, low-cost motivation methods of sterilisation and IUD insertions. The vasectomy camps of the late 1960s and early 1970s were a big success. Doctors were admirably spoken of for their speed at disposing off cases. Replication of such camps which curtailed the family size, was thought to be the panacea for the country's developmental planning and goals. Higher officials were given demonstrable prizes and perks to encourage others to achieve higher targets.

While four to six children per couple was common in the 1950s and 60s, the state wanted people to have only three children. Two sons and one daughter was thought as ideal by most of the highly-educated people in towns and cities who accepted contraception. In general population, the actual number of children could be more, given higher infant and child mortality in the late 1960s and 1970s. Couples wanted two sons and one daughter to be alive; they did not account for the number ever born. Infant and child mortality was high and its fear palpably felt. What mattered to them was the number of children surviving till they were old and gone (see Patel 1994). High child mortality was one of the main factors of resistance against fertility control among large sections of Indians. Note also, that fewer daughters compared to sons, were seen as ideal/desirable for a couple. Though the sex of the children was not stressed in the state's policies, in people's minds it was always clear. Sons were needed for family continuity, for caring for parents in their old age and for standing behind their sisters in lending social and emotional support, besides providing them gifts at life cycle rituals and rites after the parents had passed away.

Of course, there has always been a gap between what the family planning department projects as the ideal size of the family for the nation as a whole and the actual size of the family, people go in for. From the extension approach and target-cum-incentive approach phase of the 1960s onwards, the health workers had used the argument of development, unemployment, limited physical resources (land included), to convince couples that their family budget could be managed better through a small family. Population was believed to be the greatest monster that stood in the way of the nation's development. In view of this, the reproductive couple was viewed as less than a truly responsible citizen, in need of more than mère education and information. The non-compliant couple was not seen as patriotic enough. Different states and districts within states competed with one another in achieving sterilisation targets, e.g. from Maharashtra's record of 1,400 sterilisations in a camp in 1961, to 1,500 in Kerala in 1971. Yet the worry of the state and the Planning Commission in Delhi was that the country's population was growing rather than reducing. Even the three children per couple, in accordance with the small family norm, was proving to be rather on the higher side for the country to progress and develop, given the vast absolute base of the population. From an annual growth rate of 1.25 per cent in 1961, it had soared to 1.95 percent in 1971. The task at hand was to bring down the crude birth rate of 35. The target to reduce the crude birth rate to 30 had to involve local health functionaries more intensively.

The small family norm was aided enormously by Medical Termination of Pregnancy Act, 1971 (MTP). Indian women, unlike the women in the West, did not have to struggle for decades before the right to abortion was obtained. In the US, abortion was legalised in the late 1960s and implemented even later. In India, abortion was legalised in 1971. Sterilisation camps for men in late the 1960s and abortion (MTP) for women in 1971, were designed as effective means to stabilise population. Though theoretically there were certain conditions under which abortion could be obtained, in practice it was rather simple and permitted until 20 weeks of pregnancy. By 1975–76, it had become common for the health staff to motivate women to abort an unwanted and/or unintended pregnancy. During the emergency, women who went in for abortion were treated only if they agreed to have themselves sterilised or get IUD insertions. Many IUD insertions were made to women even without having been informed, let alone obtaining consent. Abortion remains a common means of fertility control and population control till date in India.

Forced sterilisations during the emergency were the result of the state's thinking wherein married couples were not heeding to government advice for a small family. The total fertility rate was still hovering around five children, while the FPP had the goal of reducing it by more than a half. During the emergency, when all civil rights were suspended, the state had the power and opportunity to pressurise and force the entire spectrum of health staff and people into compliance. The number of sterilisations rose phenomenally, with the scare of the FPP spreading like wild fire, both among government employees and the general population even though for contrary reasons. The government employees were desperate to get cases to complete their quotas to achieve targets, while people ran for protection from indiscriminate invasion on their bodies through uninformed and/or forced sterilisations. In 1973–74 there were 0.9 million sterilisations recorded in India. During the 22-month period of emergency, 11 million people, many of them unmarried, many overage, and many with less than two children, were sterilised forcibly (Bose 1988). Targets for other means of contraception had fallen substantially short during the period. Sterilisation was the main plank of the population policy document issued in April, 1976.

The emergency set off an infectious competition among officials to chase targets and people in villages became strikingly aware of the population control programme. All seven cases of sterilisation in the Rajasthan village, Mogra (Patel 1994), were conducted during the emergency period. Six of these were vasectomies and one was a tubectomy. For the first time, people in the village were pleaded by teachers, *gram sevaks*, nurses and doctors posted in the village dispensary, to agree to sterilise to save the latter's increments and even jobs (Many of Punjab's Jats had earlier accepted contraceptives from those who distributed them in the Khanna region in the 1960s, thinking the acceptance was a good sign for the suppliers and might earn them promotions, Mamdani 1972). Information about these sterilisations and their adverse after-effects spread through out the area as each village had a few cases persuaded by the health staff posted in the village schools, and health centres/dispensaries. One failed vasectomy and the adverse health effects on the woman who had been persuaded by the friendly neighbour, the wife of the school teacher, for tubectomy, generated a great deal of stigma for the first woman and heart-burning between the two women, for several years after the emergency. FPP was defined in the village only as the dubious and the undesirable sterilisation programme of the government (*raj*). Sterilisation came to be called, '*nas bandi*' (tying of tubes) '*uperason*' (though it is generic term for surgery, it is used commonly for sterilisation unless otherwise specified). It is also described as '*baccha bund kara diya*' (put a stop to having children) in rural Rajasthan, as in rural North India.

Often, health workers shared some of their monetary incentives with their cases to woo them from other workers. Some women had demanded such a share from the health workers. One of them said, 'It is we who get the cut on our stomach, why should you not share what you get just for free'. As these local level health staff/functionaries of the state's health department are usually co-villagers, their motivation is perceived as conversation and people are usually envious of them, and say, 'They are being paid just for visiting homes and chatting with people, while we work so hard for a living'. Through the practice of cuts and sharing of incentives, people had got sucked into the state programme. During the emergency, generous government funds, fixing of quotas and incentives were provided while the general health budget remained more or less constant (Qudeer 1986, mentioned in Gandhi and Shah 1991). Quotas were set up for the country as a whole, for each state, district and further to the level of each Primary Health Centre (PHC) and its sub-centres (SC) to be achieved by the village health workers (quotas did not disappear even after the emergency, see Bumiller 1990, for the pressure on health workers who often had to turn in their incentive money to those who got sterilised through them and even provide help with house work until women rested for a day or two). Reprimands, especially scolding lower staff for laxity in fulfilling targets was common, as Bumiller witnessed.

b) The Post-Emergency Phase (FWP): Small Family as Two Children Family

The inherent contradiction between the state's and the society's values surfaced as the voting populace conveyed its unacceptability of the state's values and state's force on people's bodies, especially their masculinity. The electoral defeat of the government at the following election for FPP's excesses during the emergency, was a watershed in the state's FPP. Though fertility reduction and population control remained governmental priorities, having already burnt its fingers, the FPP diverted its attention from men and turned to women. As mentioned earlier, the gender hierarchy in reproduction was exploited by the state's new stance on women as targets. It then became a female-focused programme. To make it appear people-friendly, its name was changed. From FPP it became the Family Welfare Programme (FWP) of the Department of Family Welfare in the Ministry of Health and Family Welfare of the government. The state's small family norm by then was reduced to only two children, preferably one son and one daughter, and no longer that of two sons and one daughter that had been reported in survey research. Surveys continued to report that it was common for people not to count the number of daughters when reporting about the number of children couples had.[3] 'The daughters will go away', said people when further probed; thus suggesting as it were, 'count what is going to be with us'. From tubectomies constituting 25 per cent of the sterilisations, these shot up to 80 per cent of all sterilisations in 1981–82 (Balsubramanyan

1983). As many as 500 laparoscopic sterilisations a day, in camps, were recorded and applauded. The approach for changing the number of children from three to two to define the 'small family' (*hum do humare do* and *chhota parivar sukhi parivar*, literally, the two of us and our two children, and small family a happy family)[4], shifted from extension to mass education and motivation.

Information, Education and Communication (IEC) approach was adopted to reach as many reproductive couples as possible. The ANM (auxiliary nurse midwife), the adult education worker and *angan wadi* worker in Mogra, had complained to me of the excessive demands on their time, made by the doctors in the village Sub-Centre (SC). The ANMs did not visit as many houses as they were expected to visit, but used their discretion to contact women who were pregnant or lactating, and would interact with them. Being from the village itself, they knew most such mothers and had themselves met many of them. They were not pleased with the visits they were to make to other villages. They had to be escorted by a male member of the family to make such visits. The target was to reduce TFR from 4.4 children per woman to 2.3, CBR from 33 to 21, infant mortality rate (IMR) from 127 to 80 and increase couple protection rate (CPR), i.e. contraception coverage for couples from 22 per cent to 60 per cent during the VI Plan period of 1980–85. The small family norm for controlling the country's population growth deployed more health workers at local levels. During the VII Plan period from 1985–90, the network of local level workers was spread out more extensively. There were 22,400 PHCs and 1,30,000 SCs in India by 1990. By mid-1980s, the new technology of laparoscopic sterilisation was gaining popularity with women in rural areas. Patel (1994, 1999) describes how laparoscopy in the mid 1980s became an acceptable terminal method for women who had attained the desired number and sex composition of children.

Along with the past experiences and other welfare, health and developmental efforts of the state, the mass education approach for over a few decades, the FPP had been able to bring about a certain shift in society's 'thought style' (Fleck 1979) towards the number of children per couple. From an earlier position of not wanting to enlist one's children for the fear of the supernatural[5] and state adversity in doing so, young parents in the village would argue that survival of at least two sons and a daughter were essential. For ensuring the survival of 'social optimum' number and sex composition of children, one or two more children had to be born to a couple.

Sexually active life was not considered desirable after the eldest child attained puberty and was married. Patel (1994) describes the several institutional mechanisms, views and indigenous practices to arrest fertility once the desired number and sex composition of children was attained by a couple. Once they had completed their social optimum of children, the FPP logic used by the health functionaries was acceptable to the parents. This thinking of young parents was clear to the various local level health functionaries but not to the FPP officials. That indigenous fertility mechanisms existed, did not come out in the numerous studies conducted on fertility and contraception in India (Caldwell 1982 had described it as the 'pregnant grandmother syndrome' for African communities, See also Patel 1994, 1997).[6] This mismatch between the state's and society's perception, was conducive to various pressures exercised by the state machinery, e.g. famine relief work was provided on a priority basis to those who got themselves sterilised.

The camps brought the sterilisation service to the society, at people's door step. It was a clear experience of reduction in infant and child mortality that gave mothers in rural Rajasthan, some confidence to go in for the terminal method, i.e. sterlisation/*uperason*. Of course, for most, the ideal then would have been an injection to stall conception for a few years. Several women had asked me if there was not an injection which did the trick for a few years. Three women even claimed to have got the same from a male nurse belonging to a neighbouring village, and were sad that he was no more. These women were nearing their 50s and would have liked their daughters to be judicious enough to get such an injection only after they had waited and made sure that their children had grown up well. The FPP campaign, including advertisements for oral pill, IUDs and condoms had a mixed response. A woman in Mogra had to get the IUD removed as she bled so frequently that she could not carry out even the minimum tasks a menstruating woman does, as she, in her polluted state, keeps away from the kitchen and the hearth (Patel 1994). Large scale trails of two types of injectable contraceptives (Depo-provera and Net-en), and the long acting steroids and hormonal implant, Norplant were cleared by the Indian state. Though in due course, as a consequence of vocal women's campaigns against these contraceptives, for their seriously harmful effects on women's health, they were not fully integrated into the FPP. These do find mention in some programmmes in some states alongside other contraception and IEC activities. For example, one NGO's activities under the National Advocacy Campaign on Pre-birth Elimination of Girl Child, has injectables (three month protection) among other contraceptive measures in a report of the Population Foundation of India (2003).

c) The FWP in the 1990s: The Decentralising Phase

By the 1980s, the concept of well-being of the family in the FWP was concretised through the Mother and Child Health (MCH) programme by bringing under its fold the following activities. Universal immunisation programme (UIP), post-partum programme, services of Auxiliary Nurse Midwife (ANM) oral re-hydrating therapy (ORT), and safe motherhood programme (SMP) became the prominent constituents of family planning. By the 1990s, more healthcare items were added to the programme and activities for the health workers. The child survival and safe motherhood programme(CSSM) was integrated with the existing health programmes. India Population Project –VII launched with World Bank support in 1991, encouraged these activities.

The FWP's reasoning for stressing on the family budget in raising children continued to be used to motivate couples, especially with women who were to be brought under contraception. The increase in the number of health workers at the local (peripheral) level during the VII plan period of 1985–90 were to combine public health as well as population control responsibilities. Thus at every stage targets for individual contraceptives were determined from above. Of course, targets for any year were (and are presently too) determined after looking at the previous year's achievement of targets. Such a manner of target determination from above, necessarily reflected a perception about higher levels of contraceptive needs, rather than the preference or choice of people to determine the use of individual methods. The MCH programme was, in fact, aimed at enhancing the population control efforts. Prakash (1987, mentioned in Gandhi and Shah 1991) had pointed out that even after so many years of (MCH) programmes, only about half of the pregnant women receive antenatal care. Similarly, ICDS for child welfare under the Department of women and child development, is another means for achieving

FPP targets. By March 1990, 118 million births were averted in India. Women's groups have been vocal in criticising what are euphemistically-worded programmes, under the garb of which, population control takes place. One such description regarding the 1980s is,

> The target and incentive approach affects other programmes as well as the general approach towards people, their feelings, wishes and indeed their health. Liberalisation of abortion for unwanted pregnancies, is also aimed at population control. Most MTPs in governmental hospitals are immediately inserted with an IUD. (Gandhi and Shah 1991: 115)

Not only adults, even adolescent children in Bundelkhand are aware of the activities of village health workers (VHWs/MPWs), auxiliary nurse midwives (ANMs), and anganwadi workers, in motivating parents to have a small family, i.e. fewer children, to be able to look after them well. From about two to three children (*do ya teen bacche*) in the 1970s, the small family norm for FPP shrunk to only two children (*hum do humare do*) in the 1980s, though for most parents in rural areas it remained three children with at least two sons. By the late 1990s, the small family for FPP came to mean 'a boy or girl' (*ladka ya ladki*), though it still means at least two children, if not two sons, in most parts of India. The Ministry of Health and Family Welfare now advertises for the small family as, 'Have fun with one', and 'Lets grow in quality, not in numbers'. The state's stress on indifference toward the sex of the child in the late 1990s, has ironically come when the crisis of adverse child sex ratio is at its peak. The difference between the state's meaning of the small family norm and that of the society, has remained. Even though the gap in the total number of children born per couple, has narrowed, the meaning in terms of sex of children continues to exist. Also, despite the change in nomenclature from FPP to FWP, population stabilisation is retained as the goal for the country. The aims, aspirations and the meaning of children for parents, of course, continues to differ from those for FWP of the Indian State, even though fertility and population growth have both been reducing. The average annual growth rate for the decade 1991–2001, has come down to 1.93 per cent from 2.14 per cent for the previous decade. However, the FWP would like the decline to be sharper than the one achieved in the last decade.

Target Free Approach of the 1990s: Small Family as One Child Family _____

In 1992, the universal immunisation programme was strengthened and expanded into Child Survival and Safe Motherhood (CSSM) project for infants and mothers, and covered obstetric referrals and emergencies. Several new initiatives were introduced to impart dynamism to FWP. For effective community participation, the programme of *Mahila Swasthya Sanghs* (MSS) at the village level was constituted in 1990–91.

It was in 1996, two years after the 1994 Cairo International Conference on Population and Development that the FWP adopted the target free approach (TFA) in 1996, i.e. targets for individual contraception were done away with. The small family norm was to be achieved in a more voluntary fashion. Incentives for sterilisation or other contraception were done away with, though incentives for motivators were not discontinued. Until 1996 national and state-level targets were fixed and work was accordingly planned, down to the village health workers, to primary health centres (PHCs), sub-centres (SCs) and community health centres (CHCs). Established during the IX Plan, each CHC works as a referral centre for four PHCs . The aim was to overcome target chasing, which was at the cost of quality of care and the practice of over-reporting the numeral achievements to claim higher credit. The target free approach of the FWP thought it worthwhile to be guided by the needs and prefer-ences of the citizens. Note the state's fatigue or its willingness to get closer to the grassroots to curtail population growth. Retaining the democratic ethos and respecting the choice of citizens, received primacy. The changed policy, initially called target free approach (TFA) was later renamed in 1997 as Community Needs Assessment Approach (CNAA) to give it an even more positive connotation.

To solicit extensive community involvement, voluntary organisations were encouraged to participate in the programme. NGOs have been involved with the government in tackling several health problems, such as tuberculosis, blindness, HIV/AIDS, and population stabilisation by involving in reproductive health programmes (GOI 2003). The logic is that as NGOs have better knowledge of the socio-cultural and economic status of the popula-tion, they would have a wider reach with people in the communities.

The basic guide for NGOs and health functionaries produced by the ministry of health and family welfare, GOI states,

> The Family Welfare Programme has twin objectives; firstly, to reduce the growth rate of population so as to achieve stable population at the earliest and secondly, to ensure good reproduction and child health status. (1999: 9)

The population stabilisation goal has been pursued through a few new initiatives in the 1990s. A USAID-assisted project named, Innovations in Family Planning Services in U.P. works with the specific objective of reducing TFR from 5.4 to 4 and increasing the couple protection rate (CPR) from 35 per cent to 50 per cent over the 10-year period. Targets were given up precisely to work towards population stabilisation. But soon the figures (obviously estimated 'target' figures, though not officially given to the local level health functionaries) fell to meet the expected goal of population stabilisation. In many states the numeral achievements had gone down by up to 50 per cent. Local level health workers had to be retrained to work in a target-free context.

> The goal of achieving stable population has continued undiluted and indeed targets' were given up with the specific objective of achieving faster progress in the goal of stable population. (GOI 1999: 5)

ANMs are to set their own targets on the basis of the needs worked out with the community. These needs are of course to be worked out not only to include contraception/sterilisation, but also maternal and child health needs. It is expected and explicitly stated that these needs be raised by 5–10 per cent annually.

ANMs Assess Community Needs: Some Overlapping Interests

The ANM's needs assessment requires her to be in close interaction with the local community members. To get a great deal of personal information, she has to build a certain rapport with the community members. They expect her to be helpful in health matters they consider important. Refusal to oblige the community she works in, jeopardises her position to collect the requisite information. One of them told me, 'You have to often accompany a woman to a dispensary if she requests, after all they also come to my aid when I need them. Can you clap with one hand?'

The ANMs and anganwadi workers in Bundelkhand reside in the village or in the vicinity of the villages under their charge. They keep the records of all the pregnant women; their fertility history is known to them. Their infants' and children's immunisation status and ante-natal state of pregnant women is recorded. ANMs submit their monthly records to their supervisors. A co-resident in the village as a tenant of one of the families or while residing in one's own house, if employed in the same village, can get many health details filled up for official records only through sheer local residence and social interaction. Further details are obtained by willingly providing favours in return. Being a member of the community she is liable to think and behave like one. She understands the community needs and can empathise with residents more than the higher-level officials in the health system wish or care to do. ANMs feign ignorance about any local facility for ultrasound tests. But the prompt reply is, 'People go to Jhansi and Gwalior for the test (jaanch), they don't come to us'. One ANM in a small town centre near Datiya said, 'Sometimes if there is a case of miscarriage in my area, I drop the name of the woman in the next month's record. What else can you do.' She stated softly, 'If the woman has a daughter or two already, what can you tell her?'

Another ANM, who is a widow and has only one grown-up daughter (married), did not ask anyone to use contraceptives before having a five-year old son who was strong and healthy. She was turned out from her conjugal home by her husband's brother after her husband's death. Homeless, she returned to her brother and in due course she got this job as an ANM. She lives in the village in one rented room in a large house consisting of an old couple, their three sons, their wives and children. Her brother comes often to spend the night so that she feels protected and others know that she is. Without a son, her life is a dead end. She can barely manage to eat and pay rent from what she gets irregularly as salary/honorarium for working as an ANM. When I met her in March, 2003, she had not received salary/honorarium for five months. 'How can I fulfil my obligations towards my daughter (married)? My brother has to do all those on my behalf. It is important to have fewer children. Two or three are enough. One has to educate them, but without a son what is there in life.'

As these local health workers spend most of their time with people in the villages, they develop close relations with many and know most people personally. Soliciting volunteers for contraception is done over a long drawn time period. After escorting Hansi to a town for abortion, the ANM said, 'Now she will feel obliged to listen to something I say'. The ANM had been investing in the relationship to ensure Hansi's case for sterilisation after Hansi had a at least one school-going son. One supervisor in a district was on long leave because she was transferred out of her home town to a far away town in Madhya Pradesh. This was to accommodate a local politician's relative in her place. The supervisor was critical of the corrupt practices in the health department. She elaborated it through the family disruption she had been subjected to, for the sake of someone politically connected. 'She does not even know the work properly but is given this post', complained Mrs Saxena, two of whose daughters are studying in college. And to make matters worse, 'He (pointing to her husband who sat on our side) is retired with a small pension. My son has just completed B.A. and is still unemployed'. The local health workers are better-off in empathy with the local populace. They know jolly well that they cannot displease people and yet get their job done.

FWP and the National and State (Provinces) Population Policies 2000

As stated above, the goal is population stabilisation through health care. In order to make a small family more attractive to society, there are a few schemes with monetary incentives for those who sterilise after having only two daughters and no sons. A small cash payment is also made to poor mothers when they give birth to a daughter with the aim of empowering her to spend money on her health care at a time when the family is not likely to care for the parturient woman for having produced a daughter. The saying commonly quoted in Bundelkhand is, *beta ho to taliyan, beti ho to galiayan* (greet with clapping when a son is born, and cursing when a daughter).

Late in 2005, a scheme was announced to give free education to a girl if she is the only child of her parents. I have not collected data on the implementation of these schemes. But there has been a great deal of criticism of the disincentive schemes introduced in the population policies of some states, for being anti-woman. This criticism needs a context because the 73rd amendment of the Indian constitution provides reservation to women for 1/3rd of the elected representative bodies at the local level. After a decade of revolutionary nature of the amendment and appreciation of its effects at the local level, the population policy in a few states has introduced the condition that only those women who have no more than two children are eligible to contest elections in the local bodies. All the research on women's education, gainful employment, and empowerment has been overlooked in this context of conditional candidacy. And there are reports of powerful men having a second wife to fulfil the requirement to retain the local body representation within the family.[7] On the other hand, none of the population policy documents have been revised to reverse the declining child sex ratio trend after the 2001 Census revealed the enormous deficit of girls. Whether the state is indifferent or not is not certain.

Abortion versus Foeticide: MTP and the RCH Programme

Let us revert to the pre-emergency phase of FPP to explore the close relationship between abortion and female foeticide, the former being projected as a rational biological act, while the latter is seen in myriad moral shades. Under MTP 1971, abortion could be sought by a pregnant woman if continuation of pregnancy was hazardous for her or the baby, for eugenic(*sic*) reasons, if the baby was likely to be born with serious abnormalities, if pregnancy was due to rape (to prevent the pregnant woman from stigma). The rather interesting clause in the MTP Act 1971, was the ability to seek abortion if the foreseeable social or economic environment could lead to risk or injury to mother's or baby's health. 'For example, if a woman has many children, or the pregnancy is unplanned, or if she cannot afford to support another child'. The act laid out that medical termination of pregnancy could not be conducted at any place other than a government hospital or at one approved by the government.

One of the main reasons, acknowledged by the government (GOI 1999), as to why women prefer private facilities to government hospitals, is an immediate insertion of IUD or sterilisation following MTP. Distrust of public hospitals has added to the success of private hospitals or clinics. Secondly, ultrasound involves little coercion owing to its secrecy, a culturally desirable feature of reproductive practice in Indian society. Some private clinics have state-of-the-art technology, giving painless abortions. The private practitioners' purpose is to conduct the ultrasound test for a hefty fee, and they have no pressure to meet targets, unlike public hospital staff. Private provision of sonography suits most clients as it is both non-coercive and permits utmost secrecy. The two parties are co-conspirators in this matter. Local level health workers join the game to meet their targets. The medical professionals, the family members and the pregnant women collude in secrecy. Each one of the colluders is better-off in maintaining the secret. The victim, the foetus, is not alive to accuse or seek justice.

MTP is also an important component of the RCH programme launched in October, 1997. The explicitly spelt-out purpose is to increase and improve MTP facilities and their utilisation.

> MTP can be performed in all District hospitals, sub-Divisional hospitals, CHCs, and in all PHCs where there are operation theatres and doctors trained in MTP procedures.... In view of the importance of ensuring adequate facilities for MTP in the interest of women's health, MTP equipment will be provided to well-run and competent medical clinics in the non-government sectors also provided they have operation theatres and trained doctors/nurses. (GOI 1999: 37)

The popularity of abortions in India is well known. Women had been attempting abortions on their own without modern medical expertise (Prakash 1986). While science unveiled nature's secrets through human agency, the state made them manipulable. Despite a few conditions under which MTP could earlier be sought in government-run hospitals, the conditions were simply marked for official records' sake and abortions were routinely conducted in hospitals with great ease. The pressure on health staff at all levels has been such that they are the ones who have to take a lax view of the conditions to woo targets. Since 1997, abortions have become more easy, as private medical facilities are authorised besides CHCs and PHCs, to abort. Rarely is any woman denied abortion in government hospitals. On the contrary, it adds up to the numeral targets at the aggregate level even though officially they no longer exist at the individual level. Karuna, an NGO staff described the way MTP provision is made use of by people in small towns of U.P.

> Women go for the test, i.e. foetal screening (*janch*) to a private clinic with their husbands, mothers-in-law, sisters, or with a friend. They find out the sex of the foetus. Then they go to a government hospital in a big town for abortion. People do not know them in those hospitals. So they can do it all without others getting to know of it. You just have to say I don't want another child so early, and get the abortion (MPT) done.

Several other NGO workers concurred with her report of the common practice. Singh, an NGO worker for over ten years added, 'This way neither the *janch* clinic nor the hospital suspect anything wrong. It is the cheapest way to get rid of an unwanted pregnancy (*kanya bhroon*, i.e. female foetus)'. *kanya bhroon hatya* (killing of the female foetus) was a common term used by most people in towns and cities in Budelkhand, though some women in rural Bundelkhand understood only when elaborated in a less sanskritised language. They all understood when described as, '*janch* of the baby's sex in the womb'.

The web of health workers at the local level has been like that of a spider's. Close interaction between them and the common man is essential for their own functioning and the community's health care. The health workers mingle with people beyond simply recording answers to questions from among those in the community. They share the meanings and symbols of the reproductive processes in people's lives. If they are outsiders, they soon learn the ways of the local people, as did the nurse in the Rajasthan village (Patel 1994) and the ANM in Datiya. It is a challenge for them to push the norm set by the state if it happens to differ from that of the community, which has largely been the case since the FPP's inception. By the time people begin to value the state's family size norm, the state's norm itself changes. While people grapple with the state's small family norm, get around it to have a fair deal for themselves, it is too late and too little as far as the state is considered. This leaves the people constantly lagging behind and the state blaming the society for being less enthusiastic towards the nation's developmental aspirations and goals. The boundaries of the state's regulatory mechanism are defined differently than the boundaries which the society itself embodies in its values and symbols, and the meanings it gives to its units.

Safe Motherhood, Institutional Deliveries and Sonography

Since the beginning of the 1990s, and in some parts of India from an even earlier time, ultrasound scan has become a norm in antenatal care in hospitals. There are at least two ultrasound scans during a pregnancy in government run hospitals. Three ultrasound scans are conducted in private hospitals and maternity homes. Under the programmes introduced in the 1990s, women are encouraged by local health workers and referred to PHCs/CHCs or hospitals for antenatal care. The introduction to ultrasound technology is established for women choosing institutional deliveries. Dr Gaur from Bhopal was not surprised with the popularity of ultrasound clinics even among people from remote areas in Bundlekhand. He said,

> Any woman who comes for an antenatal check-up, goes through it two or three times during a pregnancy. The frequent use has made it a joke. It is not used with discretion. In private hospitals and maternity homes, no doctor wants to take the blame, so they ask for a scan. The excessive dependence of machines is in vogue.

The ANM is expected to enhance the number of institutional deliveries and refer pregnant women for antenatal care, if there is any complication. Once at the medical facility, it is easy to pressurise the local ANM to learn the sex of the foetus. We have seen above how information about sex comes for a price.

While all levels of health workers try to persuade couples and families to limit the number of children, the family members hope and pressurise reproductive couples, especially women to have son/s. Having a son is a woman's pride and her measure. She knows it well in advance, even before she is a son's mother. Even within the family, the endless wait to have a son is not appreciated. For over twenty years now, the total number of children Indians wish to have has been decreasing as some wish to have only two but at least a son to put a stop to their fertility. This is precisely what Wadley (1993) brings out in relating fertility with different mortality figures for sons and daughters to attain a certain family composition in a U.P. village. The local health workers' and society's desire for a small family meets up at some point. If the health workers help people achieve the social optimum composition of children, they get to meet their informal targets and also keep the parents and families happy. The dual pressure on the young mother presently is ideal for getting at least a son but only two children.

How does one ensure that at least one of the first two born would be a son? All women in the reproductive age group are born in the FPP era. For example, a woman aged 49 in 2005, was born in 1956, five years after the introduction of FPP and has been exposed to its campaigns for the model of the small family. Many of the entire generation of women past their reproductive age are likely to have entered marriage around 1971(when MTP became legal). They have been used to hearing about aborting foetuses being legal and many have themselves aborted foetuses since 1971. It was washed off any moral criminality for several decades.[8] People also see and experience the importance of the son. It is an embodied experience in a woman's life. Many in the Rajasthan village, who got themselves sterilised in the mid 1980s after three or four children, now favour their daughters and daughters-in-law's decision to sterilise even after two but not before at least one son reaches the school-going age. Conscious choices combine the FPP messages with those of one's own kin and relatives regarding the small family size derived from the notion of the social optimum children. Often, the two sets of messages give different signals. And abortion is the means to marry the two. Temporary methods of contraception have been relatively less popular in rural areas, though they are favoured by the educated, middle class in urban areas. For the local health workers, both male and female workers, the focus has been more on abortion and sterilisation; both have been high on the state's priority list.

The National Health Policy (2002) declares that implementing it with the National Population Policy 2000, will be the cornerstone of the plan for India's health. After all the Department of Family Welfare falls under the Ministry of Health and Family Welfare of the government. Governments elsewhere have also had their interventions in influencing people's reproductive outcomes. For example, racial hygiene (Bock 1991) had state patronage and encouragement during the National socialist regime of Hitler in Germany that forced sterilisations on Jews, Roma and Sinti populations. Officially-funded sterilisations in the US in the 1970s, were supported by legislative measures which established family planning clinics. From 201,000 in 1970 they rose to 670,000 in 1978. Shapiro *et al.* (1983) also refer to other studies whereby the blacks considered these as genocide and eventually the stress declined after protests and U.S. Congressional hearings on the matter. But further data also show that sterilisation for poor whites had begun to catch up.

IV

Society's Varying Perceptions of the Small Family Norm

The first three decades after India's independence have been precisely the decades with highest, decadal growth rate of population. The population grew at the rate of 1.25 per cent per annum between 1951 to 61, at 1.95 per cent during 1961 to 1971 and 2.22 per cent during 1971 to 81. These were also the decades when population control was among the top priorities for the country. In India, fertility control campaigns combined the norm of a small family with the state's goal of population control. This twin goal to curtail births and control the country's population growth differed from that in China, the most populated country. Croll (1985), who has closely studied the Chinese family planning programmes, reports that in its initial stages, China dissociated fertility planning at the family level from that of the state level (population control). For India, planning a small family at the micro-level was associated directly with control of population growth of the country and with population stabilisation. Croll states,

> There were a number of birth control campaigns from the mid 1950s, which were only interrupted by the Great Leap Forward (1958–59) and the Cultural Revolution (1966–69), but these campaigns had primarily advocated family planning with the emphasis on planning fertility. Just as individuals and couples were encouraged to plan their

work, study and leisure, so they were encouraged to plan their child-bearing. Even the campaigns to raise the age of marriage were presented and rationalised in terms of the benefits to women and children, rather than fertility reduction and the consequent elimination of one or two generations every century. Thus the campaigns concentrated on delivering contraceptives and other family planning services to encourage spacing and fertility limitations for couples who had already completed their desired family size. Contraception, abortion and sterilisations became widely available to those who voluntarily chose to avail themselves of these services. (1985: 13–4)

In India, the state continued to thrust upon people, the idea that the small family was good for them as much as it was for the country. Somehow, it always remained smaller than the people's actual family. The state wanted people to see such a family size as a desirable one. People on the other hand, ignored the state's call for family planning even while the state linked the country's economic growth with that of the family's. People's experience was quite the contrary. This was evident through the quiet acceptance of free contraceptives distributed throughout the 1960s in the Khanna region in Punjab without using them. Mamdani (1972) was told that just as the forest is not made of one tree, a Jat is not made of one son. A small family for a Jat amounted to courting disaster. The sum of all the demands on the rural, peasant household and the interdependence of the young and old members, encouraged the expansion of the household. Not only was it plain and clear to people that those who had more children were usually better-off but also that those with fewer children were worse-off during the first three decades of India's rapid population growth. At least two surviving sons were considered essential during that period. During the high child mortality phase, until early, the 1980s, it was common in rural India to hear the phrase: 'One eye is no eye', implying one son is no son. Thus the state's logic of directly matching the state's resources with those of the family's, did not appeal to people. The FPP reasoned by describing the distribution of the state's resources among the population. It invoked the notion of the family budget and thinning of the pie's slices with every child added to the family. Neither the state's logic nor their own experience made much sense to people in what the state exhorted them to see. In India there clearly was the national population plan with a new model of the family size even if it hardly matched with the size, structure and composition of the family on the ground. People's calculus of supply and demand of children incorporated social, cultural and politico-economic considerations as rational. To them all these factors, child mortality included, constituted a single frame.

With a decline in infant mortality, the landed people began to think about land fragmentation among many sons as less rewarding. With the introduction of laparoscopic sterilisation technology in the 1980s, rural young couples had begun to accept sterilisation after completing their family. As discussed by Patel (1994), women in rural Rajasthan reasoned in support of sterilisation only after attaining the social optimum of children by asking, 'where is the land?' This implied that each son will have lesser land than his parents and it should not be fragmented into smaller sizes by having several surviving sons. Families with several sons were sending one or two to urban areas to explore possibilities of income sources. People in Mogra told me life in cities is tough and costly unless one has a good education and a job with a regular income. They saw household benefit in mixing their investments in both agriculture and the urban sector. They however wanted two sons, so that they could educate one to send home regular remittances through an urban job (Patel 1982). Sons are obliged to care for old parents as there is no pension for most of the elderly in India except a fraction of them who had secure public employment. But sons are important for many other purposes in routine life, and caring for parents in an all-encompassing manner. Caring for parents should therefore not be seen as mere economic provision for parents' food, clothing and shelter. To have a son or two while the old parents are alive, means a respectable life, not only within the household but outside too; and means a sensible priority.

People have controlled their fertility in the past as well, but younger parents accept sterilisation more easily than did their parents. With a decline in infant and child mortality, along with a myriad associated developments, younger couples are more confident to take the risk of putting a stop to their fertility after having fewer children. The number and sex composition of the surviving children is critical to stop reproducing further. Even in the mid 1980s, those who got themselves sterilised had assured that they had two or at least one son (Patel 1994). The other risk they take in arresting fertility earlier than their parents did is owing to a sense that life is getting harder. Both the material and human cost of raising children is rapidly rising. The demands children make on parents is on the rise what with a wide range of consumer goods in the market vying for attention. The sex composition of possible number of children can now be fine tuned more carefully with NRTs. Das Gupta and Bhat (1997) convincingly argue with supportive macro-level data that the decrease in fertility and sex bias are positively correlated.

By late 1980s and 1990s people could see for themselves that the well-off families were those where each couple had fewer children. By the mid 1980s, urban exposure, urbanisation and mass media influence (culture industry) had increased in most parts of India. A small family with three children per couple, followed by sterilisation, has been considered desirable by young Indians since the late 1980s and by the 1990s some prefer only two or even one child. Ultrasound technology has enabled them to get a firmer handle on the means to keep the family small. Of course, urban, rural, religious, and socio-economic status differences are found in what is a desirable family, but as specified earlier, such desegregation cannot be taken up here as the emerging common feature, all want fewer children than their mothers wanted, but not without a son (See Bose for more on sex ratio at parity in this volume, Jha *et al.* 2006, and for earlier evidence Sudha and Rajan 1990). Also, the religious difference in fertility in India has become a contentious issue and deserves a separate treat-ment. However, the lack of convergence between the state's small family size and that of the society's, remains across religious com-munities, notwithstanding their fertility differences. While a major-ity of the Hindus may be inching towards the state's model for the two child family, they are skewing the sex ratios terribly; the poor among the lower castes and Muslims may not yet be nearing the two child family, but they are not creating as severe demographic imbal-ances and ethical problems through the use of sonography. Further, on the whole, Muslims seem to resemble local patterns more closely (Sen 2003) than a categorically different pattern of their own. In both the cases, the state finds the society's response to its population stabilisation goal challenging, rather than appreciative, despite 55 years of effort.

Every one in north India knows that it is better to spend a hefty amount now than to raise another daughter, who is in any case going to be someone else's property and drain the family resources all her life (constant flow of gifts continues not only from parents to the daughter and her affinal family but also from the mother's brother to his sisters' conjugal family and sisters' children at least until their wedding if not later as well). Accumulating resources for dowry is the common anxiety expressed by most people in public, as well as, private conversation.

It is somewhat easier to find women, aged 40 and above, to have more than two daughters in the present times, i.e. in 2003 in the study areas. Though such women would not have liked to have three or more daughters, they accepted them until they had at least a son. The historically infamous girl child neglect in many parts of India and female infanticide among many communities might be related with parents' acceptance of a girl's birth in the absence of the possibility of knowing the sex of the foetus. Female infanticide is a historical feature of 19th and 20th century India, while female neglect is found in contemporary India, especially north India (see Wadley 1993 for a careful analysis of changes in infant and child mortality by sex, over the last 50 years, as a family composition strategy in Karimpur, a village in Uttar Pradesh). Female infanticide has been spreading to the erstwhile female tolerant region of South India as well (Bumiller 1990). Younger women today prefer to use ultrasound test and abort the female foetus to have control on the number and sex composition of their children. They are less willing to accept daughters as they come. Ultrasound technology is incorporated into the culture of non-preference not for the daughter as such, but for more than one daughter.

V

First the Family: The Order of the State Comes only Next _____

Sonography has a potential to reduce the separation between 'desirable' and 'actual' reproductive outcomes. The technology and people meet each other with a rapid speed. The technology has become desirable as it is seen to be in the specific service of the pregnant woman and her family. The formal and informal networks of the state and the community have been the conduits that have brought about this fit between ultrasound technology and their popular use. Formal organisations and informal relations work in close collaboration with each other to make this particular practice of sex determination test and female foeticide so accessible and popular. Bose's essay in the book speaks of the social context of informal relations doctors have with those having formal authority, which makes it difficult to take action against unethical practices. Health workers, be they doctors or paramedical workers, have their social circles as do other people in the community. And wherever there is any convergence of interests, aspirations and meanings between the people and the state, state measures get plucked out of the package. Until the mid-1980s I often came across the comment, 'Is Raj (state) feeding our children?' If children were not raised on state funds, people reasoned the state should not interfere in asking them to stop having children. This has been now substituted by the following commonly quoted statement, 'Will they provide for our daughters' marriage and dowry if we have more daughters?' The matters of family are considered private matters and the state's interference is little appreciated.

The normative system consists in the rules and regulations which, people should follow if their behaviour is to be accepted by their society as proper. People, in this case, husband-wife couples, should follow the norm of the social optimum composition of children to be accepted as proper in the family and society. We have seen that the state, through its FPP, set up the small family norm for the society to follow. It is the rule that is the norm, not the fact that many people do not restrict their child bearing to it. Norms should on no account be confused with the patterns of behaviour which people actually perform. When we examine the small family norm set up by the state then we are entering into an arena of a dual normative system. One norm (of the small family) set by the state and the other norm (of the social optimum composition of children per couple) embodied by the community. The actual fertility practices of members of the community are not the norm, and may in fact, differ from either of the two norms. What symbols and meanings people associate with the community/society norms, as against those set up by the state, is of significance here. People don't often dance to the state's tune. In people's structuring of the world of marriage, procreation and family, the meanings and symbols of the community differ in significance compared with those at the state level. The world in which people see themselves as living in families and households, and their domain of reproduction, relates them with one another in a primary and basic manner.

The social organisational units of the reproductive domain hold greater value for people in their day-to-day lives, both in the immediate as well as in the long run, within the family and outside it. These constitute the basic level which informs and gives shape to norms at the community level. The ties that hold a family as a unit, such as those between husband and wife, parents and sons/daughters, siblings are primary ties and for the society, they belong to the 'order of nature'. This order is united with the order of law to which marriage ties belong, before they are affirmed through procreation, in the abstract sense. Blood ties affirm conjugality through procreation. The state is clearly in the order of law. The claims people have on each other by virtue of their familial ties, such as filial, affective and conjugal, are stronger and closer than their claims with the state. Society has its values and supports the ensuing performance of its members to fulfil its norms even if it requires them to circumvent the state's norms. People's relation with the state, i.e. at the order of law, in these arenas comes only next. The state norms are appreciated as long as they assist the units into which the reproductive and familial domains function. If state norms contradict those of the community, the resistance is likely to become apparent. Non-compliance is perceived at the society's performance level because the perception of the state's world differs from that of the society. The people's (society's) world and that of the citizens' (vis-a-vis the state) world, though overlapping, are not identical. Accordingly, state norms, as a conglomerate system, find support less forthcoming from the society, unless it suits the society, or when state coercion is used, like during the emergency. Nevertheless, the government of citizens through state institutions and organs, may show some shift in people's norms. Accordingly, people do steer their family sizes closer to those the state wishes them to have. The two lines are parallel, even though the gap between them is narrowing. While one focuses on numbers, the other considers sex composition as more important. And at the same time, there are unintended consequences of state intervention, as with sonography and tilted child sex ratios. Keeping in mind all the cultural complexities of gender and reproductive political economy dimensions, it would be too simplistic to say that female foeticide is FPP's creation. But it is important to situate historically, how certain state policies and programmes have interacted with people and with citizens during this time.

Notes

1. I am thankful to Oxfam–Lucknow for the Bundelkhand data collected for research on domestic violence and sex ratio.
2. Sonography is medically considered a harmless test in the sense that it has no radiation, and no pricking is involved. No fluid is taken in a routine sonography. It involves just a probe on the abdomen where sound waves are sent, they reflect back and are picked up by the probe again. The womb can be virtually peeped into and the insides sighted. It is indeed a technological feat and empowers man over nature. The technology for foetal testing has brought down to a great extent, high-risk births, such as babies born with neural tube defects or Down's syndrome, one of the leading causes of mental retardation worldwide. The main diagnostic test for Down's syndrome is amniocentesis, which involves the sampling of amniotic fluid obtained by needling through the wall of a uterus. Amniocentesis was traditionally used to screen for certain genetic diseases. It is only done and warranted in high risk pregnancies where the mother is 1) more than 35–40 years old and is first time pregnant to rule out Down's syndrome. It is known to happen in mothers who are first time pregnant at an advanced age and 2) where there is a family history of a genetic disease. There may be a chance of its presence in the foetus. If the foetus tests positive for the genetic disease then medical termination of pregnancy is advised (an option given to the parents). The results of the test take up to one month to obtain, by which time the pregnancy will be advanced. Since the desirable time for the test is between 16–20 weeks, it is risky and painful to abort at the advanced stage of pregnancy. The test is diagnostic and usually provides definite confirmation of Down's syndrome and other chromosomal anomalies of the foetus, except in some cases of ambiguous results because of laboratory errors
3. Kalaivani in personal communication mentioned this happening in Andhra Pradesh in south India, where the term for 'insignificant', or 'some one who'll not be there in any case' is invoked in response to a query about girl children. Arima Mishra mentioned about how the term for involuntary childlessness and sonlessness is often the same in Oriya language spoken in Orissa, personal communication. Wadley (1993) describes this practice in the village Karimpur she studied in U.P. In 1992, a man in a Rajasthan city in his 60s surprised me for a split second when he mentioned about another city dwelling neighbour, a man who was a common acquaintance as childless. I was certain he had four daughters and

two of them too grown-up to lose sight of. Sonlessness and childlessness are described as synonymous and have had comparable consequences for couples.

4. Children often repeat these common slogans. All three children (two mine and one of my sister's) in a car from Jodhpur to Mount Abu in 1987 read aloud and repeated such slogans from billboards throughout most of the several hours' journey. Ursula Sharma's small grandchildren, related to her through the extended conjugal family in Chandigarh, often asked their parents if they were a happy family because they were a small family, consisting of two children (2005, personal communication).

5. Dr Zakir Hussain's, the third President of India during 1967–69, mother is reported to have once been visibly uneasy and resisted the listing of her children.

6. It was also corroborated, in personal communication by two participants at the conference, a Philippino and a Japanese demographer after I presented a paper on the fit between social optimum number and sex of children and the acceptance of laparoscopy at the International conference of East West Centre Alumni in New Delhi (Patel 1997).

7. Reported in personal communication (2004) by women representatives at a consortium in Delhi, and also a researcher working with panchayat representatives in Rajasthan.

8. I have inquired with several nurses, doctors, ANMs, colleagues and other researchers if women or couples carry any guilt feeling and/or perform rituals or penance after abortions and I was informed there is no remorse or compunction.

References

Balasubramanyan, V. 1983. 'Contraception As if Women Mattered', Bombay: CED.

Bock, G. 1991. 'Antinatalism, Maternity and Paternity in National socialist Racism', in G. Bock and P. Thane. (eds.), *Maternity and Gender Policies: Women and the Rise of the European Welfare States, 1880s–1950s*, pp. 233–55. London: Routledge.

Bose, A. 1988. *From Population to People*. Vol. 1. Delhi: B R Publishing.

Bumiller, E. 1990. *May You Be a Mother of Hundred Sons*. N.Y.: Penguin.

Caldwell, J. C. 1982. *Theory of Fertility Decline*. London: Academic Press.

Croll, E. 1985. *China's One-child Family Policy*. London: Macmillan.

Das Gupta, M. 1987. 'Selective Discrimination Against Female Children in Rural Punjab, India', *Population and Development Review*, 13 (1): 77–100.

Das Gupta, M. and P. N. Mari Bhat. 1997. 'Fertility Decline and Increased Manifestation of Sex Bias in India,' *Population Studies*, 51: 307–16.

Donzelot, J. A. 1979. *The Policing of Families*. New York: Random House.

Fleck, L. 1979/1935. *The Genesis and Development of a Scientific Fact.* Translation 1979. Chicago: Chicago University Press.

Franklin, S. 1995. 'The Anthropology of Science', in J. MacClancy (ed.), *Exotic No More: Anthropology on the Frontline*, pp. 351–58. Chicago: University of Chicago Press.

Gandhi, N. and N. Shah. 1991. *The Issues at Stake.* New Delhi: Kali for Women.

Gerschenkron, A. 1962. *Economic Backwardness in a Historical Perspective.* Cambridge: Harvard University Press.

Government of India. 1958. *Jawahar Lal Nehru: Selected Speeches. 1953–57.* Vol. 3. Delhi: Publications Division.

———. 1999. *Basic Guide to Reproductive and Child Health Programme.* New Delhi: Ministry of Health & Family Welfare.

———. 2000. *National Population Policy 2000.* New Delhi: Ministry of Health & Family Welfare.

———. 2002. *National Health Policy 2002.* New Delhi: Ministry of Health & Family Welfare.http://listserve.indnet.org/cgi/wa.cgi?A2=ind02&L=refernce &T=0&F=&S=&P=2772 dt. 9 March 2006.

———. 2003. *Guidelines for Department of Family Welfare Supported NGO Schemes.* New Delhi: Ministry of Health & Family Welfare.

Harpwood, Vivienne. 1996. *Legal Issues in Obstetrics.* Aldershot: Dartmouth.

Haney, L. A. 1998. 'Engendering the Welfare State', *Comparative Studies in Society and History*, 40: 748–67.

Inhorn, M. C. 1995. *Infertility and Patriarchy: The Cultural Politics of Gender and Family Life in Egypt.* Philadelphia: University of Pennsylvania Press.

Inhorn, Marcia C. and Balen, Frank van (eds.), 2002. *Infertility around the Globe: New Thinking on Childlessness, Gender, and Reproductive Technologies.* London: University of California Press.

Mamdani, M. 1972. *The Myth of Population Control. Family, Caste and Class in an Indian Village.* New York: Monthly Review Press.

Miller, B. 1981.[1991] *The Endangered Sex. Neglect of Female Children in Rural North India.* Ithaca, NY: Cornell University Press.

Jha, P., R. Kumar, P. Vasa, N. Dhingra, D. Thiruchelvam and R. Moinuddin. 2006. 'Low Male-to-Female Sex-ratio of Children Born in India: National Survey on 1.1 mn. Households', *The Lancet.* Published online www. thelancet.com.pub.online, 9 January 2006. DOI:10.1016/S0141–6736 (06) 6930–0.

Panigrahi, L. 1972. *British Social Policy and Female Infanticide in India.* New Delhi: Munshiram Manoharlal.

Patel, T. 1982. 'Domestic Group, Status of Women and Fertility', *Social Action*, 32 (4): 363–79.

———. 1994. *Fertility Behaviour: Population and Society in a Rajasthan Village.* Delhi: Oxford University Press.

———. 1997. 'Sterilisation Converges with the Notion of the Optimum Composition of Children', Paper presented at the International Conference of East West Population Institute held at New Delhi.

———. 1999. 'The Precious Few: Women's Agency, Household Development and Fertility in a Rajasthan Village', *Journal of Comparative Family Studies*, 30 (4): 429–51.

Patel, T. 2003. 'Science, Gender and Social Networks: The Missing Girl Child in India'. Paper presented at the Institute of Social Studies, Vasant Kunj, New Delhi, on 26 September 2003.

———. 2005. 'The Family and the State: Continuity and Change with reference to India's Population Programme'. Paper presented at the International Conference on Continuity and Change: Social Democratic Traditions in the South Asian Context, held at Jamia Millia Islamia, New Delhi, January 5–6, 2005.

Patel, T. and Purewal. 2005. 'Inequality, Population Politics and NGOs', in M. Romerao and E. Margolis (eds.), The Blackwell Companion to Social Inequality, pp. 441–65. New York: Blackwell.

Population Foundation of India. 2003. 'National Advocacy Campaign on Prebirth Elimination of Girl Child', Focus, XVII (4): 5.

Prakash, P. 1986. 'Hormonal Methods of Contraception', Economic and Political Weekly, 21 (17): 733–34.

Rudolph, L. I. and S. H. Rudolph. 1987. In Pursuit of Lakshmi. Chicago: University of Chicago Press.

Sen, A. 2003. 'Missing Women: Revisited', British Medical Journal, 327: 1297–98.

Shah, A.M., 2005. 'Sanskritisation Revisited', Sociological Bulletin, 54 (2): 238–49.

Shapiro, T. M., W. Fisher and A. Diana. 1983. 'Family Planning and Female Sterilisation in The Unites States', Social Science and Medicine, 17 (23): 1847–55.

Sudha, S. and I.S. Rajan, 1999. 'Female Demographic Disadvantage in India 1981–91: Sex Selective Abortions and Female Infanticide', Development and Change, 30 (3): 585–618.

Tarlo, E. 2000. 'Body and Space in a Time of Crisis: Sterilization and Resettlement during the Emergency in Delhi', in V. Das, A. Kleinman, M. Ramphele and P.Reynolds (eds.), Violence and Subjectivity, pp. 242–70. Berkeley: University of California Press.

Vishwanath, L.S. 2000. Social Structure and Female Infanticide in India. Delhi: Hindustan.

Wadley, S. 1993. 'Family Composition Strategies in Rural North India', Social Science and Medicine, 37 (11): 1367–76.

Wertz, D. C. and J. C. Fletcher. 1993. 'Pre-natal Diagnosis and Sex Selection in 19 Nations', Social Science and Medicine, 37 (11): 1359–66.

APPENDIX 1
Campaign Against Female Foeticide: Perspectives, Strategies and Experiences

Bijayalaxmi Nanda

The child sex ratio is calculated as the number of girls per 1,000 boys in the 0–6 year age group. The 2001 census of India reported a child sex ratio of 927 girls per 1,000 boys. Therefore, there are 73 'missing girls' for every 1,000 boys in our country, and soon it may become very difficult to make up for them. The practice of eliminating female foetuses is believed to be one of the main reasons for the adverse child sex ratio. Millions of female foetuses were, and are still being terminated, creating a serious imbalance in the child sex ratio in the country. Female foeticide seems to be more prevalent in urban areas than in the rural areas, but the gap is fast decreasing because of the easy availability of sex determination tests now in rural areas. Some of the factors responsible for this can be categorised as:

Socio-cultural

- preference for a son by family and society (as he carries forward the name of the family, is considered a source of support during old age and he also performs the last rites at the time of cremation)
- social and familial pressure on women to produce sons
- lower status of women in the society
- inheritance system where a girl child has no right to her father's property
- social evil of dowry

Economic

- child rearing cost vis-à-vis benefits that may accrue when the child becomes an adult
- cost related to marriage, especially in the form of dowry
- most women lack financial independence

Political

- the issue does not attract the attention of political parties
- weak enforcement of existing policies and laws aimed at curbing the practice
- little political interest in bringing innovative policies to deal with the problem

The practice of eliminating unwanted girls and selecting desirable boys has been aided and facilitated by the misuse of medical technologies or reproductive technologies. Commercial minded and unethical doctors have been abusing these advanced scientific techniques for selective elimination of female foetuses through sex determination. Some of the common methods of sex determination, before birth as well as before conception are:

- Amniocentesis (*Amnion*: membrane, *Kentesis*: pricking)— in this technique, amniotic fluid is drawn from the amniotic sac surrounding the foetus in the uterus through a long needle inserted into the abdomen. Foetal cells present in the fluid help in determining the sex of the foetus. It is normally performed after 15–17 weeks of pregnancy.
- Chorionic villi biopsy— this refers to the removal of elongated cells (called villi) of the Chorion, which is the tissue surrounding the foetus, through the cervix. The tissue cells are tested to determine the sex of the foetus. This technique enables sex determination between the first 6–13 weeks of pregnancy and abortion can be carried out in the first trimester itself.
- Ultra-sonography/ultrasonic–here inaudible (to humans) sound waves are used to get a visual image of the foetus on a screen. Normally, it is used to determine the foetal position or abnormalities, but it can also be used to find the sex if external genitalia of a male foetus are seen on the screen. It is normally performed around the 10th week of pregnancy. It is the most commonly and rampantly used method for sex determination.
- Pre-conception techniques to select sex–

- Ericsson method or (X and Y chromosome sperm separation)— A male child requires an XY combination of chromosomes. Sperms may have either X or Y chromosomes, but eggs have only X chromosomes. In this method, sperms are separated into those bearing X chromosomes and those bearing Y chromosomes by filtration when put in a chemical solution. The faster moving Y sperms penetrate the solution's denser bottom layers. The egg is then fertilised with a high concentration of Y sperms to produce a male.
- Pre-implantation genetic diagnosis— one of the latest technologies to be used for sex selection, it involves chromosomal analysis of a few cells taken from a test tube embryo (fertilisation is done outside the uterus) to determine the sex.

A declining sex ratio has various socio-economic and health implications. A woman's health suffers as she is forced to undergo multiple pregnancies and abortions. A decreasing number of females in society

Figure Appendix 1.1
State Average Child Sex Ratio in 1991–2001 Decade

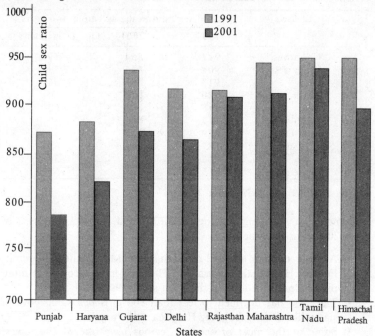

Source: Based on Provisional Populaion Totals Paper–I of 2001 and RGI (1991) C series2; Office of the Registrar General, India 2A, Mansingh Road, New Delhi 110011..

can increase sex-related crimes and violence against women. Imbalance is likely to cause a rise in social problems like dowry deaths, forced polyandry, rape, child marriages, bride-selling and kidnapping of women for marriage. For example, a recent newspaper article says that in Hathin (Haryana), two decades of female foeticide have caught up with the people. Men are resorting to the tactic of buying brides from other states like Assam and West Bengal. The price put on such a girl is much less than what people pay for cattle! After marriage, they are condemned to a life of slavery. (*Hindustan Times*, 12 July 2003, New Delhi).

It is clear from the above figure that the sex ratio in the age group 0–6 has diminished all over the country. One thing is clear that the imbalance that has been set in this early age group is difficult to be removed and would remain to haunt the population for a long time to come. To say the least, demographically, the sex ratio in the age group 0–6 does not appear to augur well for the future of the country.

Table Appendix. 1.1
Declining Child Sex Ratio in Delhi

S.No.	Districts	Child sex ratio in the age group 0–6 years		
		1991	2001	Change in points
1	North-west	913	854	-59
2	South-west	904	845	-59
3	West	913	858	-55
4	North	920	870	-50
5	East	918	868	-50
6	North-east	917	867	-50
7	New Delhi	919	882	-37
8	Central	937	902	-35
9	South	912	886	-26
	Entire state	915	865	-50

Source: UNFPA and RGI, India 2003.

Some more revealing statistics (UNFPA and Registrar General of India 2003) are given below.

- A large number of well-off states like Maharashtra, Gujarat, Punjab, Himachal Pradesh and Haryana have recorded a more than 50-point decline in the ratio since 1991
- The ratio has declined to less than 900 girls per 1,000 boys in states like Delhi, Gujarat, Haryana and Punjab
- Some of the most prosperous regions have one of the lowest ratio–south west district of Delhi–845 (a drop of 59 points from 904 girls in 1991), Ahmedabad in Gujarat–814, and Kurukshetra in Haryana–only 770

- In 1991, no state had a ratio of less than 800, but in 2001, four states (Punjab, Haryana, Himachal Pradesh, Gujarat) fell in that category
- In 2001, there are fewer districts with a child sex ratio of over 950 compared to 1991

History of the Campaigns against Sex Determination and Female Foeticide

The drive against female foeticide and sex determination techniques gained strength in the 1980s. The 1976 partial ban on sex determination tests in government hospitals had only led to the proliferation of private clinics/hospitals offering the facility. The ban was imposed because the advent of amniocentesis in 1975 caused a dramatic increase in female foeticide cases. Since then, different parts of the country have witnessed several campaigns against the misuse of science and technology to continue discrimination against women. In 1982, the Centre for Women's Development Studies (CWDS) launched the first campaign. It was initiated by Dr Veena Mazumdar and Dr Lotika Sarkar in Delhi as a protest against an advertisement for Bhandari ante-natal sex determination clinic, Amritsar, Punjab. The clinic was openly advertising its services through the press, in railway compartments and other public places. The advertisement referred to daughters as 'liabilities' to the family and a threat to the nation, and exhorted expectant parents to avail of the services of the clinics to rid themselves of this 'danger'.

More campaigns like the Forum Against Sex Determination and Sex Pre-Selection (FASDSP) in 1985 in Maharashtra and the Campaign Against Sex-Selective Abortion (CASSA), Tamil Nadu came up. FASDSP lobbied to regulate the practice of sex determination in Maharashtra by formulating a separate legislation, instead of modifying the Medical Termination of Pregnancy (MTP) Act, 1971, that had the danger of curtailing women's right to abort, the Maharashtra Regulation of Use of Prenatal Diagnostic Techniques Act, 1988, came into being.

Serious drawbacks in the state legislation and poor implementation caused the awakening of interest in the issue across the entire country. A move for an all-India ban on sex determination tests gained momentum, and the Pre-Natal Diagnostic Tests (Regulation and Prohibition of Misuse) Act, 1994, (called the PNDT Act) came into existence. Though the PNDT Act entered into force in January 1996, no evidence of decline in the practice of female foeticide came forth even after four years. Lack of concern and political will to implement the legislation by the Centre and states led to a Public Interest Litigation (PIL) in the Supreme Court (SC). The PIL was filed by three petitioners—Dr Sabu George—a social activist, *Mahila Sarvangeen Utkarsh Mandal* (MASUM), Pune, and Centre for the Enquiry of Health and Allied Themes (CEHAT), Mumbai, in February 2000. In May 2001, the SC directed the Centre to implement the PNDT Act in all its aspects and called upon all state governments to take necessary steps to implement the Act (See V. Patel 2002 and 2003). However, a further dip in the 2001 sex ratio suggests that a lot more needs to be done in this regard.

In the light of new techniques available to determine sex before conception, it was considered necessary to amend the Act. From February 14th 2003, the Pre-natal Diagnostic Techniques (Regulation and Prevention of Misuse) Amendment Act, 2002 came into force. The PNDT Act 1994 was renamed as 'the Pre-conception and Pre-natal Diagnostic Techniques (Prohibition of Sex Selection) Act, 1994.

The Delhi Students and Teachers Campaign Against Female Foeticide

The Campaign Against Female Foeticide, supported by the Centre for Women's Development Studies, was launched in Delhi in July, 2002. One of the immediate urgencies was to mobilise teachers and students of Delhi University and other educational institutions in Delhi, to build pressure on the Parliamentarians to pass the PNDT Amendment Bill. The other overarching aim of the campaign was to generate awareness about the disastrous consequences of female foeticide and to initiate a spirit of voluntarism amongst teachers and students of Delhi in order to combat this heinous practice. It was felt that sensitising students to this issue would serve a dual purpose. It would not only orient them to the issue but they would also play an important role in arresting female foeticide in their communities by acting as an advocacy group. Delhi has had an accelerated fall in child sex ratio which has declined from 915 in 1991 to 865 in 2001.

Some of the main objectives of the Campaign, therefore, are:

- To orient college teachers and students regarding the issue of female foeticide and the importance of the girl child.
- To initiate voluntarism among teachers and students and facilitate them to act as an advocacy group against female foeticide and for the cause of the girl child.

- To spread awareness about the PNDT Act in order to prevent and arrest the rampant practice of sex determination leading to female foeticide.

Many of the student volunteers did not know the meaning of female foeticide in the beginning. However, their energy and effervescence maintained the initiative, leading to a vibrant campaign.

The Campaign was initiated with a teacher's orientation meeting and then various societies within colleges like the WDC, the NSS were used to raise the issue, discuss its causes and initiate debate. Experts from all fields addressed them and apprised them of the situation. Reactions and responses have more or less been favourable, students have understood female foeticide as gender violence and shared a sense of concern, anguish and outrage. The Campaign mobilised a 'March to Parliament' on 31st July, 2002 and again in November, 2002 urging immediate passage of the PNDT Amendment Bill. More than 500 students and teachers of colleges of Delhi University and JNU joined these marches on each occasion.

Apart from this, street plays are organised regularly and films on the issue are shown in different colleges. Creative competitions like poster making, slogan writing, etc. are also organised. An inter-college choreography show depicting the theme, was held in association with CII. Some of the other noteworthy programmes include a cloth banner rally, a mobile exhibition 'Nipped in the Bud' and participation in the national campaign protesting violence against women in Delhi.

When the students were addressed their immediate response was mixed, 'yes we understand the problem and we pledge not to practise female foeticide in our married life but what else can we do?' But after sustained efforts of trying to reach them through various methods like the screening of films, using an emotive medium like the street play, presentation of the Census data, presentation of case studies, etc, their response changed to a more positive and enthusiastic ' yes, what can we do, tell us'.

So now there are about 100 volunteers spread over 19 colleges. They organise street plays on the issue, initiate debate and write papers on it and also have choreography shows on the issue. More importantly they carry the message to their homes and communities and report about their ability to convince others about the widespread occurrence of sex-selective abortions and how it affects child sex ratio and escalates gender violence. In fact, a core group of volunteers have given the names of various clinics where their relatives have had sex-selective abortions. They are monitoring the actions that are being taken.

Some of the Main Achievements of the Campaign _____

- Ability to maintain initiative and information.
- Ability to create a vibrant campaign and mobilise a large group of teachers and students.
- Effectively rallied for the passage of the PNDT amendment bill.
- Raising student voluntarism.
- Facilitating the development of a sense of ownership towards the issue.

Some of the Lessons Learnt in the Process of the Campaign are _____

1) Although it was easy to increase volunteerism amongst students, it was not the same with teachers. Teachers were hard-pressed for time and therefore found it difficult to maintain their interest and energy specifically for this cause.
2) One of the main problems faced was over the question about abortion. Some students felt that abortion should be banned thereby protecting every child's right to life. It was, however, maintained that the right to abortion must remain as an essential right to women, a right to determine their life, their body and fertility.
3) There was lesser involvement of male students who viewed this as a women's issue and not something concerning them.
4) It was difficult to have access to the women student volunteers after their marriage.
5) There was a problem in maintaining continuity and sustainability because students are a floating mass.
6) Some students felt that this awareness generation was more appropriate for slum dwellers and rural people, as teachers and students were generally gender-sensitive. Through presentations of data (specifically of Delhi), it was shown how female foeticide breaks through the rural-urban divide and is more prevalent in posh, developed, urban areas and among the educated well-off and middle class.
7) No powerful message has been sent to the unethical, medical practitioners who have a strong lobby.

Major Recommendations _____

Some of the major recommendations emerging from the various workshops and orientation programmes of the Campaign include:

- A need to do advocacy with medical students and professionals on the issue.
- Steps should be taken to bring about quick implementation of the PNDT Act against erring doctors and other perpetrators.
- Special programmes to be organised to be focused on gender equality and importance of the girl child.
- To bring about a sustained media advocacy programme on the issue.
- To bring about the enforcement of laws in respect of dowry, child marriage, sexual harassment, violence against women and child abuse.
- To bring about participation and consultation of students on this issue.

In order to make this campaign a success, there is a need to sustain the energy levels that have been created. The struggle against the patriarchal order of state and society and the elimination of gender violence can only be possible with the participation of each and every member of the civil society. The teaching-learning community has a leading role in shaping society's orientation and attitudes and must continue to protest against sex determination and sex-selection, leading to female foeticide. This is highly discriminatory, illegal, unethical and, therefore, not to be tolerated.

References

Census of India. 1991. Office of the Registrar General of India. New Delhi.
————. 2001. Office of the Registrar General of India. New Delhi.
Hindustan Times. 2003. New Delhi: 12 July.
Patel, Vibhuti. 2002. *Women's Challenges of the New Millennium*. New Delhi: Gyan Publications.
Patel, Vibhuti. 2003. 'Sons are Rising, Daughters Setting', *Humanscape*, September, 2003: 14–16.
United Nations Population Fund, Office of the Registrar General and Census Commissioner. 2003. *Missing...: Mapping the Adverse Child Sex Ratio in India*. New Delhi: Ministry of Health and Family Welfare, June.

APPENDIX 2
PNDT (Regulation and Prevention of Misuse) Act 1994

ACT NO. 57 OF 1994 _____

[20th September, 1994]

An Act to provide for the regulation of the use of pre-natal diagnostic techniques for the purpose of detecting genetic or metabolic disorders or chromosomal abnormalities or certain congenital malformations or sex linked disorders and for the prevention of the misuse of such techniques for the purpose of pre-natal sex determination leading to female foeticide; and, for matters connected there with or incidental thereto.

Be it enacted by Parliament in the Forty-fifth Year of the Republic of India as follows:—

Chapter I

Preliminary _____

1. Short title, extent and commencement:

   (1) This Act may be called the Pre-natal Diagnostic Techniques (Regulation and Prevention of Misuse) Act, 1994.
   (2) It shall extend to the whole of India except the State of Jammu and Kashmir.
   (3) It shall come into force on such date as the Central Government may, by notification in the Official Gazette, appoint.

2. Definitions: In this Act, unless the context otherwise requires,—

   (a) 'Appropriate Authority' means the Appropriate Authority appointed under section 17;

(b) 'Board' means the Central Supervisory Board constituted under section 7;

(c) 'Genetic Counselling Centre' means an institute, hospital, nursing home or any place, by whatever name called, which provides for genetic counselling to patients;

(d) 'Genetic Clinic' means a clinic, institute, hospital, nursing home or any place, by whatever name called, which is used for conducting pre-natal diagnostic procedures;

(e) 'Genetic Laboratory' means a laboratory and includes a place where facilities are provided for conducting analysis or tests of samples received from Genetic Clinic for pre-natal diagnostic test;

(f) 'Gynaecologist' means a person who possesses a post-graduate qualification in gynaecology and obstetrics;

(g) 'Medical geneticist' means a person who possesses a degree or diploma or certificate in medical genetics in the field of pre-natal diagnostic techniques or has experience of not less than two years in such field after obtaining—

(i) any one of the medical qualifications recognised under the Indian Medical Council Act, 1956 (102 of 1956); or

(ii) a post-graduate degree in biological sciences;

(h) 'Pediatrician' means a person who possesses a post-graduate qualification in pediatrics;

(i) 'Pre-natal diagnostic procedures' means all gynecological or obstetrical or medical procedures such as ultrasonography foetoscopy, taking or removing samples of amniotic fluid, chorionic villi, blood or any tissue of a pregnant woman for being sent to a Genetic Laboratory or Genetic Clinic for conducting pre-natal diagnostic test;

(j) 'Pre-natal diagnostic techniques' includes all pre-natal diagnostic procedures and pre-natal diagnostic tests;

(k) 'Pre-natal diagnostic test' means ultrasonography or any test or analysis of amniotic fluid, chorionic villi, blood or any tissue of a pregnant woman conducted to detect genetic or metabolic disorders or chromosomal abnormalities or congenital anomalies or haemoglobinopathies or sex-linked diseases;

(l) 'Prescribed' means prescribed by rules made under this Act;

(m) 'Registered medical practitioner' means a medical practitioner who possesses any recognised medical qualification as defined in clause (h) of section 2 of the Indian Medical Council Act, 1956, (102 of 1956.) and whose name has been entered in a State Medical Register;

(n) 'Regulations' means regulations framed by the Board under this Act.

Chapter II

Regulation of Genetic Counselling Centres, Genetic Laboratories and Genetic Clinics _____

3. Regulation of Genetic Counselling Centres, Genetic Laboratories and Genetic Clinics— On and from the commencement of this Act,—

   (1) no Genetic Counselling Centre, Genetic Laboratory or Genetic Clinic unless registered under this Act, shall conduct or associate with, or help in, conducting activities relating to pre-natal diagnostic techniques;

   (2) no Genetic Counselling Centre, Genetic Laboratory or Genetic Clinic shall employ or cause to be employed any person who does not possess the prescribed qualifications;

   (3) no medical geneticist, gynaecologist, paediatrician, registered medical practitioner or any other person shall conduct or cause to be conducted or aid in conducting by himself or through any other person, any pre-natal diagnostic techniques at a place other than a place registered under this Act.

Chapter III

Regulation of Pre-Natal Diagnostic Techniques _____

4. Regulation of pre-natal diagnostic techniques— On and from the commencement of this Act,—

   (1) no place including a registered Genetic Counselling Centre or Genetic Laboratory or Genetic Clinic shall be used or caused to be used by any person for conducting pre-natal diagnostic techniques except for the purposes specified in clause (2) and after satisfying any of the conditions specified in clause (3);

   (2) no pre-natal diagnostic techniques shall be conducted except for the purposes of detection of any of the following abnormalities, namely:—

    (i) chromosomal abnormalities;

    (ii) genetic metabolic diseases;

    (iii) haemoglobinopathies;

    (iv) sex-linked genetic diseases;

    (v) congenital anomalies;

    (vi) any other abnormalities or diseases as may be specified by the Central Supervisory Board;

(3) no pre-natal diagnostic techniques shall be used or conducted unless the person qualified to do so is satisfied that any of the following conditions are fulfilled, namely:—

    (i) age of the pregnant woman is above thirty-five years;

    (ii) the pregnant woman has undergone two or more spontaneous abortions or foetal loss;

    (iii) the pregnant woman had been exposed to potentially teratogenic agents such as drugs, radiation, infection or chemicals;

    (iv) the pregnant woman has a family history of mental retardation or physical deformities such as spasticity or any other genetic disease;

    (v) any other condition as may be specified by the Central Supervisory Board;

(4) no person, being a relative or the husband of the pregnant woman shall seek or encourage the conduct of any pre-natal diagnostic techniques on her except for the purpose specified in clause (2).

5. Written consent of pregnant woman and prohibition of communicating the sex of foetus.

(1) No person referred to in clause

(2) of section 3 shall conduct the pre-natal diagnostic procedures unless—

    (a) he has explained all known side and after effects of such procedures to the pregnant woman concerned;

    (b) he has obtained in the prescribed form her written consent to undergo such procedures in the language which she understands; and

    (c) a copy of her written consent obtained under clause (b) is given to the pregnant woman.

(3) No person conducting pre-natal diagnostic procedures shall communicate to the pregnant woman concerned or her relatives, the sex of the foetus by words, signs or in any other manner.

6. Determination of sex prohibited— On and from the commencement of this Act,—

(a) no Genetic Counselling Centre or Genetic Laboratory or Genetic Clinic shall conduct or cause to be conducted in its Centre, Laboratory or Clinic, pre-natal diagnostic techniques including ultrasonography, for the purpose of determining the sex of a foetus;

(b) no person shall conduct or cause to be conducted any pre-natal diagnostic techniques including ultrasonography for the purpose of determining the sex of a foetus.

Chapter IV

Central Supervisory Board _____

7. Constitution of Central Supervisory Board—

(1) The Central Government shall constitute a Board to be known as the Central Supervisory Board to exercise the powers and perform the functions conferred on the Board under this Act.

(2) The Board shall consist of—

(a) the Minister in charge of the Ministry or Department of Family Welfare, who shall be the Chairman, ex-officio;

(b) the Secretary to the Government of India in charge of the Department of Family Welfare, who shall be the Vice-Chairman, ex-officio;

(c) two members to be appointed by the Central Government to represent the Ministries of Central Government in charge of Woman and Child Development and of Law and Justice, ex-officio;

(d) the Director General of Health Services of the Central Government, ex-officio;

(e) ten members to be appointed by the Central Government, two each from amongst—

(i) eminent medical geneticists;

(ii) eminent gynaecologists and obstetricians;

(iii) eminent paediatricians;

(iv) eminent social scientists; and

(v) representatives of women welfare organisations;

(f) three women Members of Parliament, of whom two shall be elected by the House of the People and one by the Council of States;

(g) four members to be appointed by the Central Government by rotation to represent the States and the Union territories, two in alphabetical order and two in the reverse alphabetical order:

Provided that no appointment under this clause shall be made except on the recommendation of the State Government or, as the case may be, the Union territory;

(h) an officer, not below the rank of a Joint Secretary or equivalent of the Central Government, in charge of Family Welfare, who shall be the Member-Secretary, ex-officio.

8. Term of office of members.—

(1) The term of office of a member, other than an ex officio member, shall be,—

(a) in case of appointment under clause (e) or clause (f) of subsection (2) of section 7, three years; and

(b) in case of appointment under clause (g) of the said subsection, one year.

(2) If a casual vacancy occurs in the office of any other member, whether by reason of his death, resignation or inability to discharge his functions owing to illness or other incapacity, such vacancy shall be filled by the Central Government by making a fresh appointment and the member so appointed shall hold office for the remainder of the term of office of the person in whose place he is so appointed.

(3) The Vice-Chairman shall perform such functions as may be assigned to him by the Chairman from time to time.

(4) The procedure to be followed by the members in the discharge of their functions shall be such as may be prescribed.

9. Meetings of the Board—

(1) The Board shall meet at such time and place, and shall observe such rules of procedure in regard to the transaction of business at its meetings (including the quorum at such meetings) as may be provided by regulations:

Provided that the Board shall meet at least once in six months.

(2) The Chairman and in his absence the Vice-Chairman shall preside at the meetings of the Board.

(3) If for any reason the Chairman or the Vice-Chairman is unable to attend any meeting of the Board, any other member chosen by the members present at the meeting shall preside at the meeting.

(4) All questions which come up before any meeting of the Board shall be decided by a majority of the votes of the members present and voting, and in the event of an equality of votes, the Chairman, or in his absence, the person presiding, shall have and exercise a second or casting vote.

(5) Members other than ex-officio members shall receive such allowances, if any, from the Board as may be prescribed.

10. Vacancies, etc., not to invalidate proceedings of the Board. No act or proceeding of the Board shall be invalid merely by reason of—

(a) any vacancy in, or any defect in the constitution of, the Board; or

(b) any defect in the appointment of a person acting as a member of the Board; or

(c) any irregularity in the procedure of the Board not affecting the merits of the case.

11. Temporary association of persons with the Board for particular purposes.

(1) The Board may associate with itself, in such manner and for such purposes as may be determined by regulations, any person whose assistance or advice it may desire in carrying out any of the provisions of this Act.

(2) A person associated with it by the Board under sub-section (1) for any purpose shall have a right to take part in the discussions relevant to that purpose, but shall not have a right to vote at a meeting of the Board and shall not be a member for any other purpose.

12. Appointment or officers and other employees of the Board—

(1) For the purpose of enabling it efficiently to discharge its functions under this Act, the Board may, subject to such regulations as may be made in this behalf, appoint (whether on deputation or otherwise) such number of officers and other employees as it may consider necessary:

Provided that the appointment of such category of officers, as may be specified in such regulations, shall be subject to the approval of the Central Government.

(2) Every officer or other employee appointed by the Board shall be subject to such conditions of service and shall be entitled to such remuneration as may be specified in the regulations.

13. Authentication of orders and other instruments of the Board. All orders and decisions of the Board shall be authenticated by the

signature of the Chairman or any other member authorised by the Board in this behalf, and all other instruments issued by the Board shall be authenticated by the signature of the Member-Secretary or any other officer of the Board authorised in like manner in this behalf.

14. Disqualifications for appointment as member. A person shall be disqualified for being appointed as a member if, he—

   (a) has been convicted and sentenced to imprisonment for an offence which, in the opinion of the Central Government, involves moral turpitude; or
   (b) is an undischarged insolvent; or
   (c) is of unsound mind and stands so declared by a competent court; or
   (d) has been removed or dismissed from the service of the Government or a Corporation owned or controlled by the Government; or
   (e) has, in the opinion of the Central Government, such financial or other interest in the Board as is likely to affect prejudicially the discharge by him of his functions as a member; or
   (f) has, in the opinion of the Central Government, been associated with the use or promotion of pre-natal diagnostic technique for determination of sex.

15. Eligibility of member for re-appointment—Subject to the other terms and conditions of service as may be prescribed, any person ceasing to be a member shall be eligible for re-appointment as such member.

16. Functions of the Board. The Board shall have the following functions, namely:—

   (i) to advise the Government on policy matters relating to use of pre-natal diagnostic techniques;
   (ii) to review implementation of the Act and the rules made thereunder and recommend changes in the said Act and rules to the Central Government;
   (iii) to create public awareness against the practice of pre-natal determination of sex and female foeticide;
   (iv) to lay down the code of conduct to be observed by persons working at Genetic Counselling Centres, Genetic Laboratories and Genetic Clinics;
   (v) any other functions as may be specified under the Act.

Chapter V

Appropriate Authority and Advisory Committee _____

17. Appropriate Authority and Advisory Committee—

(1) The Central Government shall appoint, by notification in the Official Gazette, one or more Appropriate Authorities for each of the Union territories for the purposes of this Act.

(2) The State Government shall appoint, by notification in the Official Gazette, one or more Appropriate Authorities for the whole or part of the State for the purposes of this Act having regard to the intensity of the problem of pre-natal sex determination leading to female foeticide.

(3) The officers appointed as Appropriate Authorities under sub-section (1) or sub-section (2) shall be,—

(a) when appointed for the whole of the State or the Union territory, of or above the rank of the Joint Director of Health and Family Welfare; and

(b) when appointed for any part of the State or the Union territory, of such other rank as the State Government or the Central Government, as the case may be, may deem fit.

(4) The Appropriate Authority shall have the following functions, namely:—

(a) to grant, suspend or cancel registration of a Genetic Counselling Centre, Genetic Laboratory or Genetic Clinic;

(b) to enforce standards prescribed for the Genetic Counselling Centre, Genetic Laboratory and Genetic Clinic;

(c) to investigate complaints of breach of the provisions of this Act or the rules made thereunder and take immediate action; and

(d) to seek and consider the advice of the Advisory Committee, constituted under sub-section (5), on application for registration and on complaints for suspension or cancellation of registration.

(5) The Central Government or the State Government, as the case may be, shall constitute an Advisory Committee for each Appropriate Authority to aid and advise the Appropriate Authority in the discharge of its functions, and shall appoint one of the members of the Advisory Committee to be its Chairman.

(6) The Advisory Committee shall consist of—

(a) three medical experts from amongst gynaecologists, obstericians, paediatricians and medical geneticists;

(b) one legal expert;

(c) one officer to represent the department dealing with information and publicity of the State Government or the Union territory, as the case may be;

(d) three eminent social workers of whom not less than one shall be from amongst representatives of women's organisations.

(7) No person who, in the opinion of the Central Government or the State Government, as the case may be, has been associated with the use or promotion of pre-natal diagnostic technique for determination of sex shall be appointed as a member of the Advisory Committee.

(8) The Advisory Committee may meet as and when it thinks fit or on the request of the Appropriate Authority for consideration of any application for registration or any complaint for suspension or cancellation of registration and to give advice thereon:

Provided that the period intervening between any two meetings shall not exceed the prescribed period.

(9) The terms and conditions subject to which a person may be appointed to the Advisory Committee and the procedure to be followed by such Committee in the discharge of its functions shall be such as may be prescribed.

Chapter VI

Registration of Genetic Counselling Centres, Genetic Laboratories and Genetic Clinics

18. Registration of Genetic Counselling Centres, Genetic Laboratories or Genetic Clinics.

(1) No person shall open any Genetic Counselling Centre, Genetic Laboratory or Genetic Clinic after the commencement of this Act unless such Centre, Laboratory or Clinic is duly registered separately or jointly under this Act.

(2) Every application for registration under sub-section (1), shall be made to the Appropriate Authority in such form and in such manner and shall be accompanied by such fees as may be prescribed.

(3) Every Genetic Counselling Centre, Genetic Laboratory or Genetic Clinic engaged, either partly or exclusively, in counselling or conducting pre-natal diagnostic techniques for any of the purposes mentioned in section 4, immediately before the commencement of this Act, shall apply for registration within sixty days from the date of such commencement.

(4) Subject to the provisions of section 6, every Genetic Counselling Centre, Genetic Laboratory or Genetic Clinic engaged in counselling or conducting pre-natal diagnostic techniques shall cease to conduct any such counselling or technique on the expiry of six months from the date of commencement of this Act unless such Centre, Laboratory or Clinic has applied for registration and is so registered separately or jointly or till such application is disposed of, whichever is earlier.

(5) No Genetic Counselling Centre, Genetic Laboratory or Genetic Clinic shall be registered under this Act unless the Appropriate Authority is satisfied that such Centre, Laboratory or Clinic is in a position to provide such facilities, maintain such equipment and standards as may be prescribed.

19. Certificate of registration—

(1) The Appropriate Authority shall, after holding an inquiry and after satisfying itself that the applicant has complied with all the requirements of this Act and the rules made thereunder and having regard to the advice of the Advisory Committee in this behalf, grant a certificate of registration in the prescribed form jointly or separately to the Genetic Counselling Centre, Genetic Laboratory or Genetic Clinic, as the case may be.

(2) If, after the inquiry and after giving an opportunity of being heard to the applicant and having regard to the advice of the Advisory Committee, the Appropriate Authority is satisfied that the applicant has not complied with the requirements of this Act or the rules, it shall, for reasons to be recorded in writing, reject the application for registration.

(3) Every certificate of registration shall be renewed in such manner and after such period and on payment of such fees as may be prescribed.

(4) The certificate of registration shall be displayed by the registered Genetic Counselling Centre, Genetic Laboratory or Genetic Clinic in a conspicuous place at its place of business.

20. Cancellation or suspension of registration—

(1) The Appropriate Authority may *suo moto*, or on complaint, issue a notice to the Genetic Counselling Centre, Genetic Laboratory or Genetic Clinic to show cause why its registration should not be suspended or cancelled for the reasons mentioned in the notice.

(2) If, after giving a reasonable opportunity of being heard to the Genetic Counselling Centre, Genetic Laboratory or Genetic Clinic and having regard to the advice of the Advisory Committee, the Appropriate Authority is satisfied that there has been a breach of the provisions of this Act or the rules, it may, without prejudice to any criminal action that it may take against such Centre, Laboratory or Clinic, suspend its registration for such period as it may think fit or cancel its registration, as the case may be.

(3) Notwithstanding anything contained in sub-sections (1) and (2), if the Appropriate Authority is, of the opinion that it is necessary or expedient so to do in the public interest, it may, for reasons to be recorded in writing, suspend the registration of any Genetic Counselling Centre, Genetic Laboratory or Genetic Clinic without issuing any such notice referred to in sub-section (1).

21. Appeal. The Genetic Counselling Centre, Genetic Laboratory or Genetic Clinic may, within thirty days from the date of receipt of the order of suspension or cancellation of registration passed by the Appropriate Authority under section 20, prefer an appeal against such order to—

(i) the Central Government, where the appeal is against the order of the Central Appropriate Authority; and

(ii) the State Government, where the appeal is against the order of the State Appropriate Authority, in the prescribed manner.

Chapter VII

Offences and Penalties _____

22. Prohibition of advertisement relating to pre-natal determination of sex and punishment for contravention—

(1) No person, organisation, Genetic Counselling Centre, Genetic Laboratory or Genetic Clinic shall issue or cause to be issued

any advertisement in any manner regarding facilities of pre-natal determination of sex available at such Centre, Laboratory, Clinic or any other place.

(2) No person or organisation shall publish or distribute or cause to be published or distributed any advertisement in any manner regarding facilities of pre-natal determination of sex available at any Genetic Counselling Centre, Genetic Laboratory, Genetic Clinic or any other place.

(3) Any person who contravenes the provisions of sub-section (1) or sub-section (2) shall be punishable with imprisonment for a term which may extend to three years and with fine which may extend to ten thousand rupees.

Explanation—For the purposes of this section, 'advertisement' includes any notice, circular, label wrapper or other document and also includes any visible representation made by means of any light, sound, smoke or gas.

23. Offences and penalties—

(1) Any medical geneticist, gynaecologist, registered medical practitioner or any person who owns a Genetic Counselling Centre, a Genetic Laboratory or a Genetic Clinic or is employed in such a Centre, Laboratory or Clinic and renders his professional or technical services to or at such a Centre, Laboratory or Clinic, whether on an honorary basis or otherwise, and who contravenes any of the provisions of this Act or rules made thereunder shall be punishable with imprisonment for a term which may extend to three years and with fine which may extend to ten thousand rupees and on any subsequent conviction, with imprisonment which may extend to five years and with fine which may extend to fifty thousand rupees.

(2) The name of the registered medical practitioner who has been convicted by the court under sub-section (1), shall be reported by the Appropriate Authority to the respective State Medical Council for taking necessary action including the removal of his name from the register of the Council for a period of two years for the first offence and permanently for the subsequent offence.

(3) Any person who seeks the aid of a Genetic Counselling Centre, Genetic Laboratory or Genetic Clinic or of a medical geneticist, gynaecologist or registered medical practitioner for conducting pre- natal diagnostic techniques on any pregnant woman (including such woman unless she was compelled to undergo such diagnostic techniques) for purposes other than those specified in clause (2) of section 4, shall, be punishable

with imprisonment for a term which may extend to three years and with fine which may extend to ten thousand rupees and on any subsequent conviction with imprisonment which may extend to five years and with fine which may extend to fifty thousand rupees.

24. Presumption in the case of conduct of pre-natal diagnostic techniques— Notwithstanding anything in the Indian Evidence Act, 1872 (1 of 1872), the court shall presume unless the contrary is proved that the pregnant woman has been compelled by her husband or the relative to undergo pre-natal diagnostic technique and such person shall be liable for abetment of offence under sub-section (3) of section 23 and shall be punishable for the offence specified under that section.

25. Penalty for contravention of the provisions of the Act or rules for which no specific punishment is provided. Whoever contravenes any of the provisions of this Act or any rules made thereunder, for which no penalty has been elsewhere provided in this Act, shall be punishable with imprisonment for a term which may extend to three months or with fine, which may extend to one thousand rupees or with both and in the case of continuing contravention with an additional fine which may extend to five hundred rupees for every day during which such contravention continues after conviction for the first such contravention.

26. Offences by companies—

   (1) Where any offence, punishable under this Act has been committed by a company, every person who, at the time the offence was committed was in charge of, and was responsible to the company for the conduct of the business of the company, as well as the company, shall be deemed to be guilty of the offence and shall be liable to be proceeded against and punished accordingly:

   Provided that nothing contained in this sub-section shall render any such person liable to any punishment, if he proves that the offence was committed without his knowledge or that he had exercised all due diligence to prevent the commission of such offence.

   (2) Notwithstanding anything contained in sub-section (1), where any offence punishable under this Act has been committed by a company and it is proved that the offence has been committed with the consent or connivance of, or is attributable to any neglect on the part of, any director, manager, secretary or other officer of the company, such director, manager, secretary or

other officer shall also be deemed to be guilty of that offence and shall be liable to be proceeded against and punished accordingly.

Explanation—For the purposes of this section,—

(a) 'company' means any body corporate and includes a firm or other association of individuals, and

(b) 'director', in relation to a firm, means a partner in the firm.

27. Offence to be cognizable, non-bailable and non-compoundable— Every offence under this Act shall be cognizable, non-bailable and non-compoundable.

28. Cognizance of offences.

   (1) No court shall take cognizance of an offence under this Act except on a complaint made by—

   (a) the Appropriate Authority concerned, or any officer authorised in this behalf by the Central Government or State Government, as the case may be, or the Appropriate Authority; or

   (b) a person who has given notice of not less than thirty days in the manner prescribed, to the Appropriate Authority, of the alleged offence and of his intention to make a complaint to the court.

   Explanation—For the purpose of this clause, 'person' includes a social organisation.

   (2) No court other than that of a Metropolitan Magistrate or a Judicial Magistrate of the first class shall try any offence punishable under this Act.

   (3) Where a complaint has been made under clause (b) of subsection (1), the court may, on demand by such person, direct the Appropriate Authority to make available copies of the relevant records in its possession to such person.

Chapter VIII

Miscellaneous

29. Maintenance of records.

   (1) All records, charts, forms, reports, consent letters and all other documents required to be maintained under this Act and the rules shall be preserved for a period of two years or for such period as may be prescribed:

Provided that, if any criminal or other proceedings are instituted against any Genetic Counselling Centre, Genetic Laboratory or Genetic Clinic, the records and all other documents of such Centre, Laboratory or Clinic shall be preserved till the final disposal of such proceedings.

(2) All such records shall, at all reasonable times, be made available for inspection to the Appropriate Authority or to any other person authorised by the Appropriate Authority in this behalf.

30. Power to search and seize records, etc.—

(1) If the Appropriate Authority has reason to believe that an offence under this Act has been or is being committed at any Genetic Counselling Centre, Genetic Laboratory or Genetic Clinic, such Authority or any officer authorised thereof in this behalf may, subject to such rules as may be prescribed, enter and search at all reasonable times with such assistance, if any, as such authority or officer considers necessary, such Genetic Counselling Centre, Genetic Laboratory or Genetic Clinic and examine any record, register, document, book, pamphlet, advertisement or any other material object found therein and seize the same if such Authority or officer has reason to believe that it may furnish evidence of the commission of an office punishable under this Act.

(2) The provisions of the Code of Criminal Procedure, 1973 (2 of 1974) relating to searches and seizures shall, so far as may be, apply to every search or seizure made under this Act.

31. Protection of action taken in good faith. No suit, prosecution or other legal proceeding shall lie against the Central or the State Government or the Appropriate Authority or any officer authorised by the Central or State Government or by the Authority for anything which is in good faith done or intended to be done in pursuance of the provisions of this Act.

32. Power to make rules—

(1) The Central Government may make rules for carrying out the provisions of this Act.

(2) In particular and without prejudice to the generality of the foregoing power, such rules may provide for—

(i) the minimum qualifications for persons employed at a registered Genetic Counselling Centre, Genetic Laboratory or Genetic Clinic under clause (1) of section 3;

(ii) the form in which consent of a pregnant woman has to be obtained under section 5;

(iii) the procedure to be followed by the members of the Central Supervisory Board in the discharge of their functions under sub-section (4) of section 8;

(iv) allowances for members other than ex-officio members admissible under sub-section (5) of section 9;

(v) the period intervening between any two meetings of the Advisory Committee under the proviso to sub-section (8) of section 17;

(vi) the terms and conditions subject to which a person may be appointed to the Advisory Committee and the procedure to be followed by such Committee under sub-section (9) of section 17;

(vii) the form and manner in which an application shall be made for registration and the fee payable thereof under sub-section (2) of section 18;

(viii) the facilities to be provided, equipment and other standards to be maintained by the Genetic Counselling Centre, Genetic Laboratory or Genetic Clinic under sub-section (5) of section 18;

(ix) the form in which a certificate of registration shall be issued under sub-section (1) of section 19;

(x) the manner in which and the period after which a certificate of registration shall be renewed and the fee payable for such renewal under sub-section (3) of section 19;

(xi) the manner in which an appeal may be preferred under section 21;

(xii) the period up to which records, charts, etc., shall be preserved under sub-section (1) of section 29;

(xiii) the manner in which the seizure of documents, records, objects, etc., shall be made and the manner in which seizure list shall be prepared and delivered to the person from whose custody such documents, records or objects were seized under sub-section (1) of section 30;

(xiv) any other matter that is required to be, or may be, prescribed.

33. Power to make regulations— The Board may, with the previous sanction of the Central Government, by notification in the Official Gazette, make regulations not inconsistent with the provisions of this Act and the rules made thereunder to provide for—

(a) the time and place of the meetings of the Board and the procedure to be followed for the transaction of business at such meetings and the number of members which shall form the quorum under sub-section (1) of section 9;

(b) the manner in which a person may be temporarily associated with the Board under sub-section (1) of section 11;

(c) the method of appointment, the conditions of service and the scales of pay and allowances of the officer and other employees of the Board appointed under section 12;

(d) generally for the efficient conduct of the affairs of the Board.

34. Rules and regulations to be laid before Parliament—Every rule and every regulation made under this Act shall be laid, as soon as may be after it is made, before each House of Parliament, while it is in session, for a total period of thirty days which may be comprised in one session or in two or more successive sessions, and if, before the expiry of the session immediately following the session or the successive sessions aforesaid, both Houses agree in making any modification in the rule or regulation or both Houses agree that the rule or regulation should not be made, the rule or regulation shall thereafter have effect only in such modified form or be of no effect, as the case may be; so, however, that any such modification or annulment shall be without prejudice to the validity of anything previously done under that rule or regulation.

APPENDIX 3
PNDT (Regulation and Prevention of Misuse) Amendment Act 2002

PNDT Amendment Act 2002, Registered No. DL-33004/2003

The Gazette of India

Extraordinary

PART II – Section I

Published by Authority

No. 15
New Delhi, Monday, January 20, 2003/ Pausa 30, 1924

Ministry of Law and Justice

(Legislative Department)
New Delhi, the 20th January, 2003/Pausa 30, 1924 (Saka)

The following Act of Parliament received the assent of the President on the 17th January, 2003, and is hereby published for general information:

The Pre-natal Diagnostic Techniques (Regulation and Prevention of Misuse) Amendment Act, 2002 Known as Pcpndt Act, 2002

No. 14 of 2003
[17th January, 2003]

An Act further to amend the Pre-natal Diagnostic Techniques (Regulation and Prevention of Misuse) Act, 1994. BE it enacted by Parliament in the Fifty-third year of the Republic of India as follows:-

1. (1) This Act may be called the Pre-natal Diagnostic Techniques (Regulation and Prevention of Misuse) Amendment Act, 2002.
   (2) It shall come into force on such date as the Central Government may, by notification in the Official Gazette, appoint. Short title and commencement 57 of 1994.

2. In the Pre-natal Diagnostic Techniques (Regulation and Prevention of Misuse) Act, 1994 (hereinafter referred to as the principal Act), for the long title, the following long title shall be substituted, namely:— 'An Act to provide for the prohibition of sex selection, before or after conception, and for regulation of pre-natal diagnostic techniques for the purposes of detecting genetic abnormalities or metabolic disorders or chromosomal abnormalities or certain congenital malformations or sex-linked disorders and for the prevention of their misuse for sex determination leading to female foeticide and for matters connected therewith or incidental thereto.' Substitution of long title.

Amendment of section 1.3.

In section 1 of the principal Act, in sub-section (1), for the words and brackets 'the Pre-natal Diagnostic Techniques (Regulation and Prevention of Misuse)', the words and brackets 'the Pre-conception and Pre-natal Diagnostic Techniques (Prohibition of Sex Selection)' shall be substituted.

Amendment of section 2.4. In section 2 of the principal Act,—

(i)   after clause (b), the following clauses shall be inserted, namely:—

'(ba) "conceptus" means any product of conception at any stage of development from fertilisation until birth including extra embryonic membranes as well as the embryo or foetus;

(bb) "embryo" means a developing human organism after fertilisation till the end of eight weeks (fifty-six days);

(bc) "foetus" means a human organism during the period of its development beginning on the fifty-seventh day following fertilisation or creation (excluding any time in which its development has been suspended) and ending at the birth;';

(ii) in clause (d), the following Explanation shall be added, namely:-
'Explanation– For the purpose of this clause, "Genetic Clinic" includes a vehicle, where ultrasound machine or imaging machine or scanner or other equipment capable of determining sex of the foetus or a portable equipment which has the potential for detection of sex during pregnancy or selection of sex before conception, is used;';

(iii) in clause (e), the following Explanation shall be added, namely:—
'Explanation—For the purposes of this clause "Genetic Laboratory" includes a place where ultrasound machine or imaging machine or scanner or other equipment capable of determining sex of the foetus or a portable equipment which has the potential for detection of sex during pregnancy or selection of sex before conception, is used;';

(iv) for clause (g), the following clause shall be substituted, namely:-
'(g) "medical geneticist" includes a person who possesses a degree or diploma in genetic science in the fields of sex selection and pre-natal diagnostic techniques or has experience of not less than two years in any of these fields after obtaining–

  (i) any one of the medical qualifications recognised under the Indian Medical Council Act, 1956; or
  (ii) a post-graduate degree in biological sciences;';

(v) for clause (i), the following clause shall be substituted, namely:—
'(i) "pre-natal diagnostic procedures" means all gynaecological or obstetrical or medical procedures such as ultrasonography, foetoscopy, taking or removing samples of amniotic fluid, chorionic villi, embryo, blood or any other tissue or fluid of a man, or of a woman before or after conception, for being sent to a Genetic Laboratory or Genetic Clinic for conducting any type of analysis or pre-natal diagnostic tests for selection of sex before or after conception;';

(vi) for clause (k), the following clause shall be substituted, namely:—
'(k) "pre-natal diagnostic test" means ultrasonography or any test or analysis of amniotic fluid, chorionic villi, blood or any tissue or fluid of a pregnant woman or conceptus conducted to detect genetic or metabolic disorders or chromosomal abnormalities or congenital anomalies or haemoglobinopathies or sex-linked diseases;';

(vii) after clause (n), the following clauses shall be inserted, namely:—
'(o) "sex selection" includes any procedure, technique, test or administration or prescription or provision of anything for the purpose of ensuring or increasing the probability that an embryo will be of a particular sex;

  (p) "sonologist or imaging specialist" means a person who possesses any one of the medical qualifications recognised under the Indian Medical Council Act, 1956 or who possesses a post-graduate qualification in ultrasonography or imaging techniques or radiology;

  (q) "State Board" means a State Supervisory Board or a Union territory Supervisory Board constituted under section 16 A;

  (r) "State Government" in relation to Union territory with Legislature means the Administrator of that Union territory appointed by the President under article 239 of the Constitution.'
102 of 1956.

5. In section 3 of the principal Act, for clause (2), the following clause shall be substituted, namely:— '(2) no Genetic Counselling Centre or Genetic Laboratory or Genetic Clinic shall employ or

cause to be employed or take services of any person, whether on honorary basis or on payment who does not possess the qualifications as may be prescribed.'.

Amendment of section 3. 6. After section 3 of the principal Act, the following sections shall be inserted, namely:—

'3A. No person, including a specialist or a team of specialists in the field of infertility, shall conduct or cause to be conducted or aid in conducting by himself or by any other person, sex selection on a woman or a man or on both or on any tissue, embryo, conceptus, fluid or gametes derived from either or both of them.

3B. No person shall sell any ultrasound machine or imaging machine or scanner or any other equipment capable of detecting the sex of the foetus to any Genetic Counselling Centre, Genetic Laboratory, Genetic Clinic or any other person not registered under the Act.'. Insertion of new sections 3A and 3B. Prohibition of sex-selection. Prohibition on sale of ultrasound machine etc. to persons, laboratories, clinics etc. not registered under the Act.

7. In section 4 of the principal Act, for clauses (3) and (4), the following clauses shall be substituted, namely:—

'(3) no pre-natal diagnostic techniques shall be used or conducted unless the person qualified to do so is satisfied for reasons to be recorded in writing that any of the following conditions are fulfilled namely:—

(i) age of the pregnant woman is above thirty-five years,

(ii) the pregnant woman has undergone two or more spontaneous abortions or foetal loss;

(iii) the pregnant woman had been exposed to potentially teratogenic agents such as, drugs, radiation, infection or chemicals;

(iv) the pregnant woman or her spouse has a family history of mental retardation or physical deformities such as, spasticity or any other genetic disease;

(v) any other condition as may be specified by the Board: Provided that the person conducting ultrasonography on a pregnant woman shall keep complete record thereof in the clinic in such manner, as may be prescribed, and any deficiency or inaccuracy found therein shall amount to contravention of the provisions of section 5 or section 6 unless contrary is proved by the person conducting such ultrasonography;

(4) no person including a relative or husband of the pregnant woman shall seek or encourage the conduct of any pre-natal diagnostic techniques on her except for the purposes specified in clause (2);

(5) no person including a relative or husband of a woman shall seek or encourage the conduct of any sex-selection technique on her or him or both.'

Amendment of section 4.
Amendment of section 5.8. In section 5 of the principal Act, for sub-section (2), the following sub-section shall be substituted, namely:—

'(2) No person including the person conducting pre-natal diagnostic procedures shall communicate to the pregnant woman concerned or her relatives or any other person the sex of the foetus by words, signs, or in any other manner.'

Amendment of section 6.
9. In section 6 of the principal Act, after clause (b), the following clause shall be inserted, namely:—

'(c) no person shall, by whatever means, cause or allow to be caused selection of sex before or after conception.'

Amendment of Section 7.
10. In section 7 of the principal Act,- (i) in sub-section (2), for clause (c), the following clause shall be substituted, namely:—

'(c) three members to be appointed by the Central Government to represent the Ministries of Central Government in charge of Women and Child Development, Department of Legal Affairs or Legislative Department in the Ministry of Law, Justice, and Indian System of Medicine and Homeopathy, ex-officio;';

(ii) in clause (e), for sub-clause (ii), the following sub-clause shall be substituted, namely:—

'(ii) eminent gynaecologist and obstetrician or expert of stri-roga or prasuti-tantra.'.

Amendment of section 14.11.
In section 14 of the principal Act, for clause (f), the following clause shall be substituted, namely:—

'(f) has, in the opinion of the Central Government, been associated with the use or promotion of pre-natal diagnostic technique for determination of sex or with any sex selection technique.'.

Amendment of section 15.12. In section 15 of the principal Act, the following proviso shall be inserted, namely:—

'Provided that no member other than an ex-officio member shall be appointed for more than two consecutive terms.'.
Substitution of new section for section 16.

Functions of the Board. 13. For section 16 of the principal Act, the following section shall be substituted, namely:— '16. The Board shall have the following functions, namely:—

  (i) to advise the Central Government on policy matters relating to use of pre-natal diagnostic techniques, sex selection techniques and against their misuse;

 (ii) to review and monitor implementation of the Act and rules made thereunder and recommend to the Central Government changes in the said Act and rules.

(iii) to create public awareness against the practice of pre-conception sex selection and pre-natal determination of sex of foetus leading to female foeticide;

(iv) to lay down a code of conduct to be observed by persons working at Genetic Counselling Centres, Genetic Laboratories and Genetic Clinics;

 (v) to oversee the performance of various bodies constituted under the Act and take appropriate steps to ensure its proper and effective implementation;

(vi) any other functions as may be prescribed under the Act.'.

14. After section 16 of the principal Act, the following section shall be inserted, namely:—

'16A(1) Each State and Union territory having Legislature shall constitute a Board to be known as the State Supervisory Board or the Union territory Supervisory Board, as the case may be, which shall have the following functions:—

  (i) to create public awareness against the practice of pre-conception sex selection and pre-natal determination of sex of foetus leading to female foeticide in the State;

 (ii) to review the activities of the Appropriate Authorities functioning in the State and recommend appropriate action against them;

(iii) to monitor the implementation of provisions of the Act and the rules and make suitable recommendations relating thereto, to the Board;

(iv) to send such consolidated reports as may be prescribed in respect of the various activities undertaken in the State under the Act to the Board and the Central Government; and

 (v) any other functions as may be prescribed under the Act.

(2) The State Board shall consist of:—

  (a) the Minister in-charge of Health and Family Welfare in the State, who shall be the Chairperson, ex officio;

  (b) Secretary in-charge of the Department of Health and Family Welfare who shall be the Vice-Chairperson, ex officio;

  (c) Secretaries or Commissioners in charge of Departments of Women and Child Development, Social Welfare, Law and Indian System of Medicines and Homeopathy, ex-officio, or their representatives;

  (d) Director of Health and Family Welfare or Indian System of Medicines and Homeopathy of the State Government, ex-officio;

  (e) three women members of Legislative Assembly or Legislative Council;

  (f) ten members to be appointed by the State Government out of which two each shall be from the following categories:—

    (i) eminent social scientists and legal experts;

    (ii) eminent women activists from non-governmental organisations or otherwise;

    (iii) eminent gynaecologists and obstetricians or experts of stri-roga or prasuti-tantra;

    (iv) eminent pediatricians or medical geneticists;

    (v) eminent radiologists or sonologists;

  (g) an officer not below the rank of Joint Director in-charge of Family Welfare, who shall be the Member Secretary, ex-officio

(3) The State Board shall meet at least once in four months.

(4) The term of office of a member, other than an ex-officio member, shall be three years.

(5) If a vacancy occurs in the office of any member other than an ex-officio member, it shall be filled by making fresh appointment.

(6) If a member of the Legislative Assembly or member of the Legislative Council who is a member of the State Board, becomes Minister or Speaker or Deputy Speaker of the Legislative Assembly or Chairperson or Deputy Chairperson of the Legislative Council, she shall cease to be a member of the State Board.

(7) One-third of the total number of members of the State Board shall constitute the quorum.

(8) The State Board may co-opt a member as and when required, provided that the number of co-opted members does not exceed one-third of the total strength of the State Board.

(9) The co-opted members shall have the same powers and functions as other members, except the right to vote and shall abide by the rules and regulations.

(10) In respect of matters not specified in this section, the State Board shall follow procedures and conditions as are applicable to the Board.'. Insertion of new section 16A. Constitution of State Supervisory Board and Union territory Supervisory Board.

Amendment of section 17.15. In section 17 of the principal Act:—

(i) in sub-section (3), for clause (a), the following clause shall be substituted, namely:— '(a) when appointed for the whole of the State or the Union territory, consisting of the following three members-
  (i) an officer of or above the rank of the Joint Director of Health and Family Welfare–Chairperson;
  (ii) an eminent woman representing a women's organisation; and
  (iii) an officer of Law Department of the State or the Union territory concerned: Provided that it shall be the duty of the State or the Union territory concerned to constitute multi-member State or Union territory level Appropriate Authority within three months of the coming into force of the Pre-natal Diagnostic Techniques (Regulation and Prevention of Misuse) Amendment Act, 2002: Provided further that any vacancy occurring therein shall be filled within three months of the occurrence.';

(ii) in sub-section (4), after clause (d), the following clauses shall be inserted, namely:—

'(e) to take appropriate legal action against the use of any sex selection technique by any person at any place, *suo-moto* or brought to its notice and also to initiate independent investigations in such matter;

(f) to create public awareness against the practice of sex selection or pre-natal determination of sex;

(g) to supervise the implementation of the provisions of the Act and rules;

(h) to recommend to the Board and State Boards modifications required in the rules in accordance with changes in technology or social conditions;
  (i) to take action on the recommendations of the Advisory Committee made after investigation of complaint for suspension or cancellation of registration.';

(iii) for sub-section (7), the following sub-section shall be substituted, namely:— '(7) No person who has been associated with the use or promotion of pre-natal diagnostic techniques for determination of sex or sex selection shall be appointed as a member of the Advisory Committee.'.

16. After section 17 of the principal Act, the following section shall be inserted, namely:—

'17A. The Appropriate Authority shall have the powers in respect of the following matters, namely:—

   (a) summoning of any person who is in possession of any information relating to violation of the provisions of this Act or the rules made thereunder;

   (b) production of any document or material object relating to clause (a);

   (c) issuing search warrant for any place suspected to be indulging in sex selection techniques or pre-natal sex determination; and

   (d) any other matter which may be prescribed.'. Insertion of new section 17A.

Powers of Appropriate Authorities

17. In section 18 of the principal Act, for sub-section (1), the following sub-section shall be substituted, namely:—

'(1) No person shall open any Genetic Counselling Centre, Genetic Laboratory or Genetic Clinic, including clinic, laboratory or centre having ultrasound or imaging machine or scanner or any other technology capable of undertaking determination of sex of foetus and sex selection, or render services to any of them, after the commencement of the Pre-natal Diagnostic Techniques (Regulation and Prevention of Misuse) Amendment Act, 2002 unless such centre, laboratory or clinic is duly registered under the Act.'.

Amendment of section 18. 18. For section 22 of the principal Act, the following section shall be substituted, namely:—

'(1) No person, organisation, Genetic Counselling Centre, Genetic Laboratory or Genetic Clinic, including clinic, laboratory or centre having ultrasound machine or imaging machine or scanner or any other technology capable of undertaking determination of sex of the foetus or sex selection shall issue, publish, distribute, communicate or cause to be issued, published, distributed or communicated any advertisement, in any form, including internet, regarding facilities of pre-natal determination of sex or sex selection before conception available at such centre, laboratory, clinic or at any other place.

(2) No person or organisation including Genetic Counselling Centre, Genetic Laboratory or Genetic Clinic shall issue, publish, distribute, communicate or cause to be issued, published, distributed or communicated any advertisement in any manner regarding pre-natal determination or pre-conception selection of sex by any means whatsoever, scientific or otherwise.

(3) Any person who contravenes the provisions of sub-section (1) or sub-section (2) shall be punishable with imprisonment for a term which may extend to three years and with a fine which may extend to ten thousand rupees.

Explanation:— For the purposes of this section, "advertisement" includes any notice, circular, label, wrapper or any other document including advertisement through internet or any other media in electronic or print form and also includes any visible representation made by means of any hoarding, wall-painting, signal, light, sound, smoke or gas.'. Substitution of new section for section 22.
Prohibition of advertisement relating to pre-conception and pre-natal determination of sex and punishment for contravention. Amendment of section 23.19. In section 23 of the principal Act, for sub-sections (2) and (3), the following sub-sections shall be substituted, namely:—

'(2) The name of the registered medical practitioner shall be reported by the Appropriate Authority to the State Medical Council concerned for taking necessary action including suspension of the registration if the charges are framed by the court and till the case is disposed of and on conviction for removal of his name from the register of the Council for a period of five years for the first offence and permanently for the subsequent offence.

(3) Any person who seeks the aid of any Genetic Counselling Centre, Genetic Laboratory, Genetic Clinic or ultrasound clinic or imaging clinic or of a medical geneticist, gynaecologist, sonologist or imaging specialist or registered medical practitioner or any other person for sex selection or for conducting pre-natal diagnostic techniques on any pregnant women for the purposes other than those specified in sub-section (2) of section 4, he shall, be punishable with imprisonment for a term which may extend to three years and with fine which may extend to fifty thousand rupees for the first offence and for any subsequent offence with imprisonment which may extend to five years and with fine which may extend to one lakh rupees.

(4) For the removal of doubts, it is hereby provided, that the provisions of sub-section (3) shall not apply to the woman who was compelled to undergo such diagnostic techniques or such selection.'.

Presumption in the case of conduct of pre-natal diagnostic techniques. 20. For section 24 of the principal Act, the following section shall be substituted, namely:—
'24 Notwithstanding anything contained in the Indian Evidence Act, 1872, the court shall presume unless the contrary is proved that the

pregnant woman was compelled by her husband or any other relative, as the case may be, to undergo pre-natal diagnostic technique for the purposes other than those specified in sub-section (2) of section 4 and such person shall be liable for abetment of offence under sub-section (3) of section 23 and shall be punishable for the offence specified under that section.'.

Substitution of new section for section 24. 21. In section 28 of the principal Act, in sub-section (1), in clause (b), for the words 'thirty days', the words 'fifteen days' shall be substituted. Amendment of section 28. 22. In section 30 of the principal Act, for sub-section (1), the following sub-section shall be substituted, namely:—

'(1) If the Appropriate Authority has reason to believe that an offence under this Act has been or is being committed at any Genetic Counselling Centre, Genetic Laboratory, Genetic Clinic or any other place, such Authority or any officer authorised in this behalf may, subject to such rules as may be prescribed, enter and search at all reasonable times with such assistance, if any, as such Authority or officer considers necessary, such Genetic Counselling Centre, Genetic Laboratory, Genetic Clinic or any other place and examine any record, register, document, book, pamphlet, dvertisement or any other material object found therein and seize and seal the same if such Authority or officer has reason to believe that it may furnish evidence of the commission of an offence punishable under this Act.'. Amendment of section 30.

23. After section 31 of the principal Act, the following section shall be inserted, namely:—

'31A. (1) If any difficulty arises in giving effect to the provisions of the Pre-natal Diagnostic Techniques (Regulation and Prevention of Misuse) Amendment Act, 2002, the Central Government may, by order published in the Official Gazette, make such provisions not inconsistent with the provisions of the said Act as appear to it to be necessary or expedient for removing the difficulty: Provided that no order shall be made under this section after the expiry of a period of three years from the date of commencement of the Pre-natal Diagnostic Techniques (Regulation and Prevention of Misuse) Amendment Act, 2002.

(2) Every order made under this section shall be laid, as soon as may be after it is made, before each House of Parliament.'. Insertion of new section 31 A.

Removal of difficulties. 24. In section 32, in sub-section (2)-(i) for clause (i), the following clauses shall be substituted, namely:—

'(i) the minimum qualifications for persons employed at a registered Genetic Counselling Centre, Genetic Laboratory or Genetic Clinic under clause (2) of section 3; (ia) the manner in which the person conducting ultrasonography on a pregnant woman shall keep record thereof in the Clinic under the proviso to sub-section (3) of section 4;'

(ii) after clause (iv), the following clauses shall be inserted, namely:—

'(iva) code of conduct to be observed by persons working at Genetic Counselling Centres, Genetic Laboratories and Genetic Clinics to be laid down by the Central Supervisory Board under clause (iv) of section 16;

(ivb) the manner in which reports shall be furnished by the State and Union territory Supervisory Boards to the Board and the Central Government in respect of various activities undertaken in the State under the Act under clause (iv) of sub-section (1) of section 16A;

(ivc) empowering the Appropriate Authority in any other matter under clause (d) of section 17A;'. Amendment of section 32.

K.N. Chaturvedi
Additional Secretary to the
Government of India

APPENDIX 4
PNDT (Regulation and Prevention of Misuse) Amendment Rules 2003

PNDT Amendment Rules, 2003 Regd. No. D.L.-33004/99
The Gazette of India

Extraordinary
PART II- Section 3-Sub-section(i)

Published by Authority
No. 74 New Delhi, Friday, 14 February 2003/Magha 25, 1924

Ministry of Health and Family Welfare
(Department of Family Welfare)

Notification
New Delhi, the 14th February, 2003

The Pre-Natal Diagnostic Techniques (Regulation and Prevention of Misuse) Amendment Rules, 2003. known as PCPNDT Rules, 2003

G.S.R.109(E).-- In exercise of the powers conferred by section 32 of the Pre-Natal Diagnostic Techniques (Regulation and Prevention of Misuse) Act, 1994 (57 of 1994), the Central Government hereby makes the following amendments to the Pre-Natal Diagnostic Techniques (Regulation and Prevention of Misuse) Rules, 1996.

1. (1) These may be called the Pre-Natal Diagnostic Techniques (Regulation and Prevention of Misuse) Amendment Rules, 2003.
   (2) They shall come into force on the date of their publication in the official gazette.
2. In the Pre-Natal Diagnostic Techniques (Regulation and Prevention of Misuse) Rules, 1996 (hereinafter referred to as the said rules) in rule 1, for sub-rule (1) the following sub-rule shall be substituted, namely:—
   '(1) These Rules may be called the Pre-conception and Pre-natal Diagnostic Techniques (Prohibition of Sex Selection) Rules, 1996.'

3. In the said rules, in rule 2, clause (d) shall be omitted.

4. In the said rules, for rule 3 the following rule shall be substituted, namely:—

'3. The qualifications of the employees, the requirement of equipment etc. for a Genetic Counselling Centre, Genetic Laboratory, Genetic Clinic, Ultrasound Clinic and Imaging Centre shall be as under:

(1) Any person being or employing

    (i) a gynaecologist or a paediatrician having six months experience or four weeks training in genetic counseling or

    (ii) a medical geneticist, having adequate space and educational charts/models/equipments for carrying out genetic counselling may set up a genetic counselling centre and get it registered as a genetic counselling centre.

(2) (a) Any person having adequate space and being or employing

    (i) a Medical Geneticist and

    (ii) a laboratory technician, having a B.Sc. degree in Biological Sciences or a degree or diploma in medical laboratory course with at least one year experience in conducting appropriate prenatal diagnostic techniques, tests or procedures may set up a genetic laboratory.

  (b) Such laboratory should have or acquire such of the following equipments as may be necessary for carrying out chromosomal studies, bio-chemical studies and molecular studies:—

    (i) Chromosomal studies:

(1) Laminar flow hood with ultraviolet and fluorescent light or other suitable culture hood.

(2) Photo-microscope with fluorescent source of light.

(3) Inverted microscope.

(4) Incubator and oven.

(5) Carbon dioxide incubator or closed system with 5% CO_2 atmosphere.

(6) Autoclave.

(7) Refrigerator.

(8) Water bath.

(9) Centrifuge.

(10) Vortex mixer.

(11) Magnetic stirrer.

(12) pH Meter.

(13) A sensitive balance (preferably electronic) with sensitivity of 0.1 milligram.

(14) Double distillation apparatus (glass).

(15) Such other equipments as may be necessary.

(ii) Biochemical studies: (requirements according to tests to be carried out)

(1) Laminar flow hood with ultraviolet and fluorescent light or other suitable culture hood.

(2) Inverted microscope.

(3) Incubator and oven.

(4) Carbon dioxide incubator or closed system with 5% CO_2 atmosphere.

(5) Autoclave.

(6) Refrigerator.

(7) Water bath.

(8) Centrifuge.

(9) Electrophoresis apparatus and power supply.

(10) Chromatography chamber.

(11) Spectro-photometer and Elisa reader or Radio-immunoassay system (with gamma beta-counter) or fluorometer for various biochemical tests.

(12) Vortex mixer.

(13) Magnetic stirrer.

(14) pH meter.

(15) A sensitive balance (preferably electronic) with sensitivity of 0.1 milligram.

(16) Double distillation apparatus (glass).

(17) Liquid nitrogen tank.

(18) Such other equipments as may be necessary.

(iii) Molecular studies:

(1) Inverted microscope.

(2) Incubator.

(3) Oven.

(4) Autoclave.

(5) Refrigerators (4 degree and minus 20 degree Centigrade).

(6) Water bath.

(7) Microcentrifuge.

(8) Electrophoresis apparatus and power supply.

(9) Vertex mixer.

(10) Magnetic stirrer.

(11) pH meter.

(12) A sensitive balance (preferably electronic) with sensitivity of 0.1 milligram.

(13) Double distillation apparatus (glass).

(14) P.C.R. machine.

(15) Refrigerated centrifuge.

(16) U.V. Illuminator with photographic attachment or other documentation system.

(17) Precision micropipettes.

(18) Such other equipments as may be necessary.

(3) (1) Any person having adequate space and being or employing

(a) Gynaecologist having experience of performing at least 20 procedures in chorionic villi aspirations per vagina or per abdomen, chorionic villi biopsy, amniocentesis, cordocentesis foetoscopy, foetal skin or organ biopsy or foetal blood sampling etc. under supervision of an experienced gynaecologist in these fields, or

(b) a Sonologist, Imaging Specialist, Radiologist or Registered Medical Practitioner having Post Graduate degree or diploma or six months training or one year experience in sonography or image scanning, or.

(c) A medical geneticist may set up a genetic clinic/ultrasound clinic/ imaging centre.

(2) The Genetic Clinic/ultrasound clinic/imaging centre should have or acquire such of the following equipments, as may be necessary for carrying out the tests or procedures-

(a) Equipment and accessories necessary for carrying out clinical examination by an obstetrician or gynaecologist.

(b) An ultra-sonography machine including mobile ultrasound machine, imaging machine or any other equipment capable of conducting foetal ultrasonography.

(c) Appropriate catheters and equipment for carrying out chorionic villi aspirations per vagina or per abdomen.

(d) Appropriate sterile needles for amniocentesis or cordocentesis.

(e) A suitable foetoscope with appropriate accessories for foetoscopy, foetal skin or organ biopsy or foetal blood sampling shall be optional.

(f) Equipment for dry and wet sterilization.

(g) Equipment for carrying out emergency procedures such as evacuation of uterus or resuscitation in case of need.

(h) Genetic Works Station.'.

5. In the said rules, after rule 3 a new rule 3A shall be inserted as follows, namely:—

'3A. Sale of ultrasound machines/imaging machines:

(1) No organisation including a commercial organization or a person, including manufacturer, importer, dealer or supplier of ultrasound

machines/imaging machines or any other equipment, capable of detecting sex of foetus, shall sell distribute, supply, rent, allow or authorize the use of any such machine or equipment in any manner, whether on payment or otherwise, to any Genetic Counselling Centre, Genetic Laboratory, Genetic Clinic, Ultrasound Clinic, Imaging Centre or any other body or person unless such Centre, Laboratory, Clinic, body or person is registered under the Act.

(2) The provider of such machine/equipment to any person/body registered under the Act shall send to the concerned State/UT Appropriate Authority and to the Central Government, once in three months a list of those to whom the machine/equipment has been provided.

(3) Any organization or person, including manufacturer, importer, dealer or supplier of ultrasound machines/imaging machines or any other equipment capable of detecting sex of foetus selling, distributing, supplying or authorizing, in any manner, the use of any such machine or equipment to any Genetic Counselling Centre, Genetic Laboratory, Genetic Clinic, Ultrasound Clinic, Imaging Centre or any other body or person registered under the Act shall take an affidavit from the Genetic Counselling Centre, Genetic Laboratory, Genetic Clinic, Ultrasound Clinic, Imaging Centre or any other body or person purchasing or getting authorization for using such machine/equipment that the machine/equipment shall not be used for detection of sex of foetus or selection of sex before or after conception.'.

6. In the said rules, in rule 4 for sub-rule (1) the following sub-rule shall be substituted, namely:—

'(1) An application for registration shall be made to the Appropriate Authority, in duplicate, in Form A, duly accompanied by an Affidavit containing–

(i) an undertaking to the effect that the Genetic Centre/Laboratory/Clinic/Ultrasound Clinic/Imaging Centre/Combination thereof, as the case may be, shall not conduct any test or procedure, by whatever name called, for selection of sex before or after conception or for detection of sex of foetus except for diseases specified in Section 4(2) nor shall the sex of foetus be disclosed to any body; and

(ii) an undertaking to the effect that the Genetic Centre/Laboratory/Clinic/Combination thereof, as the case may be, shall display prominently a notice that they do not conduct any technique, test or procedure etc. by whatever name called, for detection of sex of foetus or for selection of sex before or after conception.'.

7. In the said rules, for rule 5, the following rule shall be substituted, namely:—

'5. Application Fee– (1) Every application for registration under Rule 4 shall be accompanied by an application fee of:—

(a) Rs 3000 for Genetic Counselling Centre, Genetic Laboratory, Genetic Clinic, Ultrasound Clinic or Imaging Centre.

(b) Rs 4000 for an institute, hospital, nursing home, or any place providing jointly the service of a Genetic Counselling Centre, Genetic Laboratory and Genetic Clinic, Ultrasound Clinic or Imaging Centre or any combination thereof.

Provided that if an application for registration of any Genetic Clinic/Laboratory/Centre etc. has been rejected by the Appropriate Authority, no fee shall be required to be paid on re-submission of the application by the applicant for the same body within 90 days of rejection. Provided further that any subsequent application shall be accompanied with the prescribed fee. Application fee once paid will not be refunded.

(2) The application fee shall be paid by a demand draft drawn in favour of the Appropriate Authority, on any scheduled bank payable at the headquarters of the Appropriate Authority concerned. The fees collected by the Appropriate Authorities for registration of Genetic Counselling Centre, Genetic Laboratory, Genetic Clinic, Ultrasound Clinic and Imaging Centre or any other body or person under sub-rule (1), shall be deposited by the Appropriate Authority concerned in a bank account opened in the name of the official designation of the Appropriate Authority concerned and shall be utilized by the Appropriate Authority in connection with the activities connected with implementation of the provisions of the Act and these rules.'.

8. In the said rules, in rule 9,—

(a) for sub-rule (1), the following sub-rule shall be substituted, namely:—

'(1) Every Genetic Counselling Centre, Genetic Laboratory, Genetic Clinic, Ultrasound Clinic and Imaging Centres shall maintain a register showing, in serial order, the names and addresses of the men or women given genetic counselling, subjected to pre-natal diagnostic procedures or pre-natal diagnostic tests, the names of their spouse or father and the date on which they first reported for such counselling, procedure or test.';

(b) for sub-rule (3), the following sub-rule shall be substituted, namely:—

'(3) The record to be maintained by every Genetic Laboratory, in respect of each man or woman subjected to any pre-natal diagnostic procedure/technique/test, shall be as specified in Form E.';

(c) for sub-rule (4), the following sub-rule shall be substituted, namely:—

'(4) The record to be maintained by every Genetic Clinic, in respect of each man or woman subjected to any pre-natal diagnostic procedure/technique/test, shall be as specified in Form F.';

(d) after sub-rule (7), the following sub-rule shall be inserted, namely:—

'(8) Every Genetic Counselling Centre, Genetic Laboratory, Genetic Clinic, Ultrasound Clinic and Imaging Centres shall send a complete report in respect of all pre-conception or pregnancy related procedures/techniques/tests conducted by them in respect of each month by 5th day of the following month to the concerned Appropriate Authority.'.

9. In the said rules, in rule 10,—
(a) for sub-rule (1), the following sub-rule shall be substituted, namely:—

'(1) Before conducting preimplantation genetic diagnosis, or any pre-natal diagnostic technique/test/procedure such as amniocentesis, chorionic villi biopsy, foetoscopy, foetal skin or organ biopsy or cordocentesis, a written consent, as specified in Form G, in a language the person undergoing such procedure understands, shall be obtained from her/him.';

(b) after sub-rule (1), the following new sub-rule (1A) shall be inserted, namely:—

'(1A) Any person conducting ultrasonography/image scanning on a pregnant woman shall give a declaration on each report on ultrasonography/image scanning that he/she has neither detected nor disclosed the sex of foetus of the pregnant woman to any body. The pregnant woman shall before undergoing ultrasonography/image scanning declare that she does not want to know the sex of her foetus.'.

10. In the said rules, for rule 11, the following rule shall be substituted, namely:— '11. Facilities for inspection.—

(1) Every Genetic Counselling Centre, Genetic Laboratory, Genetic Clinic, Ultrasound Clinic, Imaging Centre, nursing home, hospi-

tal, institute or any other place where any of the machines or equipments capable of performing any procedure, technique or test capable of pre-natal determination of sex or selection of sex before or after conception is used, shall afford all reasonable facilities for inspection of the place, equipment and records to the Appropriate Authority or to any other person authorised by the Appropriate Authority in this behalf for registration of such institutions, by whatever name called, under the Act, or for detection of misuse of such facilities or advertisement therefore or for selection of sex before or after conception or for detection/ disclosure of sex of foetus or for detection of cases of violation of the provisions of the Act in any other manner.

(2) The Appropriate Authority or the officer authorized by it may seal and seize any ultrasound machine, scanner or any other equipment, capable of detecting sex of foetus, used by any organisation if the organisation has not got itself registered under the Act. These machines of the organisations may be released if such organisation pays penalty equal to five times of the registration fee to the Appropriate Authority concerned and gives an undertaking that it shall not undertake detection of sex of foetus or selection of sex before or after conception.'.

11. In the said rules, in rule 12 for sub-rule (1), the following sub-rule shall be substituted, namely:—

'12. Procedure for search and seizure.—(1) The Appropriate Authority or any officer authorised in this behalf may enter and search at all reasonable times any Genetic Counselling Centre, Genetic Laboratory, Genetic Clinic, Imaging Centre or Ultrasound Clinic in the presence of two or more independent witnesses for the purposes of search and examination of any record, register, document, book, pamphlet, advertisement, or any other material object found therein and seal and seize the same if there is reason to believe that it may furnish evidence of commission of an offence punishable under the Act. Explanation:—In these Rules–

(1) "Genetic Laboratory/Genetic Clinic/Genetic Counselling Centre" would include an ultrasound centre/imaging centre/nursing home/hospital/institute or any other place, by whatever name called, where any of the machines or equipments capable of selection of sex before or after conception or performing any procedure, technique or test for pre-natal detection of sex of foetus, is used;

(2) "material object" would include records, machines and equipments; and

(3) "seize" and "seizure" would include "seal" and "sealing" respectively.'.

12. In the said rules, after rule 17, the following rules shall be inserted, namely:—

'18. Code of Conduct to be observed by persons working at Genetic Counselling Centres, Genetic Laboratories, Genetic Clinics, Ultrasound Clinics. Imaging Centres etc.

All persons including the owner, employee or any other persons associated with Genetic Counselling Centres, Genetic Laboratories, Genetic Clinics, Ultrasound Clinics, Imaging Centres registered under the Act/these Rules shall–

(i)   not conduct or associate with, or help in carrying out detection or disclosure of sex of foetus in any manner;

(ii) not employ or cause to be employed any person not possessing qualifications necessary for carrying out pre-natal diagnostic techniques/procedures, techniques and tests including ultrasonography;

(iii) not conduct or cause to be conducted or aid in conducting by himself or through any other person any techniques or procedure for selection of sex before or after conception or for detection of sex of foetus except for the purposes specified in sub-section (2) of section 4 of the Act;

(iv) not conduct or cause to be conducted or aid in conducting by himself or through any other person any techniques or test or procedure under the Act at a place other than a place registered under the Act/these Rules;

(v)   ensure that no provision of the Act and these Rules are violated in any manner;

(vi) ensure that the person, conducting any techniques, test or procedure leading to detection of sex of foetus for purposes not covered under section 4 (2) of the Act or selection of sex before or after conception, is informed that such procedures lead to violation of the Act and these Rules which are punishable offences;

(vii) help the law-enforcing agencies in bring to book the violators of the provisions of the Act and these Rules;

(viii) display his/her name and designation prominently on the dress worn by him/her;

(ix) write his/her name and designation in full under his/her signature;

(x)   on no account conduct or allow/cause to be conducted female foeticide;

(xi) not commit any other act of professional misconduct.

19. Appeals.–

(1) Anybody aggrieved by the decision of the Appropriate Authority at sub-district level may appeal to the Appropriate Authority at district level within 30 days of the order of the sub-district level Appropriate Authority.

(2) Anybody aggrieved by the decision of the Appropriate Authority at district level may appeal to the Appropriate Authority at State/UT level within 30 days of the order of the District level Appropriate Authority.

(3) Each appeal shall be disposed of by the District Appropriate Authority or by the State/Union Territory Appropriate Authority, as the case may be, within 60 days of its receipt.

(4) If an appeal is not made within the time as prescribed under sub-rule (1), (2) or (3), the Appropriate Authority under that sub-rule may condone the delay in case he/she is satisfied that appellant was prevented for sufficient cause from making such appeal.'.

13. In the said rules, Schedule I, Schedule II and Schedule III shall be omitted.

14. In the said rules, for the words 'Genetic Counselling Centre, Genetic Laboratory and Genetic Clinic', the words 'Genetic Counselling Centre, Genetic Laboratory, Genetic Clinic, Ultrasound Clinic and Imaging Centres' shall be substituted wherever they occur.

15. In the said rules, for Form A, Form B, Form C, Form D, Form E, Form F, Form G, and Form H, the following forms shall be substituted respectively, namely:—

Form A

[See rules 4(1) and 8(1)]
(To be submitted in Duplicate with supporting documents as enclosures)

Form of Application for Registration or Renewal of Registration of A Genetic Counselling Centre/Genetic Laboratory/Genetic Clinic/Ultrasound Clinc/Imaging Centre

1. Name of the applicant (Indicate name of the organisation sought to be registered)
2. Address of the applicant
3. Type of facility to be registered (Please specify whether the application is for registration of a Genetic Counselling Centre/Genetic Laboratory/Genetic Clinic/Ultrasound Clinic/Imaging Centre or any combination of these)
4. Full name and address/addresses of Genetic Counselling Centre/Genetic Laboratory/Genetic Clinic/Ultrasound Clinic/Imag-

ing Centre with Telephone/Fax number(s)/Telegraphic/Telex/E-mail address (s).

5. Type of ownership of Organisation (individual ownership/partnership/company/co-operative/any other to be specified). In case type of organization is other than individual ownership, furnish copy of articles of association and names and addresses of other persons responsible for management, as enclosure.

6. Type of Institution (Govt. Hospital/Municipal Hospital/Public Hospital/Private Hospital/Private Nursing Home/Private Clinic/Private Laboratory/any other to be stated.)

7. Specific pre-natal diagnostic procedures/tests for which approval is sought

   (a) Invasive (i) amniocentesis/chorionic villi aspiration/chromosomal/biochemical/molecular studies

   (b) Non-Invasive Ultrasonography Leave blank if registration is sought for Genetic Counselling Centre only.

8. Equipment available with the make and model of each equipment (List to be attached on a separate sheet).

9. (a) Facilities available in the Counselling Centre. (b) Whether facilities are or would be available in the Laboratory/Clinic for the following tests:

   (i) Ultrasound
   (ii) Amniocentesis
   (iii) Chorionic villi aspiration
   (iv) Foetoscopy
   (v) Foetal biopsy
   (vi) Cordocentesis

Whether facilities are available in the Laboratory/Clinic for the following:

   (i) Chromosomal studies
   (ii) Biochemical studies
   (iii) Molecular studies
   (iv) Preimplantation genetic diagnosis

10. Names, qualifications, experience and registration number of employees (may be furnished as an enclosure).

11. State whether the Genetic Counselling Centre/Genetic Laboratory/Genetic Clinic/Ultrasound clinic/Imaging centre [1] qualifies for registration in terms of requirements laid down in Rule 3]

12. For renewal applications only:

   (a) Registration No.

   (b) Date of issue and date of expiry of existing certificate of registration.

13. List of Enclosures: (Please attach a list of enclosures/supporting documents attached to this application.)

Date:

(...................)

Place:

Name, designation and signature of the person authorized to sign on behalf of the organisation to be registered.

Declaration

I, Sh./Smt./Kum./Dr........................... son/daughter/wife of .... aged.......... years resident of................................ working as (indicate designation) .... in (indicate name of the organisation to be registered) .... hereby declare that I have read and understood the Pre-natal Diagnostic Techniques (Regulation and Prevention of Misuse) Act, 1994 (57 of 1994) and the Pre-natal Diagnostic Techniques (Regulation and Prevention of Misuse) Rules, 1996, I also undertake to explain the said Act and Rules to all employees of the Genetic Counselling Centre/Genetic Laboratory/ Genetic Clinic/ultrasound clinic/imaging centre in respect of which registration is sought and to ensure that Act and Rules are fully complied with.

Date:

(...................)

Place:

Name, designation and signature of the person authorized to sign on behalf of the organisation to be registered [Seal of The Organisation Sought to be Registered]

Acknowledgement
[See Rules 4(2) and 8(1)]

The application in Form A in duplicate for grant*/renewal* of registration of Genetic Counselling Centre*/Genetic Laboratory*/Genetic Clinic*/Ultrasound Clinic*/Imaging Centre* by .... (Name and address of applicant) has been received by the Appropriate Authority .... On (date). *The list of enclosures attached to the application in Form A has been verified with the enclosures submitted and found to be correct. OR

*On verification it is found that the following documents mentioned in the list of enclosures are not actually enclosed. This acknowledgement does not confer any rights on the applicant for grant or renewal of registration.

(...................)

Signature and Designation of Appropriate Authority, or authorized person in the Office of the Appropriate Authority.

Date:

Place:

Seal

Original/Duplicate for Display

Form B

[See Rules 6(2), 6(5) and 8(2)]

Certificate of Registration (To be issued in duplicate)

1. In exercise of the powers conferred under Section 19 (1) of the Pre-natal Diagnostic Techniques (Regulation and Prevention of Misuse) Act, 1994 (57 of 1994), the Appropriate Authority .... hereby grants registration to the Genetic Counselling Centre*/Genetic Laboratory*/Genetic Clinic*/Ultrasound Clinic*/Imaging Centre* named below for purposes of carrying out Genetic Counselling/Pre-natal Diagnostic Procedures*/Pre-natal Diagnostic Tests/ultrasonography under the aforesaid Act for a period of five years ending on ....

2. This registration is granted subject to the aforesaid Act and Rules thereunder and any contravention thereof shall result in suspension or cancellation of this Certificate of Registration before the expiry of the said period of five years apart from prosecution.

   A. Name and address of the Genetic Counselling Centre*/Genetic Laboratory*/Genetic Clinic*/Ultrasound Clinic*/Imaging Centre*.

   B. Pre-natal diagnostic procedures* approved for (Genetic Clinic). Non-Invasive
     (i) Ultrasound Invasive
     (ii) Amniocentesis
     (iii) Chorionic villi biopsy
     (iv) Foetoscopy
     (v) Foetal skin or organ biopsy
     (vi) Cordocentesis
     (vii) Any other (specify)

   C. Pre-natal diagnostic tests* approved (for Genetic Laboratory)
     (i) Chromosomal studies
     (ii) Biochemical studies
     (iii) Molecular studies

   D. Any other purpose (please specify)

3. Model and make of equipments being used (any change is to be intimated to the Appropriate Authority under rule 13). Registration No. allotted

5. Period of validity of earlier Certificate of Registration. (For renewed Certificate of Registration only) From .... To ....

Signature, name and designation of The Appropriate Authority

Date:

Seal

Display One Copy of This Certificate at A Conspicuous Place at The Place of Business

Form C

[See Rules 6(3), 6(5) and 8(3)] Form for Rejection of Application for Grant/Renewal of Registration

In exercise of the powers conferred under Section 19(2) of the Prenatal Diagnostic Techniques (Regulation and Prevention of Misuse) Act, 1994, the Appropriate Authority .... hereby rejects the application for grant*/renewal* of registration of the undermentioned Genetic Counselling Centre*/Genetic Laboratory*/Genetic Clinic*/Ultrasound Clinic*/Imaging Centre*.

(1) Name and address of the Genetic Counselling Centre*/Genetic Laboratory*/Genetic Clinic*/Ultrasound Clinic*/Imaging Centre*

(2) Reasons for rejection of application for grant/renewal of registration:

Signature, name and designation of the Appropriate Authority with SEAL of Office

Date:

Place:

*Strike out whichever is not applicable or necessary.

Form D

[See rule 9(2)]

Form for Maintenance of Records by The Genetic Counselling Centre

1. Name and address of Genetic Counselling centre.
2. Registration No.
3. Patient's name

4. Age
5. Husband's/Father's name
6. Full address with Tel. No., if any
7. Referred by (Full name and address of Doctor(s) with registration No.(s) (Referral note to be preserved carefully with case papers)
8. Last menstrual period/weeks of pregnancy
9. History of genetic/medical disease in the family (specify) Basis of diagnosis:
   (a) Clinical
   (b) Bio-chemical
   (c) Cytogenetic
   (d) Other (e.g. radiological, ulrasonography)
10. Indication for pre-natal diagnosis

    A. Previous child/children with:
       (i) Chromosomal disorders
       (ii) Metabolic disorders
       (iii) Congenital anomaly
       (iv) Mental retardation
       (v) Haemoglobinopathy
       (vi) Sex linked disorders
       (vii) Single gene disorder
       (viii) Any other (specify)

    B. Advanced maternal age (35 years or above)
    C. Mother/father/sibling having genetic disease (specify)
    D. Others (specify)

11. Procedure advised[2]

    (i) Ultrasound
    (ii) Amniocentesis
    (iii) Chorionic villi biopsy
    (iv) Foetoscopy
    (v) Foetal skin or organ biopsy
    (vi) Cordocentesis
    (vii) Any other (specify)

12. Laboratory tests to be carried out

    (i) Chromosomal studies
    (ii) Biochemical studies
    (iii) Molecular studies
    (iv) Pre-implantation genetic diagnosis

13. Result of diagnosis. If abnormal give details. Normal/Abnormal
14. Was MTP advised?
15. Name and address of Genetic Clinic* to which patient is referred.

16. Dates of commencement and completion of genetic counselling.

Name, Signature and Registration No. of the Medical Geneticist/ Gynaecologist/Paediatrician administering Genetic Counselling.

Place:

Date:

Form E

[See Rule 9(3)]

Form for Maintenance of Records by Genetic Laboratory

1. Name and address of Genetic Laboratory
2. Registration No
3. Patient's name
4. Age
5. Husband's/Father's name
6. Full address with Tel. No., if any
7. Referred by/sample sent by (full name and address of Genetic Clinic) (Referral note to be preserved carefully with case papers)
8. Type of sample: Maternal blood/Chorionic villus sample/amniotic fluid/Foetal blood or other foetal tissue (specify)
9. Specify indication for pre-natal diagnosis

A. Previous child/children with

  (i) Chromosomal disorders
  (ii) Metabolic disorders
  (iii) Malformation(s)
  (iv) Mental retardation
  (v) Hereditary haemolytic anaemia
  (vi) Sex linked disorder
  (vii) Single gene disorder
  (viii) Any other (specify)

B. Advanced maternal age (35 years or above)
C. Mother/father/sibling having genetic disease (specify)
D. Other (specify)

10. Laboratory tests carried out (give details)

  (i) Chromosomal studies
  (ii) Biochemical studies
  (iii) Molecular studies
  (iv) Preimplantation gentic diagnosis

11. Result of diagnosis if abnormal give details. Normal/Abnormal
12. Date(s) on which tests carried out.

The results of the Pre-natal diagnostic tests were conveyed to
.... on .... Name, Signature and Registration No. of the Medical Geneticist/Director of the Institute.

Place:

Date:

Form F

[See Proviso to Section 4(3), Rule 9(4) and Rule 10(1A)]

Form for Maintenance of Record in Respect of Pregnant Woman by Genetic Clinic/Ultrasound Clinic/Imaging Centre

1. Name and address of the Genetic Clinic/Ultrasound Clinic/Imaging Centre.
2. Registration No.
3. Patient's name and her age
4. Number of children with sex of each child
5. Husband's/Father's name
6. Full address with Tel. No., if any
7. Referred by (full name and address of Doctor(s)/Genetic Counselling Centre (Referral note to be preserved carefully with case papers)/self referral
8. Last menstrual period/weeks of pregnancy
9. History of genetic/medical disease in the family (specify) Basis of diagnosis:
   (a) Clinical
   (b) Bio-chemical
   (c) Cytogenetic
   (d) Other (e.g. radiological, ultrasonography etc. specify)
10. Indication for pre-natal diagnosis

A. Previous child/children with:

   (i) Chromosomal disorders
   (ii) Metabolic disorders
   (iii) Congenital anomaly
   (iv) Mental retardation
   (v) Haemoglobinopathy
   (vi) Sex linked disorders
   (vii) Single gene disorder
   (viii) Any other (specify)

B. Advanced maternal age (35 years)
C. Mother/father/sibling has genetic disease (specify)
D. Other (specify)

11. Procedures carried out (with name and registration No. of Gynaecologist/Radiologist/Registered Medical Practitioner) who performed it. Non-Invasive

   (i) Ultrasound (specify purpose for which ultrasound is to done during pregnancy) [List of indications for ultrasonography of pregnant women are given in the note below] Invasive
   (ii) Amniocentesis
   (iii) Chorionic Villi aspiration
   (iv) Foetal biopsy
   (v) Cordocentesis
   (vi) Any other (specify)

12. Any complication of procedure–please specify
13. Laboratory tests recommended[3]

   (i) Chromosomal studies
   (ii) Biochemical studies
   (iii) Molecular studies
   (iv) Preimplantation genetic diagnosis

14. Result of

   (a) pre-natal diagnostic procedure (give details)
   (b) Ultrasonography Normal/Abnormal (specify abnormality detected, if any).

15. Date(s) on which procedures carried out.
16. Date on which consent obtained. (In case of invasive)
17. The result of pre-natal diagnostic procedure were conveyed to .... on ....
18. Was MTP advised/conducted?
19. Date on which MTP carried out.

Date:

Name, Signature and Registration number of the Place Gynaecologist/Radiologist/Director of the Clinic

Declaration of Pregnant Woman

I, Ms. .... (name of the pregnant woman) declare that by undergoing ultrasonography/image scanning etc. I do not want to know the sex of my foetus.

Signature/Thumb impression of pregnant woman .... 3 Strike out whichever is not applicable or not necessary

Declaraton of Doctor/Person Conducting Ultrasonography/Image Scanning

I, ... (name of the person conducting ultrasonography/image scanning) declare that while conducting ultrasonography/image scanning on Ms. .... (name of the pregnant woman), I have neither detected nor disclosed the sex of her foetus to any body in any manner.

Name and signature of the person conducting ultrasonography/image scanning/Director or owner of genetic clinic/ultrasound clinic/imaging centre.

Important Note:

(i) Ultrasound is not indicated/advised/performed to determine the sex of foetus except for diagnosis of sex-linked diseases such as Duchenne Muscular Dystrophy, Haemophilia A & B etc.

(ii) During pregnancy Ultrasonography should only be performed when indicated. The following is the representative list of indications for ultrasound during pregnancy.

(1) To diagnose intra-uterine and/or ectopic pregnancy and confirm viability.

(2) Estimation of gestational age (dating).

(3) Detection of number of foetuses and their chorionicity.

(4) Suspected pregnancy with IUCD in-situ or suspected pregnancy following contraceptive failure/MTP failure.

(5) Vaginal bleeding/leaking.

(6) Follow-up of cases of abortion.

(7) Assessment of cervical canal and diameter of internal os.

(8) Discrepancy between uterine size and period of amenorrhoea.

(9) Any suspected adenexal or uterine pathology/abnormality.

(10) Detection of chromosomal abnormalities, foetal structural defects and other abnormalities and their follow-up.

(11) To evaluate foetal presentation and position.

(12) Assessment of liquor amnii.

(13) Preterm labour/preterm premature rupture of membranes.

(14) Evaluation of placental position, thickness, grading and abnormalities (placenta praevia, retroplacental haemorrhage, abnormal adherence etc.).

(15) Evaluation of umbilical cord–presentation, insertion, nuchal encirclement, number of vessels and presence of true knot.

(16) Evaluation of previous Caesarean Section scars.

(17) Evaluation of foetal growth parameters, foetal weight and foetal well being.

(18) Colour flow mapping and duplex Doppler studies.

(19) Ultrasound guided procedures such as medical termination of pregnancy, external cephalic version etc. and their follow-up.

(20) Adjunct to diagnostic and therapeutic invasive interventions such as chorionic villus sampling (CVS), amniocenteses, foetal blood sampling, foetal skin biopsy, amnio-infusion, intrauterine infusion, placement of shunts etc.

(21) Observation of intra-partum events.

(22) Medical/surgical conditions complicating pregnancy.

(23) Research/scientific studies in recognised institutions. Person conducting ultrasonography on a pregnant women shall keep complete record thereof in the clinic/centre in Form–F and any deficiency or inaccuracy found therein shall amount to contravention of provisions of section 5 or section 6 of the Act, unless contrary is proved by the person conducting such ultrasonography.

Form G

[See Rule 10]
Form of Consent
(For invasive techniques)

I, ... wife/daughter of .... Age .... years residing at .... hereby state that I have been explained fully the probable side-effects and after effects of the pre-natal diagnostic procedures.

I wish to undergo the pre-implantation/pre-natal diagnostic technique/test/procedures in my own interest to find out the possibility of any abnormality (i.e. disease/deformity/disorder) in the child I am carrying.

I undertake not to terminate the pregnancy if the pre-natal procedure/technique/test conducted show the absence of disease/deformity/disorder. I understand that the sex of the foetus will not be disclosed to me. I understand that breach of this undertaking will make me liable to penalty as prescribed in the Pre-natal Diagnostic Techniques (Regulation and Prevention of Misuse) Act, 1994 (57 of 1994) and rules framed thereunder.

Date:

Signature of the pregnant woman.

Place:

I have explained the contents of the above to the patient and her companion (Name .... Address .... Relationship ....) in a language she/they understand.

Name, Signature and/Registration number of Gynaecologist/Medical Geneticist/Radiologist/Paediatrician/ Director of the Clinic/Centre/Laboratory

Date:

Name, Address and Registration number of Genetic Clinic/Institute

Seal

Form H

[See Rule 9(5)]

Form for Maintenance of Permanent Record of Applications for Grant/Rejection of Registration Under The Pre-natal Diagnostic Techniques (Regulation and Prevention of Misuse) Act, 1994.

1. Sl. No.
2. File number of Appropriate Authority.
3. Date of receipt of application for grant of registration.
4. Name, Address, Phone/Fax etc. of Applicant:
5. Name and address(es) of Genetic Counselling Centre*/Genetic Laboratory*/Genetic Clinic*/Ultrasound Clinic*/Imaging Centre*.
6. Date of consideration by Advisory Committee and recommendation of Advisory Committee, in summary.
7. Outcome of application (state granted/rejected and date of issue of orders- record date of issue of order in Form B or Form C).
8. Registration number allotted and date of expiry of registration.
9. Renewals (date of renewal and renewed upto).
10. File number in which renewals dealt.
11. Additional information, if any.

Name, Designation and Signature of Appropriate Authority Guidance for Appropriate Authority

(a) Form H is a permanent record to be maintained as a register, in the custody of the Appropriate Authority.
(b) * Means strike out whichever is not applicable.
(c) On renewal, the Registration Number of the Genetic Counselling Centre/Genetic Laboratory/Genetic Clinic/Ultrasound Clinic/Imaging Centre will not change. A fresh registration Number will be allotted in the event of change of ownership or management.
(e) Registration number shall not be allotted twice.
(f) Each Genetic Counselling Centre/Genetic Laboratory/Genetic Clinic/Ultrasound Clinic/Imaging Centre may be allotted a folio

consisting of two pages of the Register for recording Form H.

(g) The space provided for "additional information" may be used for recording suspension, cancellations, rejection of application for renewal, change of ownership/management, outcome of any legal proceedings, etc.

(h) Every folio (i.e. 2 pages) of the Register shall be authenticated by signature of the Appropriate Authority with date, and every subsequent entry shall also be similarly authenticated.'.

(Ms. K. Sujatha Rao)
Joint Secretary to the Government of India:
[No.N.24026/14/2002-PNDT Cell]

Footnote:— The Principal Notification was published in the Gazette of India vide No.G.S.R. 1(E) dated 1st January, 1996. This is the first amendments to the Pre-Natal Diagnostic Techniques (Regulation and Prevention of Misuse) Rules, 1996.

[1] Strike out whichever is not applicable or not necessary. All enclosures are to be authenticated by signature of the applicant.

[2] Strike out whichever is not applicable or necessary.

GLOSSARY

Afsos	sympathy, expressed upon birth of a girl, especially if she is not the first child
Amritdhari	blessed Sikh, one who has taken a religious vow
Apad	times of distress
Baragam	twelve Lewa Patidar villages
Barati	the party of people accompanying the groom for wedding
Bhag	fate/destiny/share
Boora	a sect of the sun god in Orissa
Dai	local birth attendant, traditionally the occupation of a low caste woman
Datta homa	oblations of clarified butter to fire
Dattaka	adopted son
Dera	hermitage/*ashram*, sacred place (not fully a temple) where a mystic/saint devoted to religion/sect resides and is visited by devotees/followers
Dhabas	kiosks or small sheds working as make-do restaurants
Diwali	festival of lights, fireworks and worship of *Laksmi*, the goddess of wealth; it is celebrated in October-November
Dudhapiti	customary practice of female infanticide by putting opium on the mother's nipple and feeding the baby, suffocating her in a rug, or placing the afterbirth over the infant's face
Ekadas/gols	endogamous circles
Gotra	an exogenous patrilineal clan whose members claim descent from a single mythological sage, the family name
Gurudwara	Sikh temple
Holi	festival of colours and fire worship that falls in February
Huani/huasni	generic term in Rajasthan for a daughter of the household/family

Janch	literally, test; used for ultrasound test to determine the sex of a foetus
Jethuti	daughter of the husband's elder brother
Kabari	dealer in waste or recyclable goods, also known as *kabriwallah*
kanya bhroon	female foetus, sanskritised term used in formal contexts
kanya bhroon hatya	killing of female foetus, sanskritised term used in formal contexts
Kapada	literally, clothes; but when used in a context it means menstrual period (or clothes??)
kanyadan	gift of a virgin, i.e. giving away a daughter in marriage
Karma	account based on the accumulation of good and bad deeds in past life
Karwa Chauth	a day of fasting by a wife for her husband's long life and welfare; it falls a few days before *Diwali*
khadi saree	coarse cotton sari, implying austere and simple wedding
kothi	bungalow
Kuri mar	girl-killer, implies infanticide and now foeticide too
Lifafa	literally, envelope; money given to the groom and his relatives in envelopes
Lohri	ritual of fire worship in mid-January on the eve of the winter solstice
Mehndi	literally, henna; the ritual of applying henna is getting increasingly elaborate
Nas bandi	literally, to tie the tube/cord; refers to sterilisation, i.e., to prevent conception
Niyoga	the practice of appointing a widow to a male relative with a view to beget a son for the deceased
Panchali system	polyandry, a woman married to five men
Pandits	literally, scholars, priests, refers also to Brahmins
Paraya dhan	literally, others wealth; expression used for a girl implying she belongs to others, not to her parents
Parchun	groceries
Pheriwallas	those selling wares on push-carts
Pindas	cakes of boiled rice offered to deceased ancestors in *sraddhas*

Pir	a priest/mystic at a shrine/tomb belonging to the Sufi order
Punya	religious merit
Raj	to rule, refers to the government and/or the state
Rakhi	annual ritual when a thread is tied to a boy by his sister, symbolic of his protection pledged for the sister
Sastras	the codes of sacred and social duties
Sati	literally, the truthful; the Hindu practice of a widow immolating herself on her husband's funeral pyre
Savitri	pious female protagonist of an *Upanishad* tale; her piety saved her husband from death by arguing with *Yamraj* (the harbinger of death in Hinduism)
Shakti	energy and power
Sita	the ideal wife in the epic *Ramayana*
Smritis	the law codes
Sraddhas	a ritual in propitiation of the deceased ancestors
Thaka	booking the prospective groom or bride for marriage, a ritual prior to betrothal
Uperason	generic term for surgery, it is used commonly for sterilisation unless otherwise specified

ABOUT THE EDITOR AND CONTRIBUTORS

Editor

Tulsi Patel is Professor of Sociology at the Delhi School of Economics, University of Delhi, Delhi.

She has recently been Rotating Chair, India Studies at Heidelberg University, Germany for a full semester (2005–06). An Honorary Research Associate at the Department of Sociology, University of Manchester (2001–04), she has also undertaken teaching assignments at the London School of Economics and the Royal Holloway College of the University of London (1996–97). Professor Patel has previously taught at Jamia Millia Islamia, New Delhi and Miranda House (University of Delhi).

Her areas of interest include gender, anthropology of fertility and reproduction, medical sociology, sociology of the family, and old age. She has authored *Fertility Behaviour: Population and Society in a Rajasthan Village* (1994, 2nd edn 2006) and edited *The Family in India: Structure and Practice* (2005). In addition, she has published several articles in national and international journals.

Contributors

Reema Bhatia is a Reader in the Department of Sociology, Miranda House, University of Delhi. Her area of specialisation is in the field of Sociology of Medicine. For over ten years she has been researching on health related issues and the practice of female foeticide. The section included in this book is a part of her larger research.

Ashish Bose is Honorary Professor, Institute of Economic Growth, Delhi and Distinguished Professor at the Institute of Integrated Learning in Management (IILM), New Delhi. Associated with the

Voluntary Health Association of India (VHAI), he is also Chairman, Society for Applied Research in Humanities. He was formerly President of the Indian Association for the Study of Population (IASP), Chairman of the Expert Committee on 'Analysis of Religion Data in Census', and is a member of the National Commission on Population headed by the Prime Minister.

He has written extensively on population and development. His latest book is *Beyond Demography: Dialogue with People.*

Rainuka Dagar is Regional Representative of the Altus Global Alliance in the Institute for Development and Communication (IDC), Chandigarh (India). She specialises in the area of gender justice and identity politics. She has undertaken research on forms of gender violence, construction of masculinities, gender in conflict and post-conflict contexts and the interface of gender with criminal justice system. She has edited a manual on *Women's Development and Gender Justice* (1996) Ministry of Human Resource Development, Government of India, co-authored *Victims of Militancy* (1998) UNICEF, besides authoring other articles and reports.

Rashmi Kapoor teaches at the Department of African Studies, University of Delhi. She obtained her M.A. and M.Phil. in Sociology from the Department of Sociology, Delhi School of Economics, and Ph.D. from the Department of African Studies, University of Delhi. She recently did fieldwork on social mobility in Mauritius where she has also studied child adoption. She has written extensively and published articles on the Indian diaspora in Africa (in Swahili language), child abuse and child adoption in India. She is a member of the Sudan Study Unit in the Department of African Studies, University of Delhi.

Bijayalaxmi Nanda teaches Political Science at Miranda House, University of Delhi. Her areas of interest are political theory and gender. She also coordinates a campaign against female foeticide for the Centre for Women's Development Studies (CWDS), New Delhi. She has written extensively on the issue of female foeticide for various journals and policy documents. Her recent publications include a book on *Human Rights, Gender and Environment.*

Vibhuti Patel is Director, Department of Post Graduate Studies and Research, and professor and head of the Department of Economics, SNDT Women's University, Mumbai. She is a trustee of

Anusandhan Trust and its institution, Centre for Enquiry into Health and Allied Themes (CEHAT) that filed a petition in the Supreme Court of India for effective implementation of the PNDT Act, 1994 and was responsible for PCPNDT Act, 2002. She is a trustee of VACHA, Women's Research and Action Group (WRAG) and *Satya Vijay Seva Samaj* in Mumbai. She is the Governing Board member of *Vikas Adhyayan Kendra*, Mumbai, Women Power Connect, Delhi and Institute for Community Organisation and Research, Mumbai. She has co-authored *Indian Women—Change and Challenge and Reaching for Half the Sky* and has written the book *Women's Challenges of the New Millennium* (2002).

Alpana D. Sagar, a medical doctor with training in public health, is on the faculty of the Centre of Social Medicine and Community Health, Jawaharlal Nehru University, New Delhi. She worked in the villages of Ramgarh Block, Nainital district, Kumaon, and in the Gautam Nagar slum of Delhi before moving into academics. Her research work has involved understanding the gaps between the felt needs of poor people, especially women, and the medical services provided by the Government. She is currently working on examining the organisation of public health services in India and the challenge of improving health service planning and delivery, especially for the poor. Her work has an emphasis on gender issues.

Leela Visaria is Professor and Director, Gujarat Institute of Development Research, Ahmedabad, India. Her research interests include historical demography, health, education and demographic transition. She has been published in reputed journals. She is the co-author of *Contraceptive Use and Fertility in India: A Case Study of Gujarat* (1995) and co-editor of a volume *Maternal Education and Child Survival: Pathways and Evidence* (1997). She has also co-authored a book *India in the 21st Century* (2004). Since 1996 she is the coordinator of HealthWatch, a network of non-governmental organisations (NGOs), researchers and women activists.

L. S. Vishwanath is an M.A. in History from St. Stephen's College, Delhi and Ph.D in Sociology from the Department of Sociology, Delhi University. Till his retirement in August 2005, he was the Professor and Head of the Department of History, Pondicherry University. He was also the Director of the Centre for Canadian Studies in the same University. His publications include the book *Female Infanticide and Social Structure* and articles in reputed journals.

INDEX